INTRODUCTION TO

Healthcare

Quality

Management

Patrice L. Spath

INTRODUCTION TO
Healthcare
Quality
Management

THIRD EDITION

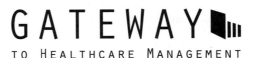

GATEWAY
TO HEALTHCARE MANAGEMENT

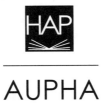

AUPHA

Health Administration Press, Chicago, Illinois
Association of University Programs in Health Administration, Washington, DC

Library of Congress Cataloging-in-Publication Data

Names: Spath, Patrice, author.
Title: Introduction to healthcare quality management / Patrice L. Spath.
Description: Third edition. | Chicago, Illinois : Health Administration Press
    (HAP) ; Washington, DC : Association of University Programs in Health
    Administration (AUPHA), [2018] | Includes bibliographical references and
    index.
Identifiers: LCCN 2018000148 (print) | LCCN 2018000573 (ebook) | ISBN
    9781567939866 (ebook) | ISBN 9781567939873 (xml) | ISBN 9781567939880
    (epub) | ISBN 9781567939897 (mobi) | ISBN 9781567939859 (alk. paper)
Subjects: LCSH: Medical care—Quality control. | Quality assurance. | Medical
    care—Quality control—Measurement. | Quality assurance—Measurement.
Classification: LCC RA399.A1 (ebook) | LCC RA399.A1 S64 2018 (print) | DDC
    362.1068—dc23
LC record available at https://lccn.loc.gov/2018000148

Acquisitions editor: Jennette McClain; Manuscript editor: Adin Bookbinder; Project manager: Andrew Baumann; Cover designer: James Slate; Layout: PerfecType

Found an error or a typo? We want to know! Please e-mail it to hapbooks@ache.org, mentioning the book's title and putting "Book Error" in the subject line.

For photocopying and copyright information, please contact Copyright Clearance Center at www.copyright.com or at (978) 750-8400.

Health Administration Press
A division of the Foundation of the
    American College of Healthcare Executives
300 S. Riverside Plaza, Suite 1900
Chicago, IL 60606-6698
(312) 424-2800

Association of University Programs
    in Health Administration
1730 M Street, NW
Suite 407
Washington, DC 20036
(202) 763-7283

I dedicate this book to my son Gordon and my daughter Karen,
who have always filled my life with pleasure and love.

BRIEF CONTENTS

DETAILED CONTENTS

FOREWORD TO THE THIRD EDITION

In forewords to the previous two editions of this book, I reported my unscientific study on the number of Google hits retrieved by searching for "healthcare quality books" (19.3 million in 2009 and 202 million in 2012) and the extreme reduction in results when the term was modified to "healthcare quality textbooks" (1.89 million and 2.24 million). Now, the pendulum appears to be swinging the other way, as this year's exercise yielded 138 million hits for "healthcare quality books" and 26.1 million hits for "healthcare quality textbooks." Certainly, there could be many explanations for these changes, but my preference is to conclude that health professionals, and educators in training programs for health professionals, recognize the need for well-vetted resources to prepare current and future practitioners for high-quality performance in the delivery and management of healthcare services. These resources, which often are classified as "textbooks," must address the conceptual foundations of healthcare quality as well as provide examples of and instruction in effective techniques used in healthcare organizations to ensure the delivery of reliable, high-quality care.

In this third edition, *Introduction to Healthcare Quality Management* continues to be a dependable resource for employed health professionals and for students in health professions programs to develop the knowledge and skills that underlie the reliable, high-quality job performance required by members of healthcare teams in a dynamic, regulated environment. Patrice Spath effectively addresses the enduring principles of healthcare quality management—measurement, assessment, and improvement—but, more important, describes and explains the evolving techniques and approaches used by healthcare providers to evaluate their performance and communicate their organization's clinical, safety, and patient satisfaction outcomes to their stakeholders.

Regulation in healthcare continues to increase, and this third edition has expanded coverage of industry standards and current policy initiatives such as value-based reimbursement. Case studies, examples, and links to trustworthy industry websites explain these issues in context.

Current professional practice also increasingly engages patients and their families at all points on the continuum of the care experience, which requires interpersonal skills that are insufficiently taught in most clinical training programs. This edition of the book helps fill that gap with new content covering discharge planning and case management, as well as healthcare quality from the perspective of consumers. It also features a new chapter devoted to managing the quality of population health care. Again, case studies and examples provide an applied learning approach that helps the student or working professional build needed job skills.

The conceptual framework of this edition illustrates how to integrate the key principles of quality management across enterprise-wide programs and activities. Spath explains the principles and illustrates them with examples. She then discusses accountability activities, such as utilization management and patient safety, that organizations use to demonstrate for regulators and consumers their ability to deliver safe, high-quality healthcare.

Some supplemental and instructional resources also are incorporated into the text, and additional resources are available to instructors who adopt this book for their course (see page xx). Notably, the discussion questions at the end of each chapter encourage not only application and self-assessment but also continued exploration of the topics addressed through references to external resources, such as websites. A guide to resources for additional study is essential for a quality management textbook because techniques and approaches are dynamic. Organizations learn from their quality measurement and analysis experiences, and the industry culture encourages sharing this experiential learning. In many cases, self-reported solutions can be transferrable to other organizations facing similar challenges.

As with previous editions, this textbook provides health professions students with core knowledge that will enable them to adapt to organization-specific models as informed, educated, and valued employees. Additionally, it is an excellent resource for employed health professionals to review important quality management principles and explore new techniques for measuring and communicating performance in their organizations.

Donna J. Slovensky, PhD, RHIA, FAHIMA
Professor and Senior Associate Dean
School of Health Professions
University of Alabama at Birmingham

PREFACE

The healthcare quality management basics—measurement, assessment, and improvement—have not changed appreciably in decades. Terminology used to describe various aspects has undergone some modifications, and specific practices have evolved, but the underlying principles are unchanged. In 1976, Jacobs, Christoffel, and Dixon wrote about measuring patient care inputs, processes, and outcomes using an improvement methodology known as Performance Evaluation Procedure audits. In 1980, Skillicorn detailed quality and patient safety improvements at San Jose Hospital following implementation of a problem-oriented, multidisciplinary approach combined with increased individual accountability. And a population-based approach to measuring and managing quality of ambulatory services was described in 1995 by Goldfield. These are just a few examples of the quality management evolution over the past few decades.

Since the first edition of this book was published in 2009, the principles of healthcare quality management have essentially stayed the same while the practices have continued to progress. External influences have always affected quality management in provider organizations; however, these forces are stronger than ever before. Value-based reimbursement and public reporting of provider-specific performance data are two of the many factors driving changes in quality management practices.

Updates for the third edition of this book cover topics such as new quality management regulations and standards, healthcare application of improvement models adopted from other industries, and how to manage the quality of population health improvement initiatives. This edition also includes more case studies from varied provider sites, new clinical and nonclinical examples, and many additional websites to expand your learning experiences.

As in past editions of this book, the material is intended for people with little or no clinical experience. The examples are primarily focused on the provision of health services, not the diagnosis and treatment of medical conditions. When topics of a clinical nature are discussed, explanatory notes and examples are added to help clarify the information. The language of quality management can also be a barrier to learning. For this reason, various analogies from common life situations are used to illustrate concepts. For example, measuring healthcare quality is similar to measuring one's weight on a scale. A simple, familiar analogy is often the best way to explain what may appear at first to be a complex topic.

CONTENT OVERVIEW

Chapter 1 introduces students to the concepts of healthcare quality from the viewpoint of various stakeholders. Consumers' perceived value of a product or service differs when the modality being purchased is healthcare services. The Institute of Medicine definition of healthcare quality and important quality characteristics also are covered in chapter 1. *How* the quality of these characteristics is managed is covered throughout the remainder of the book.

The three interconnected building blocks of quality management—measurement, assessment, and improvement—are discussed in chapter 2. Students are exposed to the history of industrial quality improvement, starting in the 1940s with the works of Walter Shewhart, W. Edwards Deming, Kaoru Ishikawa, and other quality pioneers. Quality management principles and practices that originated in manufacturing are now being successfully applied in healthcare provider organizations. The chapter concludes with a discussion of the ever-increasing external forces causing providers to strengthen their quality focus.

The building blocks of quality management are elaborated in chapters 3 through 7. Each chapter explains how to measure, assess, and improve quality. Chapter 3 describes the four categories of measures: structure, process, outcome, and patient experience. The chapter also covers current regulations and accreditation standards affecting the provider's choice of measures and how to create worthwhile measures of importance to the organization. Case studies illustrate how measures are used for quality management purposes, including how clinical decision-making is evaluated.

Measurement does not directly lead to improvements in quality. Two additional steps are needed: data compilation and assessment, which are discussed in chapter 4. Assessment of measurement data is performed to determine whether performance is acceptable, and it starts with data compilation and display. The chapter illustrates both tabular and graphic reporting formats and includes case studies showing how to create these reports and use them to evaluate results. Statistical process control (SPC), a performance assessment technique introduced in the 1940s by Shewhart, also is covered in this chapter. Examples show how SPC can be applied to healthcare measurement results.

Measurement and assessment ultimately lead to the last step—improvement. The fundamentals of quality improvement are covered in chapters 5 through 7. Chapter 5 describes various improvement models, including an expanded discussion in this third edition of Lean and Lean Six Sigma because these are becoming more commonplace in provider organizations. Chapter 5 also includes a case study that helps the reader to understand improvement model steps.

Chapter 6 covers the tools used to improve performance, including the traditional quantitative and qualitative tools used to measure quality and the improvement tools used in Lean and Six Sigma projects.

Often teams are formed to conduct improvement projects, and chapter 7 describes the responsibilities of various team members and project management functions.

Patient safety, high reliability, and utilization management are three components of healthcare quality that are of particular interest to regulators, payers, and consumers. For this reason, one chapter is devoted to each of these topics. Chapter 8 applies the building blocks of measurement, assessment, and improvement to the principles and practices of patient safety. Two specialized safety improvement models—failure mode and effects analysis, and root cause analysis—are covered in depth, accompanied by case study illustrations.

Chapter 9 explains what a reliable process is and how to create one. Techniques used for years in high-reliability industries are now being applied to healthcare processes to reduce failures and achieve reliable quality. A number of mistake-proofing strategies for clinical and nonclinical activities also are covered in this chapter.

Reducing the cost of healthcare services by using utilization management techniques continues to be challenging for payers and provider organizations. Chapter 10 describes a number of cost-control techniques, including several new payment models that incentivize providers to become more cost sensitive. The practices of discharge planning and case management also are covered in this chapter, as well as regulatory and accreditation requirements.

A new trend affecting quality management activities in provider organizations is population health care. For this reason, this third edition devotes a full chapter to this topic. Chapter 11 describes the concept of population health care and explains why new reimbursement strategies are influencing provider organizations to become involved in these initiatives. The chapter also discusses the application of the building blocks of quality management (measurement, assessment, and improvement) as they relate to population health care, and it includes two case studies illustrating the application of population health quality management activities.

Effective leadership direction and a supportive culture are cornerstones of a successful quality program. Chapter 12 provides an overview of quality program structures and key players in measurement, assessment, and improvement activities. This chapter concludes with a discussion of organizational dynamics that affect the achievement of quality goals.

SUPPLEMENTAL AND INSTRUCTIONAL RESOURCES

Each chapter concludes with student discussion questions. Some questions encourage contemplation and further dialogue on select topics, and some give students a chance to apply the knowledge they have gained. Others promote continued learning through discovery and use of information available on the Internet.

A book at least twice this size would be needed to cover every current topic associated with healthcare quality management. For this reason, only basic principles and practices are described in this book. In some instances, supplemental learning materials may be needed to delve deeper into a subject or to become familiar with a quality-related topic that is not addressed in the text. The lists of websites at the end of each chapter have been greatly expanded from the second edition to provide even more learning opportunities. For rapidly changing topics, such as alternative reimbursement models and externally imposed performance measurement requirements, current journal articles may be the best information sources.

Patrice L. Spath, MA, RHIT

REFERENCES

Goldfield, N. 1995. "The Measurement and Management of the Quality of Ambulatory Services: A Population-Based Approach." In *The Epidemiology of Quality*, edited by V. A. Kazandjian, 171–96. Gaithersburg, MD: Aspen Publishers.

Jacobs, C. M., T. H. Christoffel, and N. Dixon. 1976. *Measuring the Quality of Patient Care: The Rationale for Outcome Audit*. Cambridge, MA: Ballinger Publishing.

Skillicorn, S. A. 1980. *Quality and Accountability: A New Era in American Hospitals*. San Francisco: Editorial Consultants.

INSTRUCTOR RESOURCES

This book's Instructor Resources include a test bank, PowerPoint slides, answers to the in-book questions, and a PDF of the American College of Healthcare Executives and IHI/NPSF Lucian Leape Institute guide *Leading a Culture of Safety: A Blueprint for Success*.

For the most up-to-date information about this book and its Instructor Resources, go to ache.org/HAP and browse for the book's title or author name.

This book's Instructor Resources are available to instructors who adopt this book for use in their course. For access information, please e-mail hapbooks@ache.org.

CHAPTER 1

FOCUS ON QUALITY

After reading this chapter, you will be able to

➤ recognize factors that influence consumers' perception of quality products and services;

➤ explain the relationship between cost and quality;

➤ identify quality characteristics important to healthcare consumers, purchasers, and providers; and

➤ give examples of the varied dimensions of healthcare quality.

KEY WORDS

- ➤ Cost-effectiveness
- ➤ Defensive medicine
- ➤ Healthcare quality
- ➤ High-value healthcare
- ➤ Institute for Healthcare Improvement (IHI)
- ➤ IHI Triple Aim framework
- ➤ National Academy of Medicine

- ➤ National Quality Strategy
- ➤ Providers
- ➤ Purchasers
- ➤ Quality
- ➤ Quality assurance
- ➤ Reliability
- ➤ Value

Since opening its first store in 1971, Starbucks Coffee Company has developed into an international corporation with more than 23,000 locations worldwide. The company's dedication to providing a quality customer experience is a major contributor to its success. Starbucks's customers expect to receive high-quality, freshly brewed coffee in a comfortable, secure, and inviting atmosphere. In almost every customer encounter, Starbucks meets or exceeds those expectations. This consistency does not occur by chance. Starbucks puts a lot of behind-the-scenes work into its customer service. From selecting coffee beans that meet Starbucks's exacting standards of quality and flavor to ensuring baristas are properly trained to prepare espresso, every part of the process is carefully managed.

Providing high-quality healthcare services also requires much work behind the front lines. Every element in the complex process of healthcare delivery must be carefully managed. This book explains how healthcare organizations manage the quality of their care delivery to meet or exceed customers' expectations. These expectations include delivering an excellent patient care experience, providing only necessary healthcare services, and doing so at the lowest cost possible.

WHAT IS QUALITY?

Quality
Perceived degree of excellence.

In its broadest sense, **quality** is an attribute of a product or service. The perspective of the person evaluating the product or service influences her judgment of the attribute. No universally accepted definition of quality exists; however, its definitions share common elements:

◆   Quality involves meeting or exceeding customer expectations.

◆   Quality is dynamic (i.e., what is considered quality today may not be good enough to be considered quality tomorrow).

◆   Quality can be improved.

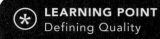

LEARNING POINT
Defining Quality

A quality product or service is one that meets or exceeds expectations. Expectations can change, so quality must be continuously improved.

RELIABILITY

An important aspect of quality is **reliability**. From an engineering perspective, reliability refers to the ability of a device, system, or process to perform its prescribed function without failure for a given time when operated correctly in a specified environment (Crossley 2007). Reliability ends when a failure occurs. For instance, your laptop computer is considered reliable when it functions properly during normal use. If it stops functioning—fails—you have an unreliable computer.

Consumers want to experience quality that is reliable. Patrons of Starbucks pay a premium to get the same taste, quality, and experience at every Starbucks location (Clark 2008). James Harrington, past president of the American Society for Quality, cautioned manufacturers to focus on reliability more than they have in recent years to retain market share. First-time buyers of an automobile are often influenced by features, cost, and perceived quality. Repeat buyers cite reliability as the primary reason for sticking with a particular brand (Harrington 2009).

Reliability can be measured. A reliable process performs as expected a high proportion of the time. An unreliable process performs as expected a low proportion of the time. Unfortunately, many healthcare processes fall into the unreliable category. Healthcare processes that fail to consistently perform as expected a high proportion of the time contribute to medical errors that cause up to 400,000 annual deaths in the United States and even more serious harm events (DuPree and Chassin 2016). Healthcare consumers are no different from consumers of other products and services; they expect quality services that are reliable.

Reliability
The measurable capability of a process, procedure, or health service to perform its intended function in the required time under commonly occurring conditions.

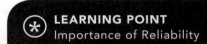

LEARNING POINT
Importance of Reliability

A necessary ingredient of quality is reliability, loosely defined as the probability a system will perform properly over a defined time span. It may be possible to achieve reliability without quality (e.g., consistently poor service), but quality can never be achieved without reliability.

COST–QUALITY CONNECTION

Value
A relative measure that describes a product's or service's worth, usefulness, or importance.

We expect to receive **value** when purchasing products or services. We do not want to find broken or missing parts when we unwrap new merchandise. We are disheartened when we receive poor service at a restaurant. We become downright irritated when our banks fail to record a deposit and our debit card withdrawals are denied.

How you respond to disappointing situations depends on how you are affected by them. With a product purchase, if the merchandise is expensive, you will likely contact the store immediately to arrange an exchange or a refund. If the product is inexpensive, you may chalk it up to experience and vow never to do business with the company again. At a restaurant, your expectations increase as the price of the food goes up. Yet, if you are adversely affected—for example, you get food poisoning—you will be an unhappy customer no matter the cost of the meal. The same is true for banks that make mistakes. No one wants the hassle of reversing a bank error, even if the checking account is free. Unhappy clients tend to move on to do business with another bank.

Cost and quality affect the customer experience in all industries. But in healthcare, these factors are harder for the average consumer to evaluate than in other types of business. Tainted restaurant food is easier to recognize than an unskilled surgeon is. As for cost, everyone agrees that healthcare is expensive, yet if someone else is paying for it—an insurance company, the government, or a relative—the cost factor becomes less important to the consumer. If your surgery does not go well, however, you'll be an unhappy customer regardless of what it cost.

In all industries, multiple dynamics influence the cost and quality of products and services. First, prices may be influenced by how much the consumer is willing to pay. For example, one person may pay a premium to get the latest and most innovative electronic gadget, whereas another person may wait until the price comes down before buying it. This phenomenon is also evident in service industries. Rosemont College, a private coeducational institution in Bryn Mawr, Pennsylvania, reduced tuition to attract students. For the 2016–2017 academic year, the college dropped tuition from $32,620 to $18,500, and room and board costs from $13,400 to $11,500. These cost reductions resulted in a 64 percent increase in applications without any change in academic offerings (Hope 2017).

Second, low quality—say, poor customer service or inferior products—eventually causes a company to lose sales. The US electronics and automotive industries faced this outcome in the early 1980s when American consumers

> ⊛ **LEARNING POINT**
> Cost–Quality Connection
>
> The cost of a product or service is indirectly related to its perceived quality. A quality healthcare experience is one that meets a personal need or provides some benefit (either real or perceived) and is provided at a reasonable cost.

started buying more Japanese products (Walton 1986). Business and government leaders realized that an emphasis on quality was necessary to compete in a more demanding, and expanding, world market.

CONSUMER–SUPPLIER RELATIONSHIP

The consumer–supplier relationship in healthcare is influenced by different dynamics. For example, consumers may complain about rising healthcare costs, but most are not in a position to delay healthcare services until the price comes down. If you break your arm, you immediately go to a doctor or an emergency department to be treated. You are not likely to shop around for the best price or postpone treatment if you are in severe pain.

In most healthcare encounters, the insurance companies or government-sponsored payment systems (such as Medicare and Medicaid) are the consumer's agent. When healthcare costs are too high, they drive the resistance against rising rates. These groups act on behalf of consumers in an attempt to keep healthcare costs down. They exert their buying power by negotiating with healthcare providers for lower rates. In addition, they monitor billing claims for overuse of services and will not pay the providers—the suppliers—for services considered medically unnecessary. If a doctor admits you to the hospital to put a cast on your broken arm, your insurance company will question the doctor's decision to treat you in an inpatient setting. Your broken arm needs treatment, but the cast can be put on in the doctor's office or emergency department. Neither you nor the insurance company should be charged for the higher costs of hospital care if a less expensive and reasonable treatment alternative is available.

The connection between cost and quality is value. Most consumers purchase a product or service because they will, or perceive they will, derive some personal benefit from it. Healthcare consumers—whether patients or health plans—want providers to meet their needs at a reasonable cost (in terms of money, time, ease of use, and so forth). When customers believe they are receiving value for their dollars, they are more likely to perceive their healthcare interactions as quality experiences.

HEALTHCARE QUALITY

What is **healthcare quality**? Each group most affected by this question—consumers, purchasers, and providers—may answer it differently. Most consumers expect quality in the delivery of healthcare services: Patients want to receive the right treatments and experience good outcomes; everyone wants to have satisfactory interactions with caregivers; and consumers want the physical facilities where care is provided to be clean and pleasant, and

Healthcare quality
"Degree to which health services for individuals and populations increase the likelihood of desired health outcomes and are consistent with current professional knowledge" (IOM 1990, 4).

they want their doctors to use the best technology available. Consumer expectations are only part of the definition, however. Purchasers and providers may view quality in terms of other attributes.

IDENTIFYING THE STAKEHOLDERS IN QUALITY CARE

Purchasers are individuals and organizations that pay for healthcare services either directly or indirectly. If you pay out of pocket for healthcare services, you are both a consumer and a purchaser. Purchaser organizations include government-funded health insurance programs, private health insurance plans, and businesses that subsidize the cost of employees' health insurance. Purchasers are interested in the cost of healthcare and many of the same quality characteristics that are important to consumers. People who are financially responsible for some or all of their healthcare costs want to receive value for the dollars they spend. Purchaser organizations are no different. Purchasers view quality in terms of **cost-effectiveness**, meaning they want value in return for their healthcare expenditures.

Providers are individuals and organizations that offer healthcare services. Provider individuals include doctors, nurses, technicians, and clinical support and clerical staff. Provider organizations include hospitals, skilled nursing and rehabilitation facilities, outpatient clinics, home health agencies, and all other institutions that provide care.

In addition to the attributes important to consumers and purchasers, providers are concerned about legal liability—the risk that unsatisfied consumers will bring suit against the organization or individual. This concern can influence how providers define quality. Suppose you have a migraine headache, and your doctor orders a CT (computed tomography) scan of your head to be 100 percent certain there are no physical abnormalities. Your physician may have no medical reason to order the test, but he is taking every possible measure to avert the prospect that you will sue him for malpractice. In this scenario, your doctor is practicing **defensive medicine**—ordering or performing diagnostic or therapeutic interventions to safeguard the provider against malpractice liability (Minami et al. 2017). Because these interventions incur additional costs, providers' desire to avoid lawsuits can be at odds with purchasers' desire for cost-effectiveness.

DEFINING HEALTHCARE QUALITY

Before efforts to improve healthcare quality can be undertaken, a common definition of quality

---

Purchasers
Individuals and organizations that pay for healthcare services either directly or indirectly.

Cost-effectiveness
The minimal expenditure of dollars, time, and other elements necessary to achieve a desired healthcare result.

Providers
Individuals and organizations licensed or trained to give healthcare.

Defensive medicine
Diagnostic or therapeutic interventions conducted primarily as a safeguard against malpractice liability.

? DID YOU KNOW?

In a consumer message to Congress in 1962, President John F. Kennedy identified the right to be informed as one of four basic consumer rights. He said that a consumer has the right "to be protected against fraudulent, deceitful, or grossly misleading information, advertising, labeling, and other practices, and to be given the facts he needs to make an informed choice" (Kennedy 1962). Consumers have come to expect this right as they purchase goods and services in the marketplace.

is needed to work from, one that encompasses the priorities of all stakeholder groups—consumers, purchasers, and providers. The Institute of Medicine (IOM), a nonprofit organization that provides science-based advice on matters of medicine and health (and now called the **National Academy of Medicine**), brought the stakeholder groups together to create a workable definition of healthcare quality. In 1990, the IOM committee charged with designing a strategy for healthcare **quality assurance** published this definition:

> Quality of care is the degree to which health services for individuals and populations increase the likelihood of desired health outcomes and are consistent with current professional knowledge (IOM 1990, 4).

In 2001, the IOM Committee on Quality of Health Care in America further clarified the concept of healthcare quality in its report *Crossing the Quality Chasm: A New Health System for the 21st Century.* The committee identified six dimensions of US healthcare quality (listed in critical concept 1.1), which influence the improvement priorities of all stakeholder groups.

National Academy of Medicine

A private, nonprofit organization created by the federal government to provide science-based advice on matters of medicine and health. Formerly called the Institute of Medicine (IOM).

Quality assurance

Evaluation activities aimed at ensuring compliance with minimum quality standards. (*Quality assurance* and *quality control* may be used interchangeably to describe actions performed to ensure the quality of a product, service, or process.)

⚠ CRITICAL CONCEPT 1.1
Six Healthcare Quality Dimensions

1. Safe—Care intended to help patients should not harm them.

2. Effective—Care should be based on scientific knowledge and provided to patients who could benefit. Care should not be provided to patients unlikely to benefit from it. In other words, underuse and overuse should be avoided.

3. Patient centered—Care should be respectful of and responsive to individual patient preferences, needs, and values, and patient values should guide all clinical decisions.

4. Timely—Care should be provided promptly when the patient needs it.

5. Efficient—Waste, including equipment, supplies, ideas, and energy, should be avoided.

6. Equitable—The best possible care should be provided to everyone, regardless of age, sex, race, financial status, or any other demographic variable.

Source: Adapted from IOM (2001).

The IOM healthcare quality dimensions, together with the 1990 IOM quality-of-care definition, encompass what are commonly considered attributes of healthcare quality. Donald Berwick, MD (2005), then president of the **Institute for Healthcare Improvement (IHI)**, put this description into consumer terms when he wrote about his upcoming knee replacement and what he expected from his providers:

Institute for Healthcare Improvement (IHI)
An independent, nonprofit organization driving efforts to improve healthcare throughout the world.

- ◆ Don't kill me (no needless deaths).

- ◆ Do help me and don't hurt me (no needless pain).

- ◆ Don't make me feel helpless.

- ◆ Don't keep me waiting.

- ◆ Don't waste resources—mine or anyone else's.

The attribute of reliability is also important in healthcare quality. It is not enough to meet consumer expectations 90 percent of the time. Ideally, healthcare services consistently meet expectations 100 percent of the time. Unfortunately, healthcare today does not maintain consistently high levels of quality over time and across all services and settings (Burstin, Leatherman, and Goldmann 2016). Quality continues to vary greatly from provider to provider, and inconsistent levels of performance are still seen within organizations. In addition to the goal of achieving ever-better performance, healthcare organizations must strive for reliable quality.

High-value healthcare
Low-cost, high-quality healthcare.

When consumers define healthcare quality, they include **high-value healthcare** that achieves good outcomes at reasonable prices. Currently, the cost–quality ratio is far from ideal. Quality shortfalls exist in areas such as treatment effectiveness, care coordination, patient safety, and person-centered care (AHRQ 2016). Poorly designed processes can create quality problems and unnecessarily increase costs throughout the healthcare system. For example, when previous test results or health records are not available to the doctor during a patient's appointment, inaccurate diagnoses or duplicate testing can occur. In a recent survey, nearly 20 percent of patients in the United States reported that records or test results had not been available at an appointment in the past two years, or that duplicate tests had been ordered (Osborn et al. 2016). Better value in healthcare cannot be attained until the quality shortfalls are greatly reduced.

National Quality Strategy
Document prepared by the Agency for Healthcare Research and Quality on behalf of the US Department of Health and Human Services that helps healthcare stakeholders across the country—patients; providers; employers; health insurance companies; academic researchers; and local, state, and federal governments—prioritize quality improvement efforts, share lessons, and measure collective success.

SELECTING IMPROVEMENT AIMS

The **National Quality Strategy**, led by the Agency for Healthcare Research and Quality (AHRQ) on behalf of the US Department of Health and Human Services, was first published in 2011 as the National Strategy for Quality Improvement in Health Care (AHRQ 2017). The purpose of the National Quality Strategy is to guide and assess local, state, and national improvement efforts. It was developed with input from more than 300 individuals, groups, organizations, and other stakeholders representing all parts of the healthcare sector and the public.

When setting national aims, the National Quality Strategy adapted the **IHI Triple Aim framework** (Berwick, Nolan, and Whittington 2008). This framework detailed an interrelated approach for achieving optimal health system performance by simultaneously making improvements in three dimensions (care, health, and cost) that IHI called the "Triple Aim." The three broad aims of the National Quality Strategy are similar (AHRQ 2017):

- ◆ Better Care: Improve the overall quality, by making healthcare more patient-centered, reliable, accessible, and safe.

- ◆ Healthy People/Healthy Communities: Improve the health of the US population by supporting proven interventions to address behavioral, social, and environmental determinants of health in addition to delivering higher-quality care.

- ◆ Affordable Care: Reduce the cost of quality healthcare for individuals, families, employers, and government.

To advance these aims, the National Quality Strategy focuses on six priorities (AHRQ 2017):

1. Making care safer by reducing harm caused in the delivery of care.

2. Ensuring that each person and family is engaged as partners in their care.

3. Promoting effective communication and coordination of care.

4. Promoting the most effective prevention and treatment practices for the leading causes of mortality, starting with cardiovascular disease.

5. Working with communities to promote wide use of best practices to enable healthy living.

6. Making quality care more affordable for individuals, families, employers, and governments by developing and spreading new healthcare delivery models.

IHI Triple Aim framework
A framework developed by the Institute for Healthcare Improvement (IHI) that encourages implementation of strategies for simultaneously enhancing the experience and outcomes of the patient, improving the health of the population, and reducing per capita cost of care for the benefit of communities (IHI 2017).

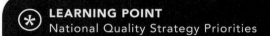

(*) **LEARNING POINT**
National Quality Strategy Priorities

The National Quality Strategy focuses on six priorities:

1. Patient safety
2. Person- and family-centered care
3. Communication and coordination of care
4. Preventive care
5. Community health
6. Care affordability

Each year, AHRQ publishes a report detailing the state of healthcare quality in the United States and the country's progress toward meeting the aims and priorities of the National Quality Strategy. At the end of this chapter is a website where the current National Quality Strategy report can be found.

CONCLUSION

Customers' perceptions and needs determine whether a product or service is "excellent." Quality involves understanding customer expectations and creating a product or service that reliably meets those expectations. Achieving high quality can be elusive because customer needs and expectations are always changing. To keep up with the changes, quality must be constantly managed and continuously improved.

Healthcare organizations are being challenged to improve the quality, reliability, and value of services. As shown in chapter 2, they can achieve this goal through a systematic quality management process.

FOR DISCUSSION

1. In your opinion, which companies provide superior customer service? Which companies provide average or mediocre customer service? Name the factors most important to you when judging the quality of a company's customer service.

2. Think about your most recent healthcare encounter. What aspects of the care or service were you pleased with? What could have been done better?

3. How does the reliability of healthcare services affect the quality of care you receive? What type of healthcare service do you find to be the least reliable in delivering a quality product? What type do you find the most reliable?

4. Which National Quality Strategy priority is most important to you as a healthcare consumer, and why? Which priority do you believe is most important to providers, and why? Which priority do you believe is most important to health insurance companies, and why? Which priority do you believe will be the most difficult to achieve, and why?

WEBSITES

- American Hospital Association's Health Research & Educational Trust
  www.hret.org

- American Public Health Association
  www.apha.org

- American Society for Quality
  www.asq.org

- Hospitals in Pursuit of Excellence, sponsored by the American Hospital Association
  www.hpoe.org

- Institute for Healthcare Improvement
  www.ihi.org

- Joint Commission Center for Transforming Healthcare
  www.centerfortransforminghealthcare.org

- National Academy of Medicine (formerly called the Institute of Medicine)
  https://nam.edu

- National Quality Strategy
  www.ahrq.gov/workingforquality

REFERENCES

Agency for Healthcare Research and Quality (AHRQ). 2017. "About the National Quality Strategy." Published March. www.ahrq.gov/workingforquality/about/index.html.

———. 2016. *2015 National Healthcare Quality and Disparities Report and 5th Anniversary Update on the National Quality Strategy*. Accessed October 22, 2017. www.ahrq.gov/research/findings/nhqrdr/nhqdr15/index.html.

Berwick, D. M. 2005. "My Right Knee." *Annals of Internal Medicine* 142 (2): 121–25.

Berwick, D. M., T. W. Nolan, and J. Whittington. 2008. "The Triple Aim: Care, Health and Cost." *Health Affairs* 27 (3): 759–69.

Burstin, H., S. Leatherman, and D. Goldmann. 2016. "Evaluating the Quality of Medical Care." *Journal of Internal Medicine* 279 (2): 154–59.

Clark, T. 2008. *Starbucked: A Double Tall Tale of Caffeine, Commerce, and Culture*. New York: Back Bay Books.

Crossley, M. L. 2007. *The Desk Reference of Statistical Quality Methods*, 2nd ed. Milwaukee, WI: ASQ Quality Press.

DuPree, E. S., and M. R. Chassin. 2016. "Organizing Performance Management to Support High-Reliability Healthcare." In *America's Healthcare Transformation: Strategies and Innovations*, edited by R. A. Phillips, 3–16. New Brunswick, NJ: Rutgers University Press.

Harrington, H. J. 2009. "Nice Car . . . When It Runs." *Quality Digest* 29 (2): 12.

Hope, J. 2017. "Consider How Lowering Tuition Paid Off in Enrollment Boost for Small College." *Enrollment Management Report* 18 (5): 6–7.

Institute for Healthcare Improvement (IHI). 2017. "IHI Triple Aim Initiative." Accessed October 22. www.ihi.org/Engage/Initiatives/TripleAim/Pages/default.aspx.

Institute of Medicine (IOM). 2001. *Crossing the Quality Chasm: A New Health System for the 21st Century*. Washington, DC: National Academies Press.

———. 1990. *Medicare: A Strategy for Quality Assurance: Volume I*, edited by K. N. Lohr. Washington, DC: National Academies Press.

Kennedy, J. F. 1962. "Special Message to the Congress on Protecting the Consumer Interest, March 15, 1962." Accessed October 22, 2017. www.presidency.ucsb.edu/ws/?pid=9108.

Minami, C. A., C. R. Sheils, E. Pavey, J. W. Chung, J. J. Stulberg, D. D. Odell, A. D. Yang, D. J. Bentrem, and K. Y. Bilimoria. 2017. "Association Between State Medical Malpractice Environment and Postoperative Outcomes in the United States." *Journal of the American College of Surgeons* 224 (3): 310–18.

Osborn, R., D. Squires, M. M. Doty, D. O. Sarnak, and E. C. Schneider. 2016. "In New Survey of Eleven Countries, US Adults Still Struggle with Access to and Affordability of Health Care." *Health Affairs* 35 (12): 2327–36.

Walton, M. 1986. *The Deming Management Method*. New York: Putnam Publishing Group.

CHAPTER 2

QUALITY MANAGEMENT BUILDING BLOCKS

LEARNING OBJECTIVES

After reading this chapter, you will be able to

➤ explain the three primary quality management activities: measurement, assessment, and improvement;

➤ recognize quality pioneers' contributions to, and influence on, the manufacturing industry;

➤ identify factors that prompted healthcare organizations to adopt quality practices originally developed for use in other industries; and

➤ describe external forces that influence quality management activities in healthcare organizations.

KEY WORDS

- Accreditation
- Accreditation standards
- Assessment
- Baldrige National Quality Award
- Conditions of Participation
- Criteria
- Data
- Harm
- Health maintenance organization (HMO)
- High-reliability organizations (HROs)
- Improvement

- Measurement
- Misuse
- Overuse
- Performance expectations
- Performance improvement
- Quality Assurance and Performance Improvement (QAPI) program
- Quality circles
- Quality control
- Quality management
- Quality planning
- Statistical thinking
- Underuse

Quality management
A way of doing business that continuously improves products and services to achieve better performance.

Overuse
Provision of healthcare services that do not benefit the patient, are not clearly indicated, or are provided in excessive amounts or in an unnecessary setting.

Underuse
Failure to provide appropriate or necessary services, or provision of an inadequate quantity or lower level of service than that required.

Quality does not develop on its own. For quality to be achieved, a systematic evaluation and improvement process must be implemented. In the business world, this process is known as **quality management**. Quality management is a way of doing business that ensures continuous improvement of products and services to achieve better performance. According to the American Society for Quality (2017), the goal of quality management in any industry is to achieve maximum customer satisfaction at the lowest overall cost to the organization while continuing to improve the process.

The authors of the 2001 Institute of Medicine (IOM) report *Crossing the Quality Chasm* recommend eliminating overuse, underuse, and misuse of services to achieve maximum customer service in healthcare (Berwick 2002). **Overuse** occurs when a service is provided even though no evidence indicates it will help the patient—for example, prescribing antibiotics for patients with viral infections. **Underuse** occurs when a service that would have been medically beneficial to the patient is not provided—for example, performing a necessary diagnostic test. **Misuse** occurs when a service is not carried out properly—for example, operating on the wrong part of the patient's body.

QUALITY MANAGEMENT ACTIVITIES

Quality management may appear to be a difficult and bewildering undertaking. While the terminology used to describe the process can be puzzling at first, the basic principles should be familiar to you. Quality management involves **measurement**, **assessment**, and **improvement**—activities people perform almost every day.

Consider this example: Most people must manage their finances. You must *measure*—that is, keep track of your bank deposits and debits—to know where you stand financially. Occasionally, you have to *assess* your current financial situation—that is, inquire about your account balance—to determine your financial "health." Can you afford to go out to dinner, or are you overdrawn? Periodically, you must make *improvements*—that is, get a part-time job to earn extra cash or remember to record debit card withdrawals—so you do not incur unexpected overdraft charges.

The three primary quality management activities—measurement, assessment, and improvement—evolve in a closely linked cycle (see exhibit 2.1). Healthcare organizations track performance through various measurement activities to gather information about the quality of patient care and support functions. Results are evaluated in the assessment step by comparing measurement **data** with **performance expectations**. If expectations are met, organizations continue to measure and assess performance. If expectations are not met, they proceed to the improvement phase to investigate reasons for the performance gap and implement changes on the basis of their findings. The quality management cycle does not end at this point, however. Performance continues to be evaluated through measurement activities.

The financial management example used earlier to explain quality management vocabulary also may help clarify basic quality management techniques. For instance, when you review your expenditures on leisure activities over the last six months, you are *monitoring performance*—looking for *trends* in your spending habits. If you decide to put 10 percent of your income into a savings account each month, you are setting a *performance goal*. Occasionally, you check to see whether you have achieved your goal; in other words, you are *evaluating performance*. If you need to save more money, you implement an *improvement plan*. You design a new savings strategy, implement that strategy, and periodically check your progress. Application of these techniques to healthcare quality management is covered in later chapters.

Misuse
Incorrect diagnoses, medical errors, and other sources of avoidable complications.

Measurement
Collection of information for the purpose of understanding current performance and seeing how performance changes or improves over time.

Assessment
Use of performance information to determine whether an acceptable level of quality has been achieved.

Improvement
Planning and making changes to current practices to achieve better performance.

Data
Numbers or facts that are interpreted for the purpose of drawing conclusions.

Performance expectations
Minimum acceptable or desired level of quality.

EXHIBIT 2.1
Cycle of
Measurement,
Assessment, and
Improvement

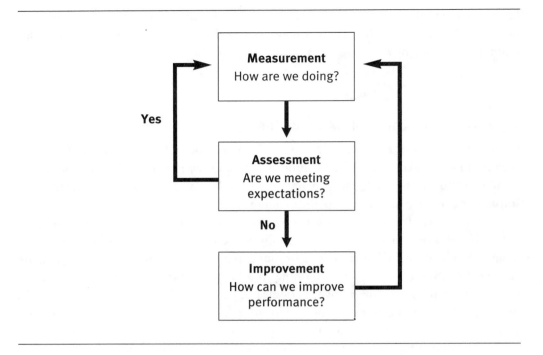

CASE STUDY

The following case study illustrates the quality management cycle of measurement, assessment, and improvement in a community health center.

The medical director of a community health center receives information about the center's patients who have used emergency department (ED) services. The information is used to *measure* the number of patients seeking ED care for nonemergent conditions that would have been better handled in the community health center. Patients who use the ED for nonemergent care are less likely to receive needed ongoing care and education about their condition. This can lead to repeat ED visits for patients and poor long-term outcomes.

In an *assessment* of the measurement data, the medical director discovered that in a six-month period 52 percent of the ED visits for the center's patients were for a non-emergent condition. *Improvements* were made to ensure the center's patients get the right care in the right place. The improvements included expanding the center's hours, creating the position of access coordinator to educate the center's patients about nonemergency services in the community, and working with the local 911 dispatcher to identify patients who need something other than emergency care. The medical director continues to measure ED use by the center's patients to evaluate the success of the improvements.

QUALITY MANAGEMENT MILESTONES IN INDUSTRY AND HEALTHCARE

The concept of quality management is timeless. To stay in business, manufacturing and service industries have long sought better ways of meeting customer expectations. Healthcare professionals live by the motto *primum non nocere*—first, do no **harm**. To fulfill this promise, discovering better ways to care for patients has always been a priority. Although the goal—quality products and services—is the same regardless of the industry, methods for achieving this goal in healthcare have evolved differently than in other fields.

Harm
An outcome that negatively affects a patient's health or quality of life.

INDUSTRIAL QUALITY EVOLUTION

The contemporary quality movement in the manufacturing industry can be traced to the work of three men in the 1920s at Western Electric Company in Cicero, Illinois. Walter Shewhart, W. Edwards Deming, and Joseph Juran learned and applied the science of quality improvement to the company's production lines (ASQ 2017). Shewhart used statistical methods to measure variations in the telephone equipment manufacturing process. Waste was reduced and product quality was improved by controlling undesirable process variation. Shewhart is referred to as the father of statistical quality control, a method we explore in chapter 4.

Deming (1994) learned Shewhart's methods and made the measurement and control of process variation a key element of his philosophy of quality management:

- ◆ Organizations are a set of interrelated processes with a common aim.

- ◆ Process variation must be understood.

- ◆ How new knowledge is generated must be understood.

- ◆ How people are motivated and work together must be understood.

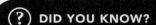

? DID YOU KNOW?

In the 1950s, W. Edwards Deming, a professor and management consultant, transformed traditional industrial thinking about quality control by emphasizing employee empowerment, performance feedback, and measurement-based quality management.

Following World War II, Japanese manufacturing companies invited Deming to help them improve the quality of their products. Over a period of several years, as a result of Deming's advice, many low-quality Japanese products became world class. The Deming model for continuous improvement is described in chapter 5.

Juran combined the science of quality with its practical application, providing a framework for linking finance and management. The components of that framework, the Juran Quality Trilogy, are as follows (Girdler et al. 2016):

Quality planning
Setting quality objectives and specifying operational processes and related resources needed to fulfill the objectives.

Quality control
Operational techniques and activities used to fulfill quality requirements. (*Quality control* and *quality assurance* may be used interchangeably to describe actions performed to ensure the quality of a product, service, or process.)

Quality circles
Small groups of employees organized to solve work-related problems.

◆ **Quality planning**—define customers and how to meet their needs

◆ **Quality control**—keep processes working well

◆ Quality improvement—learn, optimize, refine, and adapt

In the 1950s, Juran, like Deming, helped jump-start product improvements at Japanese manufacturing companies. Whereas Deming focused on measuring and controlling process variation, Juran aimed to develop the managerial aspects supporting quality. One of Juran's management principles—focusing improvements on the "vital few" sources of the problems—is described in chapter 4.

Another individual who had a significant impact on contemporary quality practices in industry was Kaoru Ishikawa, a Japanese engineer who incorporated the science of quality into Japanese culture. He was one of the first people to emphasize the importance of involving all members of the organization in this process, rather than only management-level employees. Ishikawa believed that top-down quality goals could be accomplished only through bottom-up methods (Best and Neuhauser 2008). To support his belief, he introduced the concept of **quality circles**—groups of 3 to 12 frontline employees who meet regularly to analyze production-related problems and propose solutions (Ishikawa 1990).

Ishikawa stressed that employees should be trained to use data to measure and improve processes that affect product quality. One of the data collection and presentation techniques he recommended for process improvement purposes is covered in chapter 6. The science of industrial quality focuses on improving the quality of products by improving the production process. Improving the production process means removing wasteful practices, standardizing production steps, and controlling variation from expectations. These methods have been proven effective and remain fundamental to industrial quality improvement. The work of Shewhart, Deming, and Ishikawa laid the foundation for many of the modern quality philosophies that underlie the improvement models described in chapter 5.

Following World War II, US manufacturers were under considerable pressure to meet production schedules, and product quality became a secondary consideration. Recognizing the consequences of these lags in quality, in the 1970s US executives visited Japan to discover ways to improve product quality. During these visits, Americans learned about the quality philosophies of Deming, Juran, and Ishikawa; the science of industrial quality; and the concept of quality control as a management tool. In 1980, NBC aired a television program titled *If Japan Can . . . Why Can't We?*, which described how Japanese manufacturers had adopted Deming's approach to continuous improvement, most notably his focus on variation control (Butman 1997). As a result, many US companies began to emulate the Japanese approach. Several quality gurus emerged, each with his own interpretation of quality management. During the 1980s, Juran, Deming, Philip Crosby, Armand Feigenbaum, and others received widespread attention as philosophers of quality in the manufacturing and service industries.

In 1987, President Ronald Reagan signed into law the Malcolm Baldrige National Quality Improvement Act (Spath 2005). This national quality program, managed by the US Department of Commerce's National Institute of Standards and Technology, established **criteria** for performance excellence that organizations can use to evaluate and improve their quality. Many of these criteria originated from the quality philosophies and practices advanced by Shewhart, Deming, Juran, and Ishikawa. The annual **Baldrige National Quality Award** was also created to recognize US companies that meet the program's stringent standards. For the first ten years of the award's existence, eligible companies were limited to three categories: manufacturing, service, and small business. In 1998, two categories—education and healthcare—were added. In 2002, SSM Health Care, based in St. Louis, became the first healthcare organization to win the Baldrige National Quality Award. The core values and concepts of the 2017–2018 Baldrige Performance Excellence Framework (Health Care) are summarized in critical concept 2.1.

Criteria
Standards or principles by which something is judged or evaluated.

Baldrige National Quality Award
Recognition conferred annually by the Baldrige Performance Excellence Program to US organizations, including healthcare organizations, that demonstrate performance excellence.

> ⚠ **CRITICAL CONCEPT 2.1** Interrelated Core Values and Concepts in the Baldrige Performance Excellence Framework (Health Care)
>
> **Systems Perspective:** Successful management of organization-wide performance requires synthesis, alignment, and integration. Synthesis means looking at the organization as a whole while incorporating key organizational attributes such as core competencies, strategic objectives, action plans, and work systems. Alignment means using the key organizational linkages to ensure consistency of plans, processes, measures, and actions. Integration means ensuring the individual performance management components operate in a fully interconnected, unified, and mutually beneficial manner to deliver anticipated results.
>
> **Visionary Leadership:** Senior leaders set a vision for the organization, create a focus on patients and other customers, demonstrate clear and visible organizational values and ethics, and set high expectations for the workforce. The needs of all stakeholders should be considered when establishing the vision, values, and expectations. Leaders should also ensure ongoing organizational success through creation of strategies, systems, and methods for building knowledge and capabilities, stimulating innovation, requiring accountability, and achieving performance excellence.
>
> *(continued)*

! CRITICAL CONCEPT 2.1   Interrelated Core Values and Concepts in the
Baldrige Performance Excellence Framework (Health Care) *(continued)*

Patient Focus: The delivery of health care services must be patient and customer focused—meaning that judgment of satisfaction and value considers all characteristics of
patient care delivery (medical and non-medical) and all modes of customer access and
support that contribute value to your patients and other customers. Patient-focused excellence has both current and future components: understanding the desires of patients
and other customers today and anticipating future desires and health care marketplace
potential.

Valuing People: The success of an organization depends a great deal on the knowledge,
skills, creativity, and motivation of its staff members. Valuing people means committing
to their satisfaction, development, and well-being and creating a safe, trusting and co-
operative environment. An engaged workforce benefits from meaningful work, clear organizational direction, the opportunity to learn, and accountability for performance. To
accomplish overall goals, successful organizations also build external partnerships with
people and with other organizations.

Organizational Learning and Agility: Organizational learning refers to continuous improvement of existing approaches and processes and adaptation to change, leading to
new goals and approaches. Learning is embedded in the operation of the organization.
Organizations must ensure timely design of new health care delivery systems and programs and allow for opportunities to continuously improve so patients' individual needs
are met. Organizational learning and agility is also achieved through strategic partnerships or alliances with other health care organizations.

Focus on Success: A focus on success now and into the future requires a willingness to
make long term commitments to key stakeholders—patients and families, staff, communities, employers, payers, and health profession students. Important for an organization
in the strategic planning process is the anticipation of changes in health care delivery,
resource availability, patient and other stakeholder expectations, technological devel-
opments, new partnering opportunities, evolving regulatory requirements, community/
societal expectations, and new thrust by competitors.

(continued)

CRITICAL CONCEPT 2.1 Interrelated Core Values and Concepts in the Baldrige Performance Excellence Framework (Health Care) *(continued)*

Management for Innovation: Innovation creates new value for stakeholders by making meaningful changes to improve an organization's health care services, programs, processes, operations, health care delivery model, and business model. To promote innovation an organization needs a supportive environment, a process for identifying strategic opportunities, and a desire to pursue intelligent risks. Innovation is important for all aspects of operations and all work systems and work processes. Successful organizations use both innovation and continuous incremental improvement approaches to improve performance.

Management by Fact: Measurement and analysis of performance are needed for an effective health care and administrative management system. Measures are derived from the organization's strategy and provide critical data and information about key processes, outputs, and results. The measures selected should best represent the factors that lead to improved health care outcomes; improved patient, other customer, operational, financial, and societal performance; and healthier communities. Analysis involves extracting larger meaning from data and information to support evaluation, decision-making, improvement, and innovation.

Societal Responsibility and Community Health: Leaders need to emphasize the responsibility all aspects of the organization's operations have to the public and to the improvement of community health. Leaders should be role models for the organization and its workforce in the protection of public health, safety, and the environment. Also, the organization should emphasize resource conservation and waste reduction. The organization should meet all local, state, and federal laws and regulatory requirements and should seek to excel beyond minimal compliance.

Ethics and Transparency: The leaders should stress ethical behavior in all stakeholder transactions and interactions with the governing body monitoring ethical conduct. Senior leaders should be role models of ethical behavior and clearly articulate ethical principles and expectations to the workforce. Transparency is characterized by consistently candid and open communication on the part of leadership and management and by the sharing of clear and accurate information. Ethical behavior and transparency build trust in the organization and its leaders.

(continued)

> **! CRITICAL CONCEPT 2.1** Interrelated Core Values and Concepts in the
> Baldrige Performance Excellence Framework (Health Care) *(continued)*
>
> **Delivering Value and Results:** An organization's performance measurements need to focus on key results. Results should focus on creating and balancing value for all stakeholders—patients, their families, staff, the community, payers, businesses, health profession students, suppliers and partners, stockholders, and the public. Thus results need to be a composite of measures that include not just financial results, but also health care and process results; patient, other customer, and workforce satisfaction and engagement results; and leadership, strategy, and societal performance.
>
> *Source*: Adapted from National Institute of Standards and Technology (NIST), *2017–2018 Baldrige Excellence Framework: A Systems Approach to Improving Your Organization's Performance (Health Care)*, 40–44. Gaithersburg, MD: US Department of Commerce, National Institute of Standards and Technology. Copyright © 2017.

HEALTHCARE QUALITY EVOLUTION

Until the 1970s, the fundamental philosophy of healthcare quality management was based on the pre–Industrial Revolution craft model: Train the craftspeople (e.g., physicians, nurses, technicians), license or certify them, supply them with an adequate structure (e.g., facilities, equipment), and then let them provide health services (Merry 2003). In 1913, the American College of Surgeons (ACS) was founded to address variations in the quality of medical education. A few years later, it developed the hospital standardization program to address the quality of facilities in which physicians worked. Training improvement efforts were also under way in nursing; the National League for Nursing Education released its first standard curriculum for schools of nursing in 1917.

Around the time of Shewhart's work in the 1920s, licensing and certification requirements for healthcare providers and standards for facilities, equipment, and other aspects of healthcare became more stringent. During the time Deming and Juran were advising Japanese manufacturers, the ACS hospital standardization program was turned over to The Joint Commission (2016), the United States' oldest and largest healthcare accreditation group, which currently evaluates and accredits more than 21,000 healthcare organizations and programs across the nation. The program's **accreditation standards** set a minimum bar for healthcare quality. While the standards stressed the need for physicians and other professional staff to evaluate care provided to individual patients, none of the quality practices espoused by Deming and Juran were initially required of hospitals. The standards

Accreditation standards
Levels of performance excellence that organizations must attain to become credentialed by a competent authority.

centered on structural requirements and eliminating incompetent people, not measuring and controlling variation in healthcare processes.

The Joint Commission accreditation standards served as a model for provider quality requirements of Medicare, the federal healthcare program for the elderly passed by Congress in 1965. Throughout the 1970s, quality requirements in healthcare—whether represented by accreditation standards, state licensing boards, or federal regulations—focused largely on structural details and on the disciplinary actions taken against poorly performing hospitals and physicians (Brennan and Berwick 1996).

The quality revolution affecting other industries in the 1980s also affected healthcare services. In 1980, The Joint Commission added a quality assurance (QA) standard loosely based on the work of Deming and Juran (Affeldt 1980). The QA standard required accredited facilities to implement an organization-wide program to

1. identify important or potential problems or concerns with patient care,

2. objectively assess the cause and scope of the problems or concerns,

3. implement decisions or actions designed to eliminate the problems,

4. monitor activities to ensure desired results are achieved and sustained, and

5. document the effectiveness of the overall program to enhance patient care and ensure sound clinical performance (Joint Commission 1979).

In the early 1980s, following years of rapid increases in Medicare and other publicly funded healthcare expenditures, the government established external groups (known as *peer review organizations*) to monitor the costs and quality of care provided in hospitals and outpatient settings (IOM 2006). These groups used many of the same principles found in The Joint Commission's 1980 QA standard.

Throughout the 1980s and 1990s, healthcare quality management was increasingly influenced by the industrial concepts of continuous improvement and statistical quality control, largely in response to pressure from purchasers to slow the growth of healthcare expenditures. Seeking alternative methods to improve healthcare quality and reduce costs, regulatory and accreditation groups turned to other industries for solutions. Soon, the quality practices from other industries were being applied to health services.

Application of innovative quality practices found to be successful in other settings is still a

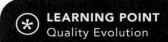

LEARNING POINT
Quality Evolution

The methods and principles guiding healthcare quality improvement efforts have evolved at a different pace than have those guiding quality improvement efforts in other industries. Several factors account for this difference. Healthcare is catching up by applying the best quality management practices of the manufacturing and service industries that can be adapted to the patient care environment.

high priority in healthcare. Healthcare costs have continued to grow considerably faster than the economy. National health spending in 2016 grew by 4.8 percent from the previous year and was estimated to be 18.1 percent of the gross national product. National health expenditures totaled $1.378 trillion in 2000, almost doubled to $2.6 trillion in 2010, and reached $3.4 trillion in 2016 (Holahan et al. 2011; Keçhan et al. 2017).

Today, many of the fundamental ideas behind quality improvement in the manufacturing and service industries shape healthcare quality management efforts. For example, The Joint Commission leadership standard incorporates concepts from the Baldrige Criteria for Performance Excellence, and the performance improvement standard requires use of statistical tools and techniques to analyze and display data. Professional groups, such as the Medical Group Management Association (MGMA), teach members to apply **statistical thinking** to healthcare practices to understand and reduce inappropriate and unintended process variation (MGMA 2017; Kumar 2017). The Institute for Healthcare Improvement (2017) sponsors improvement projects aimed at standardizing patient care practices and minimizing inappropriate variation.

Healthcare facilities have begun using high-reliability concepts to help achieve their safety, quality, and efficiency goals (Chassin and Loeb 2011). **High-reliability organizations (HROs)** experience fewer accidents than would be anticipated given the high-risk nature of the work because they have developed ways of managing the unexpected better than most organizations (Weick and Sutcliffe 2015). Early adopters of HRO philosophies were industries whose past failures had extremely catastrophic consequences (e.g., commercial airplane crashes, nuclear reactor meltdowns). Safety managers in aviation and nuclear power realized they needed to (1) identify the weak danger signals, (2) strengthen those signals, (3) address the dangers while maintaining functionality, and (4) avoid future disasters. Now, the naval and commercial aviation field and the nuclear power–generation processes are considered highly reliable. The complex systems in these organizations consistently perform nearly error free, thereby avoiding potentially catastrophic failures. Case studies illustrating the adaptation of industrial quality science and high-reliability concepts to health services improvement are found throughout this book.

Some industrial quality improvement techniques are not transferrable to healthcare. The manufacturing industry, for example, deals with machines and processes designed to be meticulously measured and controlled. At the heart of healthcare are patients whose behaviors and conditions vary from individual to individual and change over time. These factors create unpredictability that presents healthcare providers with challenges not found in other industries (Hines et al. 2008). Also, unlike the manufacturing industry, healthcare is "predominantly designed to be capacity-led, and hence there is limited ability to influence demand or make full use of freed-up resources" (Radnor, Holweg, and Waring 2012, 364).

In addition to adopting the quality practices of other industries focused on reducing waste and variation, healthcare organizations still use some components of the pre–Industrial Revolution craft model to manage quality. Adequate training and continuous monitoring are essential to building and maintaining a competent provider staff. Structural details

Statistical thinking
A philosophy of learning and action based on the following fundamental principles: All work occurs in a system of interconnected processes, variation exists in all processes, and understanding and reducing variation are keys to success.

High-reliability organizations (HROs)
Entities or businesses with systems in place that are exceptionally consistent in accomplishing their goals and avoiding potentially catastrophic errors.

remain important; considerable attention in healthcare is given to maintaining adequate facilities and equipment.

EXTERNAL FORCES AFFECTING HEALTHCARE QUALITY MANAGEMENT

Healthcare organizations, like all businesses, do not operate in a vacuum. Many external forces influence business activities, including quality management. Government regulations and the activities of accreditation groups and of large purchasers of health services exert a major influence on the operation of healthcare organizations.

GOVERNMENT REGULATIONS

Regulations are issued by governments at the local, state, and national levels to protect the health and safety of the public. Regulation is often enforced through licensing. For instance, to maintain its license, a restaurant must comply with state health department rules and periodically undergo inspection.

Just as the restaurant owner must follow state health department rules or risk closure, organizations that provide healthcare services or offer health insurance must follow government regulations, usually at the state level. Regulations differ from state to state. If a healthcare organization receives money from the federal government for providing services to consumers, it must comply with federal regulations in addition to state regulations. Both state and federal regulations include quality management requirements (discussed in more detail later). For example, licensing regulations in all states require that hospitals have a system for measuring, evaluating, and reducing patient infection rates. Similar requirements are found in federal regulations (CMS 2016b).

ACCREDITATION GROUPS

Accreditation is a voluntary process by which the performance of an organization is measured against nationally accepted standards of performance. Accreditation standards are based on government regulations and input from individuals and groups in the healthcare industry. Healthcare organizations seek accreditation because it

◆ enhances public confidence,

◆ is an objective evaluation of the organization's performance, and

◆ stimulates the organization's quality improvement efforts.

The Joint Commission's standards have always included quality measurement, assessment, and improvement requirements. All other groups that accredit healthcare

Accreditation
A self-assessment and external assessment process used by healthcare organizations to gauge their level of performance in relation to established standards and implement ways to continuously improve.

organizations and programs also require quality management activities. Exhibit 2.2 lists healthcare accreditation groups and the organizations or programs they accredit. Accreditation is an ongoing process, and visits are made to healthcare organizations at regularly scheduled or unannounced intervals to monitor their compliance with accreditation requirements. While accreditation is considered voluntary, an increasing number of purchasers and government entities mandate it.

EXHIBIT 2.2
Healthcare
Accreditation
Groups

Accreditation Group	Organizations and Programs Accredited
AABB (formerly American Association of Blood Banks) (www.aabb.org)	Freestanding and provider-based blood banks, transfusion services, and blood donation centers
Accreditation Association for Ambulatory Health Care (www.aaahc.org)	Ambulatory healthcare clinics and surgery centers, urgent care facilities, community health centers, medical home organizations, multispecialty group practices, university student health centers, and a wide range of other outpatient services
Accreditation Commission for Health Care (www.achc.org)	Home health, hospice, and private duty; DMEPOS (durable medical equipment, prosthetics, orthotics, and suppliers) agencies
American Association for Accreditation of Ambulatory Surgery Facilities (www.aaaasf.org)	Ambulatory surgery facilities, oral/maxillofacial facilities, outpatient physical therapy clinics, and rural health clinics
American College of Surgeons (www.facs.org)	Cancer programs at hospitals and freestanding treatment centers, breast centers, oncology medical homes, and stereotactic breast biopsy services
Center for Improvement in Healthcare Quality (www.cihq.org)	Hospitals
Commission for the Accreditation of Birth Centers (www.birthcenteraccreditation.org)	Birth centers
Commission on Accreditation of Medical Transport Systems (www.camts.org)	Rotorwing, fixed wing, and ground medical transport systems
Commission on Accreditation of Rehabilitation Facilities (www.carf.org)	Freestanding and provider-based medical rehabilitation and human service programs, such as behavioral health, child and youth services, and opioid treatment and continuing care retirement communities and aging services networks
Commission on Laboratory Accreditation of the College of American Pathologists (www.cap.org)	Freestanding and provider-based laboratories, forensic drug testing services, biorepository facilities, and reproductive laboratory services

(continued)

Accreditation Group	Organizations and Programs Accredited
Community Health Accreditation Partner (www.chapinc.org)	Community-based health services, including home health agencies, hospices, home medical equipment providers, and private duty home care services
Compliance Team (www.thecomplianceteam.org)	Rural health clinics, patient-centered medical homes, immediate care clinics, and sleep care management; DMEPOS agencies, private duty, ocularist/anaplastologist, and pharmacy services
Diagnostic Modality Accreditation Program of the American College of Radiology (www.acr.org)	A variety of services in freestanding and provider-based imaging facilities, including radiology and nuclear medicine
DNV GL-Healthcare (www.dnvglhealthcare.com)	Hospitals
Foundation for the Accreditation of Cellular Therapy (www.factwebsite.org)	Cellular therapy and cord blood banking services
Global Healthcare Accreditation Program (www.globalhealthcareaccreditation.com)	Medical travel program organizations
Healthcare Facilities Accreditation Program (www.hfap.org)	Hospitals; clinical laboratories; ambulatory care/surgery, mental health, substance abuse, and physical rehabilitation facilities; and primary stroke centers
Healthcare Quality Association on Accreditation (www.hqaa.org)	Durable medical and home medical equipment providers and services
Institute for Medical Quality (www.imq.org)	Surgery centers and various types of ambulatory facilities
Intersocietal Accreditation Commission (www.icanl.org)	Freestanding and provider-based nuclear medicine, nuclear cardiology, positron emission tomography, and superficial vein services
Joint Commission (www.jointcommission.org)	General, psychiatric, children's, and rehabilitation hospitals; critical access hospitals; medical equipment services, hospice services, and other home care organizations; nursing homes and other long-term care facilities; behavioral healthcare organizations and addiction services; rehabilitation centers, group practices, office-based surgeries, and other ambulatory care providers; independent or freestanding laboratories; and medical homes
National Commission on Correctional Health Care (www.ncchc.org)	Healthcare services in jails, prisons, and juvenile confinement facilities

EXHIBIT 2.2
Healthcare
Accreditation
Groups
(*continued*)

(*continued*)

Exhibit 2.2
Healthcare
Accreditation
Groups
(continued)

Accreditation Group	Organizations and Programs Accredited
National Committee for Quality Assurance (www.ncqa.org)	Health plans, managed behavioral healthcare organizations, disease management programs, case management programs, wellness and health promotion programs, and accountable care organizations
Public Health Accreditation Board (www.phaboard.org)	Tribal, state, local, and territorial public health departments
URAC (American Accreditation HealthCare Commission, Inc.) (www.urac.org)	Health plans, credential-verification organizations, independent review organizations, medical homes, mail service pharmacies, and others; also accredits specific functions in healthcare organizations (e.g., case management, pharmacy benefit management, consumer education and support, disease management)

LARGE PURCHASERS

The largest purchaser of healthcare services is the government. For 2017, the Centers for Medicare & Medicaid Services (CMS) was projected to spend more than $718 billion on patient care for Medicare enrollees, and in that same year, federal and state governments combined were projected to spend more than $586 billion on Medicaid enrollees (Keehan et al. 2017). Healthcare organizations participating in these government-funded insurance programs must comply with the quality management requirements found in state and federal regulations (see next section). For example, home health agencies that care for Medicare patients must report to CMS on the quality of care they provide, including information on patients' physical and mental health and their ability to perform basic daily activities (CMS 2016a).

> **(?) DID YOU KNOW?**
>
> There is an increasing link between quality and revenue for healthcare facilities. In early 2015, the US Department of Health and Human Services (2015) set a goal of linking 90 percent of Medicare payments to quality or value.

Conditions of Participation
Federal regulations that determine an entity's eligibility for involvement in a particular activity.

QUALITY MANAGEMENT REQUIREMENTS

Quality management requirements for each provider category are cited in federal regulations called **Conditions of Participation**. These regulations form a contract between the government purchaser and the provider. If a provider wants to participate in a federally funded insurance program, it must abide by the conditions spelled out in myriad regulations.

For example, CMS requires nursing homes to implement a **Quality Assurance and Performance Improvement (QAPI) program**, which involves the coordinated application of two mutually reinforcing aspects of a quality management system: quality assurance (QA) and **performance improvement** (PI). This systematic, comprehensive, and data-driven approach to maintaining and improving safety and quality in nursing homes is intended to involve all nursing home caregivers in practical and creative problem solving (CMS 2016c). This program consists of five key elements of effective quality management: design and scope; governance and leadership; feedback, data systems, and monitoring; performance improvement projects; and systematic analysis and systemic action (CMS 2016c).

Some other regulations and accreditation standards affecting quality management activities are detailed in later chapters. However, these requirements change often, and healthcare organizations must keep up to date on the latest rules. The websites listed in exhibit 2.2 and those found at the end of this chapter contain information on current regulations and accreditation standards affecting healthcare quality management activities.

Private insurance companies also pay a large amount of health services costs in the United States. For 2017, private insurance plans were projected to pay more than $1.208 billion to providers for the care of their enrollees (Keehan et al. 2017). For the most part, these plans rely on government regulations and accreditation standards to define basic quality management requirements for healthcare organizations. However, some private insurance companies have additional quality measurement and improvement requirements for participating providers. For example, outpatient clinics that provide care for patients in a **health maintenance organization (HMO)** may be required to report to the health plan the percentage of calls received by the clinic that are answered by a live voice within 30 seconds. The HMO uses this information, along with other data, to measure the quality of customer service in the clinic.

The measurement, assessment, and improvement requirements of private insurance companies are detailed in provider contracts. If a provider wants to participate in a health plan, it must agree to abide by the rules in the contract, some of which place quality management responsibilities on the provider.

Quality Assurance and Performance Improvement (QAPI) program
This CMS requirement for nursing homes involves the coordinated application of two mutually reinforcing aspects of a quality management system: quality assurance (QA) and performance improvement (PI).

Performance improvement
A method for analyzing performance problems and enacting improvements to ensure good performance.

Health maintenance organization (HMO)
Public or private organization providing comprehensive medical care to subscribers on the basis of a prepaid contract.

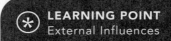

LEARNING POINT
External Influences

The measurement, assessment, and improvement activities in healthcare organizations are influenced by three external forces: accreditation standards, government regulations, and purchaser requirements.

CONCLUSION

Quality management activities in healthcare organizations are constantly evolving. These changes often occur in reaction to external forces, such as regulation or accreditation standard revisions and pressures to control costs. Healthcare quality management is also influenced by other industries. Improvement strategies used to enhance the quality of products and services are frequently updated as new learning emerges. Since their inception in 1982, the criteria of the Malcolm Baldrige National Quality Award have undergone several revisions. Healthcare quality management changed in 1998 when the Baldrige Criteria were adapted for use by healthcare organizations. In addition, the science of quality management, once reserved for the manufacturing industry, is now used in healthcare organizations.

The rules and tools of healthcare quality management will continue to evolve, but the basic principles of measurement, assessment, and improvement will remain the same. For instance, many people sort household garbage into two bins—one for recyclable materials and one for everything else. Garbage collection rules have changed, yet the basic principle—removing garbage from the house—is the same. Thirty years ago, people never would have imagined they'd be using wireless devices to make phone calls. The tool has changed, but the basic principle—communicating—has not.

Why should healthcare organizations be involved in quality management activities? Foremost, quality management is the right thing to do. Providers have an ethical obligation to patients to provide the best quality care possible. In addition, all stakeholders—consumers, purchasers, regulators, and accreditation groups—require continuous improvement. Competition among healthcare organizations is growing in intensity, and demand for high-quality services is increasing. Healthcare organizations that study and implement quality management techniques attract more patients than organizations that do not engage in such activities.

FOR DISCUSSION

1. Describe how you use the cycle of measurement, assessment, and improvement (see exhibit 2.1) to evaluate and make changes in your personal life.

2. How do quality practices that originated in the manufacturing industry differ from the traditional quality practices of healthcare organizations?

3. How would applying the core values and concepts of the Baldrige Performance Excellence Framework (Health Care) improve healthcare quality? (See critical concept 2.1.)

4. Consider the healthcare encounter you described in chapter 1 (see "For Discussion" question 2). If wasteful practices had been eliminated or steps in the process had been standardized, would you have had a different encounter? How would it have changed?

WEBSITES

- Agency for Healthcare Research and Quality, *Becoming a High Reliability Organization: Operational Advice for Hospital Leaders*
  https://archive.ahrq.gov/professionals/quality-patient-safety/quality-resources/tools/hroadvice/hroadvice.pdf

- Baldrige Performance Excellence Program
  www.nist.gov/baldrige

- Centers for Medicare & Medicaid Services
  www.cms.gov

- The Commonwealth Fund
  www.commonwealthfund.org

- Electronic Code of Federal Regulations, Title 42—Public Health
  www.ecfr.gov

- Foundation for Health Care Quality
  www.qualityhealth.org

- Juran Institute
  www.juran.com

- National Alliance of Healthcare Purchaser Coalitions
  www.nationalalliancehealth.org

- National Association of County and City Health Officials
  www.naccho.org

- National Public Health Performance Standards
  www.cdc.gov/nphpsp/index.html

- Occupational Safety and Health Administration, Regulations for Healthcare Facilities
www.osha.gov/SLTC/healthcarefacilities/
- The W. Edwards Deming Institute
http://deming.org

REFERENCES

Affeldt, J. E. 1980. "The New Quality Assurance Standard of the Joint Commission on Accreditation of Hospitals." *Western Journal of Medicine* 132 (6): 166–70.

American Society for Quality (ASQ). 2017. "Quality Glossary." Accessed October 27. www.asq.org/glossary/q.html.

Berwick, D. M. 2002. "A User's Manual for the IOM's 'Quality Chasm' Report." *Health Affairs* 21 (3): 80–90.

Best, M., and D. Neuhauser. 2008. "Kaoru Ishikawa: From Fishbones to World Peace." *Quality and Safety in Health Care* 17 (2): 150–52.

Brennan, T. A., and D. M. Berwick. 1996. *New Rules: Regulation, Markets, and the Quality of American Health Care*. San Francisco: Jossey-Bass.

Butman, J. 1997. *Juran: A Lifetime of Influence*. New York: Wiley and Sons.

Centers for Medicare & Medicaid Services (CMS). 2016a. "Home Health Quality Initiative." Accessed October 27, 2017. www.cms.gov/Medicare/Quality-Initiatives-Patient-Assessment-Instruments/HomeHealthQualityInits/.

———. 2016b. "Hospital Conditions of Participation: Infection Control, 42 CFR 482.42." Accessed October 27, 2017. www.gpo.gov/fdsys/pkg/CFR-2016-title42-vol5/xml/CFR-2016-title42-vol5-part482.xml#seqnum482.42.

———. 2016c. "QAPI Description and Background." Accessed October 27, 2017. www.cms.gov/Medicare/Provider-Enrollment-and-Certification/QAPI/qapidefinition.html.

Chassin, M. R., and J. M. Loeb. 2011. "The Ongoing Quality Improvement Journey: Next Stop, High Reliability." *Health Affairs* 30 (4): 559–68.

Deming, W. E. 1994. *The New Economics: For Industry, Government, Education,* 2nd ed. Cambridge, MA: MIT Center for Advanced Educational Services.

Girdler, S. J., C. D. Glezos, T. M. Link, and S. Alok. 2016. "The Science of Quality Improvement." *JBJS Reviews* 4 (8): 1–8.

Hines, S., K. Luna, J. Lofthus, M. Marquard, and D. Stelmokas. 2008. *Becoming a High Reliability Organization: Operational Advice for Hospital Leaders.* AHRQ Publication No. 08-0022. Rockville, MD: Agency for Healthcare Research and Quality.

Holahan, J., L. Blumberg, S. McMorrow, S. Zuckerman, T. Waidmann, and K. Stockley. 2011. *Containing the Growth of Spending in the U.S. Health System.* Urban Institute Health Care Policy Center. Published October 5. www.urban.org/publications/412419.html.

Institute for Healthcare Improvement. 2017. "Education." Accessed October 27. www.ihi.org/education/.

Institute of Medicine (IOM). 2006. *Medicare's Quality Improvement Organization Program: Maximizing Potential.* Washington, DC: National Academies Press.

———. 2001. *Crossing the Quality Chasm: A New Health System for the 21st Century.* Washington, DC: National Academies Press.

Ishikawa, K. 1990. *Introduction to Quality Control,* translated by J. H. Loftus. New York: Productivity Press.

Joint Commission. 2016. "Facts About The Joint Commission." Published July 8. www.jointcommission.org/facts_about_the_joint_commission.

———. 1979. *Accreditation Manual for Hospitals, 1980 Edition.* Oakbrook Terrace, IL: The Joint Commission.

Keehan, S. P., D. A. Stone, J. A. Poisal, G. A. Cuckler, A. M. Sisko, S. D. Smith, A. J. Madison, C. J. Wolfe, and J. M. Lizonitz. 2017. "National Health Expenditure Projections, 2016–25: Price Increases, Aging Push Sector to 20 Percent of Economy." *Health Affairs* 36 (3): 3553–63.

Kumar, N. 2017. "Using Data Analytics Techniques to Evaluate Performance." In *Applying Quality Management in Healthcare: A Systems Approach*, edited by P. L. Spath and D. L. Kelly, 167–201. Chicago: Health Administration Press.

Medical Group Management Association (MGMA). 2017. "MGMA Online Courses." Accessed October 27. www.mgma.com/education-certification/education/online/mgma -online-education.

Merry, M. D. 2003. "Healthcare's Need for Revolutionary Change." *Quality Progress* 23 (9): 31–35.

National Institute of Standards and Technology (NIST). 2017. *2017–2018 Baldrige Excellence Framework: A Systems Approach to Improving Your Organization's Performance (Health Care)*. Gaithersburg, MD: US Department of Commerce, National Institute of Standards and Technology.

Radnor, Z. J., M. Holweg, and J. Waring. 2012. "Lean in Healthcare: The Unfilled Promise?" *Social Science & Medicine* 74 (3): 364–71.

Spath, P. L. 2005. *Leading Your Healthcare Organization to Excellence: A Guide to Using the Baldrige Criteria*. Chicago: Health Administration Press.

US Department of Health and Human Services. 2015. "Better, Smarter, Healthier: In Historic Announcement, HHS Sets Clear Goals and Timeline for Shifting Medicare Reimbursements from Volume to Value." Press release, March 25. www.hhs.gov/about /news/2015/03/25/better-smarter-healthier-health-care-payment-learning-and-action -network-kick-off-to-advance-value-and-quality-in-health-care.html.

Weick, K. E., and K. M. Sutcliffe. 2015. *Managing the Unexpected: Sustained Performance in a Complex World*, 3rd ed. San Francisco: Jossey-Bass.

CHAPTER 3

MEASURING PERFORMANCE

LEARNING OBJECTIVES

After reading this chapter, you will be able to

➤ apply structure, process, and outcome measures to evaluate quality;

➤ describe common performance measures of healthcare services;

➤ demonstrate the steps involved in developing performance measures;

➤ identify national groups influencing healthcare performance measurement priorities;

➤ recognize how healthcare organizations select performance measures;

➤ describe the difference between measures of healthcare services and measures of clinical decision-making; and

➤ identify the role of balanced scorecards in performance measurement.

➤ Activity-level measures

➤ Agency for Healthcare Research and Quality (AHRQ)

➤ Average

➤ Balanced scorecards (BSCs)

➤ Check sheet

➤ Clinical practice guidelines

➤ Customer service

➤ Denominator

➤ Electronic clinical quality measures (eCQMs)

➤ Evidence-based measures

➤ Healthcare Effectiveness Data and Information Set (HEDIS)

➤ Interrater reliability

➤ Line graph

➤ Measures

➤ Metrics

➤ National Quality Forum (NQF)

➤ Numerator

➤ ORYX performance measurement

➤ Outcome measures

➤ Patient experience measures

➤ Performance

➤ Performance measures

➤ Process measures

➤ Quality indicators

➤ Ratio

➤ Reliable

➤ Sample

➤ Structure measures

➤ System-level measures

➤ Valid

➤ Validity

Measures
Instruments or tools used to gather information.

The purpose of measurement is to gather information. For example, the dashboard on my car displays lots of data. I can see how much gasoline is left in my tank, how fast I am traveling, and so on. These **measures** provide me with information about my car and my current driving situation. I decide how to use this information. Do I need to refill my gas tank soon, or can I wait a day or two? Do I need to slow down, or can I speed up a bit? My reaction to the information is partially based on personal choices, such as my willingness to risk running out of gas or incurring a speeding ticket.

It is also influenced by external factors, such as the distance to the nearest gas station and the speed limit.

Information must be accurate to be useful. If the "check engine" light on my dashboard malfunctions—blinks when the engine is functioning properly—I quickly learn to ignore it. Information also must tell me something I want to know; otherwise, I do not pay attention to it. For instance, I do not understand why a dial on my car's dashboard shows the engine RPM (revolutions per minute). This information may be important to someone, but I do not find it useful.

If the information is accurate and useful to me, I need to be able to interpret it. On more than one occasion, my car's speedometer display has mysteriously changed from miles per hour to kilometers per hour, leaving me wondering how fast I'm going. If I want to compare information, the **metrics** must be consistent. Evaluating the gasoline efficiency of two automobiles would be challenging if one rating is reported in miles per gallon and the other in liters per kilometer.

The purpose of measurement in quality management is similar to the purpose of dashboard indicators. Companies measure costs, quality, productivity, efficiency, customer satisfaction, and so on because they want information. They use this information to understand current **performance**, identify where improvement is needed, and evaluate how changes in work processes affect performance. Like the information displayed on a car dashboard, the data must be accurate, useful, easy to interpret, and reported consistently.

MEASUREMENT IN QUALITY MANAGEMENT

As shown in exhibit 3.1, measurement is the starting point of all quality management activities. The organization uses measurement information to determine how it is performing. In the next step, assessment, the organization judges whether its performance is acceptable. If its performance is acceptable, the organization continues to measure it to ensure performance does not deteriorate. If its performance is not acceptable, the organization advances to the improvement step. In this step, process changes are made. After the changes are in place for a specified time, the organization continues measuring to determine whether the changes are producing the desired result.

CASE STUDY

The following case study illustrates the use of measurement information for quality management purposes.

The Redwood Health Center is a multispecialty clinic that employs ten care providers—nine physicians and one nurse practitioner. Quality customer service is a priority for every staff person in the clinic.

Metrics
Any type of measurement used to gauge a quantifiable component of performance.

Performance
The way in which an individual, a group, or an organization carries out or accomplishes its important functions and processes.

EXHIBIT 3.1
Cycle of
Measurement,
Assessment, and
Improvement

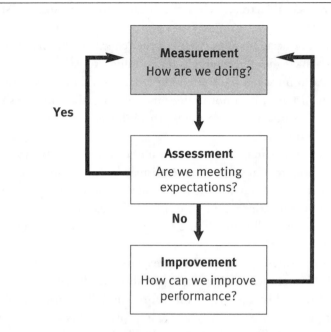

MEASUREMENT: HOW ARE WE DOING?

Customer service
A series of activities
designed to attend to
customers' needs.

To judge **customer service**, the clinic regularly measures patient satisfaction. A locked, ballot-style feedback box is located in the waiting area. It is clearly labeled: "Please tell us how we're doing. Your feedback will help us make things better." Next to the box is a container holding pens and pencils and a stack of blank feedback forms. The one-page feedback form includes the following questions:

1. What is the date of your clinic visit?

2. How would you rate the *quality of the medical care* you've received? (Please circle one.)
    (poor) 0 - 1 - 2 - 3 - 4 - 5 - 6 - 7 - 8 - 9 - 10 (perfect)

3. How would you rate the *quality of the customer service* you've received? (Please circle one.)
    (poor) 0 - 1 - 2 - 3 - 4 - 5 - 6 - 7 - 8 - 9 - 10 (perfect)

4. What did you like *best* about this visit?

5. What did you like *least* about this visit?

6. Please suggest one or more ways we could make things better.

At the end of each week, the clinic manager collects the feedback forms from the locked box. The results are tabulated and shared with the clinic staff every month.

At one monthly meeting, the clinic manager reports that many patients have complained about the amount of time they must wait before they are seen by a care provider. The providers expect clinic staff to bring patients to the exam room within ten minutes of the patient's arrival. To determine whether this goal is being met, the clinic gathers data on patient wait times for three weeks. Patients are asked to sign in and indicate their arrival time on a sheet at the registration desk. The medical assistant then records the time each patient is brought to an exam room.

ASSESSMENT: ARE WE MEETING EXPECTATIONS?

Patient wait time data for the three weeks are tallied. On most days, patient wait times are ten minutes or less. However, the average wait times are longer than ten minutes on Monday afternoons and Thursdays. Further investigation shows that the clinic serves a large number of walk-in patients on Monday afternoons. The clinic's nurse practitioner does not work on Thursdays, so physicians must see more patients on those days.

IMPROVEMENT: HOW CAN WE IMPROVE PERFORMANCE?

The wait time data help the clinic pinpoint where improvements are needed. The clinic manager meets with the care providers to discuss ways of changing the current process to reduce bottlenecks and improve customer satisfaction. The physicians ask that fewer patients be scheduled for appointments on Monday afternoons to give them more time to see walk-in patients. The nurse practitioner agrees to work on Thursday mornings.

MEASUREMENT: HOW ARE WE DOING?

To test whether these changes have improved outcomes, the clinic continues to gather feedback on overall patient satisfaction and periodically collects and analyzes patient wait time data.

LEARNING POINT
Measurement and Quality Management

Measurement is an element of all quality management activities. Performance is measured to determine current levels of quality, identify improvement opportunities, and evaluate whether changes have improved performance.

Performance measures
Quantitative tools used to evaluate an element of patient care; also called *quality measures*.

MEASUREMENT CHARACTERISTICS

Measurement is a tool—usually in the form of a number or statistic—used to monitor the quality of some aspect of healthcare services. These numbers are called **performance**

measures or **quality indicators**. Measurement data can be communicated in many ways. Examples of measures and the most common numbers or statistics used to report data for healthcare quality management purposes are shown in exhibit 3.2.

A measure expressed as a percentage is generally more useful than a measure expressed as an absolute number, because a percentage more clearly communicates a measure's prevalence in a population. For example, the percentage of nursing home residents who develop an infection is more meaningful than the number of nursing home residents who develop an infection. To provide even more information, both the percentage and number of residents who develop an infection can be reported.

An **average**, sometimes called an *arithmetic mean*, is the sum of a set of quantities divided by the number of quantities in the set. For instance, we can calculate the average nurse salary by adding up all the nurses' salaries and dividing by the number of nurses. In some situations, however, averages can be misleading. If a few of the numbers in the data set are unusually large or small (called *outliers*), they are commonly excluded when calculating an average. The excluded outliers are examined separately to determine why they occurred.

EXHIBIT 3.2
Measurement
Data for
Healthcare Quality
Management
Purposes

Number/Statistic	Measure Example
Absolute number	• Number of patients served in the health clinic • Number of patients who fall while in the hospital • Number of billing errors
Percentage	• Percentage of nursing home residents who develop an infection • Percentage of newly hired staff who receive job training • Percentage of prescriptions filled accurately by pharmacists
Average	• Average patient length of stay in the hospital • Average overall score on patient satisfaction surveys • Average charges for laboratory tests
Ratio	• Nurse-to-patient ratio • Cost-to-charge ratio • Technician-to-pharmacist ratio

A **ratio** is used to compare two things. For instance, the nurse-to-patient ratio reports the number of hospital patients cared for by each nurse. In the same month, one hospital unit may report a ratio of 1 nurse for every 5.2 patients, while another unit reports a ratio of 1 nurse for every 4.5 patients and yet another reports a ratio of 1 nurse for every 4.8 patients. A consistently calculated ratio facilitates comparison between units.

Regardless of how a measure is communicated, to be used effectively for quality management purposes it must be accurate, useful, easy to interpret, and consistently reported.

Ratio
One value divided by another; the value of one quantity in terms of the other.

ACCURACY

Performance measures must be accurate. Accuracy relates to the correctness of the numbers. For example, in the case study, the time the patient entered the clinic must be precisely recorded on the registration sign-in sheet. Otherwise, the wait time calculation will be wrong. Accuracy also relates to the **validity** of the measure. Is the measure gathering the information it is supposed to be gathering? For example, the clinic asks patients to provide feedback on its performance. One question on the feedback form is, "How would you rate the quality of the customer service you've received?" Each patient who rates the clinic's customer service may have something different in mind when answering the question. Because of these differences, the feedback is not a **valid** measure of just one aspect of clinic performance—for example, just the patient registration process. However, the average customer service rating is a good measure of patients' satisfaction with overall clinic performance.

Validity
The degree to which data or results of a study are correct or true.

Valid
Relevant, meaningful, and correct; appropriate to the task at hand.

USEFULNESS

Performance measures must be useful. Measurement information must tell people something they want to know. Computers have made data collection easier, but volume and variety do not necessarily translate to relevance. For instance, the computerized billing system of a health clinic contains patient demographic information (e.g., age, address, next of kin, insurance coverage). The clinic manager could use this information to report several performance measures, such as the percentage of patients with prescription drug insurance benefits or the percentage of patients who live more than 20 miles from the clinic. Although this information might be interesting, it won't be helpful for evaluating performance unless it is important or relevant to those using the information.

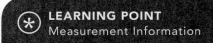

⊛ LEARNING POINT
Measurement Information

Measurement data are most commonly reported as discrete numbers, percentages, averages, and ratios. The number or statistic used to report the data can influence the interpretation of the measurement information.

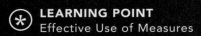

LEARNING POINT
Effective Use of Measures

Measurement provides information for quality management purposes. For the measures to be used effectively, they must be accurate, useful, easy to interpret, and reported consistently.

Line graph
A graph in which trends are highlighted by a line connecting data points.

Ease of Interpretation

Performance measures must be easy to interpret. Suppose the clinic manager in the case study reported the wait times for each patient on each day of the week. An excerpt from the report for one day is shown in exhibit 3.3.

The purpose of performance measurement is to provide information, not to make people sort through lots of data to find what they want to know. Having to read through several pages of wait time data to identify improvement opportunities would be tedious. A much better way to report the patient wait time data is illustrated in exhibit 3.4. Using a **line graph**, the clinic manager displays the average wait times for the morning and afternoon of each day of the week. The clinic's providers can easily identify trends and improvement opportunities from the graph.

Consistent Reporting

Performance measures must be uniformly reported to make meaningful comparisons between the results from one period and the results from another period. For example, suppose the clinic manager starts calculating patient wait time information differently.

Exhibit 3.3
Excerpt from Larger Report of Wait Time Data for Each Patient

Monday	
Patient 1	12 minutes
Patient 2	9 minutes
Patient 3	17 minutes
Patient 4	7 minutes
Patient 5	9 minutes
Patient 6	13 minutes
Patient 7	21 minutes
Patient 8	11 minutes
Patient 9	7 minutes
Patient 10	8 minutes

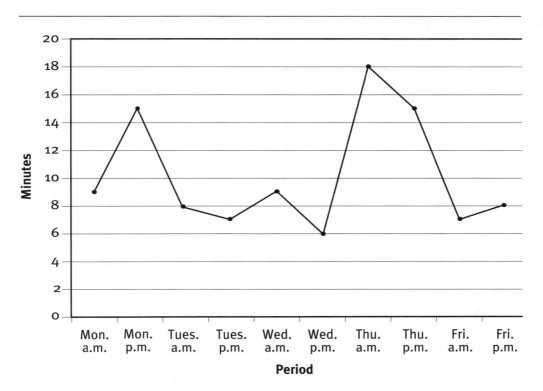

Exhibit 3.4
Line Graph
Showing Average
Patient Wait Times

He changes the wait time end point from the time the patient leaves the reception area to the time the patient is seen by a care provider. This slight change in the way wait times are calculated could dramatically affect performance results. The care providers would see an increase in average wait times and interpret it as a problem when in fact the increase was caused by the different measurement criteria, not a change in performance. This new measure can still be used, but it should be reported separately, as shown in exhibit 3.5.

MEASUREMENT CATEGORIES

Hundreds of measures can be used to evaluate healthcare performance. These measures are grouped into four categories:

◆   Structure measures

◆   Process measures

◆   Outcome measures

◆   Patient experience measures

EXHIBIT 3.5
Line Graph
Showing Two
Measures of
Patient Wait Times

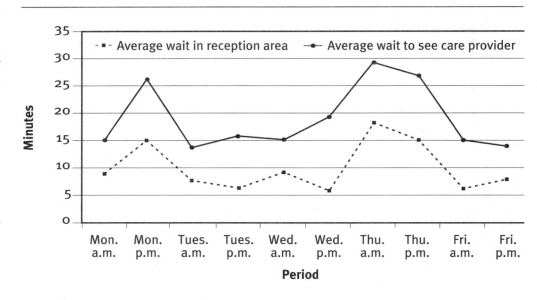

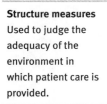

Structure measures
Used to judge the
adequacy of the
environment in
which patient care is
provided.

Process measures
Used to judge whether
patient care and
support functions are
properly performed.

Outcome measures
Used to judge the
results of patient care
and support functions.

**Patient experience
measures**
Patient-reported
information used
to judge "whether
something that should
happen in a health care
setting (such as clear
communication with
a provider) actually
happened or how often
it happened" (AHRQ
2016).

Structure, process, and outcome measurement categories were first conceptualized in 1966 by Avedis Donabedian, MD (1980). His research in quality assessment resulted in a widely accepted healthcare measurement model that is still used today. Donabedian contended that the three measurement categories—structure, process, and outcome—represent different characteristics of healthcare service. To fully evaluate healthcare performance, Donabedian recommended that performance in each dimension be measured.

Structure measures are used to judge the adequacy of the environment in which patient care is provided. **Process measures** are used to judge whether patient care and support functions are properly performed. **Outcome measures** are used to judge the results of patient care and support functions.

Donabedian classified patient satisfaction into the outcome category. Increased attention to patient-centered healthcare has placed greater emphasis on measuring more than satisfaction. This has led to the development of **patient experience measures** (LaVela and Gallan 2014). Measures of patient experience are based on patient-reported information. Patients are asked to judge "whether something that should happen in a health care setting (such as clear communication with a provider) actually happened or how often it happened" (AHRQ 2016).

Performance measures for most departments in a healthcare facility, whether the functions are directly involved in patient care or not, would fall into these same four categories. Exhibit 3.6 provides examples of structure, process, outcome, and patient/customer experience measures that could be used to evaluate the performance of an organization's emergency department (ED) and human resources (HR) department.

Measurement Category	Performance Measures for an ED	Performance Measures for an HR Department
Structure	Number of hours per day that a person skilled in reading head CT scans is available	Number of certified HR professionals in the department
Process	Percentage of ED patients ≤13 years old with a current weight in kilograms documented in the ED record	Percentage of facility job positions for which HR has conducted a market salary survey within the past three years
Outcome	Median time from ED arrival to ED departure for patients admitted to the hospital	Median time from an applicant's contingent offer of employment until all background checks have been completed for the applicant
Patient/Customer Experience	Percentage of parents who reported whether they were kept informed about their child's care in the emergency room	Percentage of department managers who reported whether HR staff provided very helpful recommendations for handling employee discipline issues

EXHIBIT 3.6
Structure, Process, Outcome, and Patient/Customer Experience Performance Measures

STRUCTURE MEASUREMENT

Measures of structure evaluate the physical and organizational resources available to support healthcare delivery—the organization's capacity or potential for providing quality services. As such, measures of structure are indirect measures of performance. For example, an HR department may be staffed with certified professionals, but staff could misfile personnel records. An ED might have someone available 24 hours a day to interpret special tests, but that person could misread the results. To ensure quality, measures of process and outcome also must be taken.

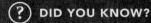

? DID YOU KNOW?

Performance measurement in healthcare is not a recent phenomenon. As early as 1754, the Pennsylvania Hospital in Philadelphia was collecting and analyzing patient outcomes data, tabulated by diagnostic group.

PROCESS MEASUREMENT

Measures of process evaluate whether activities performed during the delivery of services are performed satisfactorily. For instance, if an HR department has a policy requiring issuance of ID badges to new hires before their first day of employment, we would measure whether this policy was being followed. If an ED expects that all patients who present with symptoms of an ischemic stroke have a computed tomography (CT) scan within 25 minutes of arrival, we would measure caregivers' compliance with this expectation to determine whether their performance is acceptable.

In healthcare quality management, process measures are the most commonly used category of metrics. They provide important information about performance at all levels in the organization. However, good performance does not automatically translate to good results. In the previous ED example, even if all patients with symptoms of a stroke have a CT scan within 25 minutes of arrival, some may not recover. For this reason, another dimension of healthcare quality—outcome—must be measured.

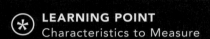

LEARNING POINT
Characteristics to Measure

To gain an understanding of current performance, healthcare organizations must measure four characteristics: structure, process, outcome, and patient experience. For example, if a manager of outpatient physical rehabilitation services wants to measure each characteristic of the unit's performance, he might ask the following questions:

- *Structure*: Is the unit staffed with a sufficient number of registered physical therapists?
- *Process*: How consistently do therapists measure and document a patient's level of pain?
- *Outcome*: How much improvement did patients have in their physical functional health after receiving therapy?
- *Patient experience*: How many patients report that their therapist clearly explained the treatment plan?

OUTCOME MEASUREMENT

Measures of outcome evaluate the results of healthcare services—the effects of structure and process. A common outcome measure is patients' health status following treatment to determine whether the interventions were successful. Healthcare facilities also measure patient mortality (death) and complication rates to identify opportunities for improvement. In addition, outcome measures are used to evaluate the use of healthcare services. Average length of hospital stay and average cost of treatment are two examples of outcome measures that examine the use of services.

Although measuring health service outcomes is important, the results can be affected by factors beyond providers' control. For example, patient mortality rates at one hospital may be higher than rates at other hospitals because the hospital cares for more terminally ill cancer patients than the others do. This healthcare organization may do all the right things but appears to be an underperformer because of the population it serves. When evaluating measurement data, many factors affecting patient outcomes must be considered.

Outcome measures can also be used to evaluate performance in departments that do not provide direct patient care. For instance, the average time between an insurance company's request for copies of a patient's health record and receipt of the record is an outcome measure for the health information management department.

PATIENT EXPERIENCE MEASURES

Measures of patient experience are a combination of process and outcome measures. For instance, a survey of hospitalized patients asks if staff always explained medicines before giving them. The task of explaining medicines to patients is part of the hospital's medication administration process. In answering this survey question, patients are providing their perspective on whether this process is working well. An outcome-related measure on this survey asks if the patient's pain was always well controlled (CMS 2017c).

The **Agency for Healthcare Research and Quality (AHRQ)** started a multiyear initiative in October 1995 to support and promote the measurement of consumers' experiences with healthcare. The initial focus was on health plans, and it has now been expanded to address a wide range of healthcare services. The Consumer Assessment of Healthcare Providers and Systems (CAHPS) program is designed to meet the information needs of healthcare consumers, purchasers, health plans, providers, and policy makers. The survey instruments and tools generated by this initiative are found on the CAHPS website (www.cahps.ahrq.gov).

In addition to experiencing direct care services, patients interact with administrative areas such as registration and billing services. Some providers add questions about administrative services to the CAHPS survey or get patient perception feedback in other ways. Patient experiences interacting with one business function—billing services—has been linked to overall satisfaction. The 2014 Connance Annual Consumer Impact Study found that 95 percent of patients who reported being satisfied with the billing process were likely to return to that hospital for another procedure. Facilities interested in improving performance should measure patient experiences with both clinical and administrative services.

Agency for Healthcare Research and Quality (AHRQ)
The health services research arm of the US Department of Health and Human Services; the lead federal agency for research on healthcare quality, costs, outcomes, and patient safety.

> ### (?) DID YOU KNOW?
>
> In the early 1980s marketing researchers in service industries (e.g., hotels, restaurants) began measuring the quality of service encounters against the customer's expectations.

SELECTING PERFORMANCE MEASURES

Healthcare organizations use two tiers of measures to evaluate performance: system-level measures and activity-level measures. The percentage of health clinic patients who are satisfied with the quality of customer service is an example of a **system-level measure**. This measure is a snapshot of overall clinic performance.

System-level measures
Data describing the overall performance of several interdependent processes or activities.

Because many activities in a health clinic influence the quality of customer service, performance also needs to be evaluated at the activity level to assess patient satisfaction. The percentage of time reception staff telephone patients to remind them of upcoming clinic appointments is an example of an **activity-level measure**.

Consider how the performance of an automobile is evaluated. A common measure of car performance is the number of miles the car can travel per gallon of gasoline. This system-level measure, miles per gallon, is just a snapshot of the car's overall performance, however. Many actions affect an automobile's fuel economy. Activity-level measures can be used to evaluate these actions. For example, average time between engine tune-ups is an activity-level measure of an action that affects car performance. By using a combination of system- and activity-level measures, the owner can judge not only overall fuel economy but also actions (or lack thereof) that might be affecting it.

A mix of system- and activity-level measures allows a healthcare organization to judge whether overall performance goals are being met and where frontline improvements may be needed. The relationship between performance goals and system- or activity-level measures in two healthcare settings is shown in exhibit 3.7.

Activity-level measures
Data describing the performance of one process or activity.

MEASUREMENT PRIORITIES

The system- and activity-level measures used by a healthcare organization for quality management purposes are influenced by external and internal factors. On the external side, numerous government regulations, accreditation standards, and purchaser requirements directly affect measurement activities. The number and type of measures used to evaluate performance vary in proportion to the number of external requirements the organization must meet. For example, critical concept 3.1 lists 9 of the more than 50 different performance measures that Medicare-certified home health agencies were required to use for quality management purposes in 2017. The quality measurement categories specific to the home health industry are process measures, outcome measures, and potentially avoidable events. The potentially avoidable events reported are outcome measures in the sense that they represent a change in health status between start or resumption of care and discharge or transfer to an inpatient facility (CMS 2017e).

The performance measurement requirements of the federal government, the largest purchaser of healthcare services, continue to increase in response to quality improvement and cost-containment efforts. Like most purchasers, the Centers for Medicare & Medicaid Services (CMS) is interested in obtaining the most value for its healthcare expenditures. The measures of performance required of healthcare organizations help purchasers assess value in terms of the six Institute of Medicine (IOM 2001) quality aims described in chapter 1: Healthcare should be safe, effective, patient centered, timely, efficient, and equitable. In addition, CMS considers the current National Quality Strategy when selecting measures.

Setting	Organization-wide Performance Goal	System-Level Measure	Activity-Level Measures
University student health center	Inform and educate students on wellness and prevention issues relevant to their age group	Percentage of incoming freshmen who are vaccinated for meningococcal meningitis within three months of first semester	• Number of hours the vaccination clinic is open each month • Percentage of incoming freshmen who receive written information about the meningococcal meningitis vaccine • Percentage of incoming freshmen who complete and return the vaccination survey
Hospital	Reduce incidence of hospital-acquired infections	Percentage of patients who develop an infection while in the hospital	• Rate of staff compliance with hand-hygiene procedures • Percentage of central vein line catheter insertions done according to protocol • Percentage of staff immunized for influenza

EXHIBIT 3.7
Performance Goals and Measures in Two Healthcare Settings

Electronic clinical quality measures (eCQMs) Data from EHR and/or health information technology systems to measure healthcare quality. These data are used by CMS in a variety of quality-reporting and incentive programs (CMS 2017a).

Clinical quality measurement expectations were part of the Health Information Technology for Economic and Clinical Health (HITECH) Act, enacted as part of the American Recovery and Reinvestment Act of 2009. The HITECH Act established financial incentives for Medicare-eligible hospitals and healthcare professionals to adopt electronic health records (EHRs) and use the technology in a meaningful way (CMS 2012). A core objective of EHR use is the ability to electronically report performance measurement data to CMS or to the state. The **electronic clinical quality measures (eCQMs)** to be reported periodically change with new measures added and some retired. Starting in 2017, the measures to be reported electronically by Medicare-eligible healthcare professionals were

CRITICAL CONCEPT 3.1
2017 Performance Measures for Medicare-Certified Home Health Agencies

Process measures

- Percentage of home health episodes of care in which the start or resumption of care date was either on the physician-specified date or within two days of the referral date or inpatient discharge date, whichever is later.

- Percentage of home health episodes of care during which patients received influenza immunization for the current flu season.

- Percentage of home health quality episodes in which patients had a multifactor fall risk assessment at the start or resumption of care.

Outcome measures

- Percentage of home health episodes of care that ended with the patient being admitted to the hospital.

- Percentage of home health episodes of care during which the patient got better at bathing self.

- Percentage of home health episodes of care during which patients are confused less often.

Potentially avoidable events

- Percentage of residents or patients with pressure ulcers that are new or worsened.

- Percentage of home health episodes of care during which patients developed a bladder or urinary tract infection.

- Percentage of home health quality episodes during which the patient's ability to take his or her medicines correctly (by mouth) got much worse.

Source: CMS (2017e).

transitioned to the new Quality Payment Program that is part of the Medicare Access and CHIP Reauthorization Act of 2015 (MACRA) legislation (CMS 2017f). Current information about the eCQMs and CMS measurement expectations for various projects can be found on the websites listed at the end of this chapter.

The number of performance measures providers are required to report to CMS and other groups has exploded in the last ten years. Costs associated with gathering, reporting, and analyzing measurement data are significant for providers, and often the data are not useful for improvement purposes (Schuster, Onorato, and Meltzer 2017). This has led to increasing calls to limit the number of performance measures to a small set of high-priority measures (Blumenthal and McGinnis 2015).

State licensing regulations often require healthcare organizations to evaluate structural issues, such as compliance with building safety and sanitation codes. Licensing regulations may also include specific requirements for process and outcome measures related to patient care. A list of clinical performance data that must be collected by ambulatory surgical treatment centers in Illinois is shown in critical concept 3.2.

Certain state and federal regulations apply only to specific healthcare units, such as radiology and laboratory departments. These regulations contain many quality control requirements with corresponding system- and activity-level performance measurement obligations. For instance, any facility that performs laboratory testing on human specimens must adhere to the quality standards of the Clinical Laboratory Improvement Amendments, passed by Congress in 1988 to ensure the accuracy, reliability, and timeliness of patient test results regardless of where the test is performed (US Food and Drug Administration 2014).

The standards of healthcare accreditation groups often contain system- and activity-level performance measurement requirements. Accreditation standards may duplicate those mandated by government regulations and purchasers. However, some measurement requirements found in accreditation standards are unique. For example,

---

✱ LEARNING POINT
Examples of eCQMs Reported to CMS by Hospitals

These are some of the eCQMs for 2018 reporting for the Hospital Inpatient Quality Reporting Program and the Medicare and Medicaid EHR Incentive programs for Eligible Hospitals and Critical Access Hospitals:

- Median elapsed time from ED arrival to ED departure for patients discharged from the ED
- The number of mothers undergoing elective vaginal deliveries or elective cesarean births between 37 and 39 weeks' gestation
- The proportion of newborns screened for hearing loss before hospital discharge
- Acute myocardial infarction patients with ST-segment elevation on the electrocardiogram taken closest to arrival time who receive primary percutaneous coronary intervention (PCI) during the hospital stay with a time from hospital arrival to PCI of 90 minutes or less

Source: Adapted from CMS (2017d).

> **⚠ CRITICAL CONCEPT 3.2** Illinois Regulations for Data Collection in Ambulatory Surgical Treatment Centers
>
> Each ambulatory surgical treatment center (ASTC) shall collect, compile and maintain the following clinical statistical data at the facility:
>
> 1. The total number of surgical cases treated by the ASTC;
>
> 2. The number of each specific surgical procedure performed;
>
> 3. The number and type of complications reported, including the specific procedure associated with each complication;
>
> 4. The number of patients requiring transfer to a hospital for treatment of complications. The procedure performed and the complication that prompted each transfer shall be listed;
>
> 5. The number of deaths, including the specific procedure that was performed; and
>
> 6. The results of the monitoring of the ASTC's hand hygiene program.
>
> *Source*: Reprinted from Illinois General Assembly, Joint Committee on Administrative Rules (2014).

ORYX performance measurement
Performance measurement project sponsored by The Joint Commission.

Healthcare Effectiveness Data and Information Set (HEDIS)
Health plan performance measurement project sponsored by the National Committee for Quality Assurance.

hospitals accredited by The Joint Commission (2017) are expected to collect data on the timeliness of diagnostic testing and reporting (an activity-level measure) to determine how quickly important test results are communicated to the patient's doctor and where improvement opportunities may exist. Some accredited organizations also must participate in the **ORYX performance measurement** reporting project, which involves gathering and sharing measurement data with The Joint Commission. Measurement activities currently required of accredited organizations can be found on The Joint Commission's website (www.joint commission.org). As much as possible, The Joint Commission coordinates its core measurement requirements with the measurement activities mandated by CMS to lighten the workload for organizations subject to the regulations and standards of both groups.

Health plans accredited by the National Committee for Quality Assurance (NCQA) must participate in the **Healthcare Effectiveness Data and Information Set (HEDIS)** measurement project. HEDIS measures address a broad range of health and customer service issues, including the following (NCQA 2017):

- Asthma medication use

- Persistence of beta-blocker treatment after a heart attack

- Controlling high blood pressure

- Comprehensive diabetes care

- Breast cancer screening

- Antidepressant medication management

- Childhood and adolescent immunization status

- Childhood and adult weight/body mass index assessment

In 2017, HEDIS included 91 measures across 7 domains of care. Health plans accredited by NCQA are not required to gather information for all the HEDIS measures. In addition to NCQA-accredited health plans, government-funded health plans, such as Medicaid and the Indian Health Service, are required to gather HEDIS measurement data. More than 90 percent of US health plans use HEDIS measures to evaluate performance on important dimensions of care and service (NCQA 2017). Information about the current HEDIS measures can be found on the NCQA website (http://ncqa.org).

A growing number of external groups are mandating that healthcare organizations gather specific performance measures for quality management purposes. When selecting performance measures, organizations must consider the most current measurement directives of relevant government regulations, accreditation bodies, and purchasers.

Externally mandated measurement requirements do not always address all of an organization's internal quality priorities. The service elements an organization wants to measure may differ from the measurement priorities of external groups. Consider a home health agency with a particularly large hospice patient population. Hospice patients have a limited life expectancy and require comprehensive clinical and psychosocial support as they enter the terminal stage of an illness or a condition. The measures required of Medicare-certified home health agencies do not address some of the performance issues unique to hospice patients and their families. Consequently, the home health agency must identify and gather its own performance measures of hospice services in addition to collecting the measures required to maintain Medicare certification.

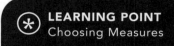

LEARNING POINT
Choosing Measures

Healthcare organizations measure many aspects of performance. Some of the measures are mandated by external regulatory, licensing, and accreditation groups. Some are chosen to evaluate performance issues important to the organization. And some measures serve both purposes: The measure is required by an external group *and* provides performance information important to the organization.

Exhibit 3.8 lists examples of performance measures that the Redwood Health Center, the subject of the case study presented earlier in the chapter, uses to evaluate various aspects of quality, with explanations as to why the clinic selected them.

EXHIBIT 3.8
Clinic Measures of Performance and Their Purposes

Data are gathered for the following measures because the clinic is required to share results with Medicare and two managed care organizations. Also, care providers want to know the clinic's performance in these measures compared with the performance of other clinics in the state.

- Percentage of patients with diabetes who have an annual eye examination
- Percentage of pregnant patients screened for HIV (human immunodeficiency virus)
- Percentage of adult patients who receive an influenza immunization annually
- Percentage of patients with newly diagnosed osteoporosis who receive counseling on vitamin D and calcium intake and exercise

Data are gathered for the following measures because care providers want to know whether these important aspects of patient care are in compliance with internal expectations.

- Number of patients who call back after an office visit to clarify instructions
- Percentage of charts that have patient medication allergies prominently displayed
- Percentage of visits that involve an interpreter (not a family member) to communicate with patients who do not speak English
- Percentage of Pap smear samples that are nondiagnostic as a result of improper collection techniques

Data are gathered for the following measures because care providers and the clinic administrator want to know about patient experiences with the clinic's services.

- Percentage of patients completing the satisfaction survey who indicated they would refer a friend or family member to the clinic
- Percentage of patients who reported whether their provider included them in decisions about their treatment or care
- Number of complaints received about an insufficient number of handicap parking spaces
- Percentage of patients who reported how often they were able to get care quickly

Data are gathered for the following measures because care providers and the clinic administrator want to know whether the clinic is providing efficient, customer-friendly services in a timely manner.

(continued)

- Average number of days between patient request for an annual physical examination and first available physician appointment
- Average number of days between patient request for a non–urgent care visit and first available physician or nurse practitioner appointment
- Average visit cycle time: total patient time in the clinic from walk-in to walk-out
- Percentage of phone calls abandoned (customer hangs up while on hold)

Data are gathered for the following measures because the clinic administrator and the business office manager want to know how well the clinic is faring financially and what can be done to improve net revenues and speed up collection of outstanding accounts.

- Percentage by which revenues exceed expenses
- Percentage of bills returned to the clinic because of outdated patient demographic information
- Percentage of patients who have a copayment and are asked for this payment at the time of service
- Average supply cost per patient office visit

Data are gathered for the following measures because the state health department requires the clinic to evaluate the safety of the environment.

- Average temperature of the clinic medication/supply refrigerator
- Percentage of smoke detectors, fire alarms, and sprinklers in compliance with local fire codes during biannual inspection
- Number of medication samples found to be outdated during quarterly inspection of medication sample cabinet
- Percentage of equipment maintenance checks performed within two weeks of deadline

EXHIBIT 3.8
Clinic Measures of Performance and Their Purposes
(continued)

CONSTRUCTING MEASURES

Measures to be reported to external groups have already been constructed and the measurement specifications shared with providers. Measures used by a provider to evaluate internal quality priorities also need to be systematically constructed. These three steps should be followed to ensure each measure yields information that is accurate, useful, easy to interpret, and consistently reported:

1. Identify the topic of interest.

2. Develop the measure.

3. Design the data collection system.

These steps can be time consuming but are essential to ensuring that the measures are useful for quality management purposes.

IDENTIFY THE TOPIC OF INTEREST

The first step to constructing a performance measure is to determine what you want to know. Consider just one function—for example, taking patient X-rays in the radiology department. This function involves several steps:

1.   The patient's doctor orders the X-ray exam.

2.   The radiology department schedules the exam.

3.   The patient registers on arrival in the radiology department.

4.   The X-ray exam is performed.

5.   The radiologist interprets the X-rays.

6.   The radiologist informs the patient's doctor of the X-ray results.

To select performance measures for X-ray procedures, consider IOM's (2001) six dimensions of healthcare quality and the corresponding performance questions listed in exhibit 3.9. Answers to these questions can help the radiology department gauge its performance in each quality dimension. The department will determine which quality characteristics it will need to measure regularly and which questions will provide the most useful answers for measurement purposes. Factors the radiology manager will take into consideration when selecting performance measures for the department are summarized in exhibit 3.10. Aspects of service that will be measured to answer performance questions must be stated explicitly. Without this knowledge, measures cannot be developed.

DEVELOP THE MEASURE

Once performance questions have been identified, the next step is to define the measures that will be used to answer the questions. Suppose the radiology manager chooses to address the question of timely reporting of X-ray exam results to patients' doctors. The department policy states that results are to be telephoned, e-mailed, or faxed within 48 hours of an exam. To turn the question into a performance measure, the manager determines the percentage of results communicated to doctors within 48 hours of completion of an outpatient X-ray exam.

To ensure she knows what information this measure will provide, the manager rewrites the measure in terms of the data that will be used to calculate it, as follows:

$$\frac{\text{Number of outpatient exam results reported to doctor within 48 hours}}{\text{Total number of exams performed}} \times 100$$

By writing the performance measure in fundamental measurement units, the manager is able to identify the data she needs to generate the measure. The top number in the fraction is the **numerator**, and the bottom number is the **denominator**. To calculate the percentage of results communicated to the doctor within 48 hours of exam completion, the top number is divided by the bottom number and then multiplied by 100.

Examples of performance measures, along with the numerators and denominators that would help answer some of the questions in exhibit 3.9, are provided in exhibit 3.11.

Numerator
The number written above the line in a common fraction, which signifies the number to be divided by the denominator.

Denominator
The number written below the line in a common fraction, which functions as the divisor of the numerator.

Exhibit 3.9
Quality Dimensions and Performance Questions for Radiology Services

Quality Dimension	Performance Questions
Safe	• How many patients react adversely to the X-ray dye? • Are pregnant patients adequately protected from radiation exposure?
Effective	• Are significant (e.g., life threatening) X-ray findings quickly communicated to the patient's doctor? • How often are presurgery X-ray findings confirmed at the time of surgery?
Patient centered	• Do patients often complain about a lack of privacy in the X-ray changing rooms? • How many patients are greeted by the receptionist upon arrival in the department?
Timely	• How long do patients wait in the reception area before an exam? • Are outpatient X-ray results reported to the patient's doctor in a timely manner?
Efficient	• How often must X-ray exams be repeated because the first exam was not performed properly? • How often is equipment unavailable because of unscheduled downtime?
Equitable	• Do uninsured patients receive the same level of service as insured patients do? • How often is the mobile mammography unit available to people living in rural areas?

EXHIBIT 3.10
Factors to
Consider When
Selecting
Performance
Measures

	Yes	No
Is the measure mandated by government regulations or accreditation standards?	_____	_____
Is reimbursement linked to good performance in this measure?	_____	_____
Is the organization's performance in this measure available to the public?	_____	_____
Does the measure evaluate an aspect of service that is linked to one of the organization's improvement goals?	_____	_____
Does the measure evaluate an aspect of service that is linked to one of the department's improvement goals?	_____	_____
Are affected physicians and staff members likely to be supportive of initiatives aimed at improving performance in this measure?	_____	_____
Are resources available to collect, report, and analyze the measurement results?	_____	_____
Is the information gained from this measurement worth the costs associated with collecting, reporting, and analyzing the measurement results?	_____	_____

Some performance measures, typically structure measures, do not have denominators. For instance, health plans usually want to know whether a hospital is accredited. Evidence of accreditation is a structure measure. Only two measurement results are possible—the hospital is accredited or it is not accredited. As another example, a common measure of a healthcare organization's compliance with environmental safety is the number of fire drills it conducts each year. This measure is an absolute number; a denominator is not necessary.

DESIGN THE DATA COLLECTION SYSTEM

Reliable
Yielding the same or compatible results in different situations.

To ensure that useful and accurate performance information is gathered, valid and **reliable** data sources must be identified. Recall that a valid data source is one that contains the correct information needed to create the performance measure. A reliable data source is one that consistently contains the information needed to create the performance measure. Reliable data are not necessarily valid. For example, clinic medical technicians may consistently document a patient's weight, but if the scale does not function properly, the data in the patient's record are invalid.

EXHIBIT 3.11
Performance
Questions and
Measures for
the Radiology
Department

Performance Question	Measure	Numerator	Denominator
How many patients react adversely to the X-ray dye?	Percentage of patients who react adversely to the X-ray dye	Number of patients who react adversely to the X-ray dye	Total number of patients receiving an X-ray dye injection
Are pregnant patients adequately protected from radiation exposure?	Percentage of women of childbearing age who are asked about pregnancy status before X-ray exam	Number of women of childbearing age asked about their pregnancy status before X-ray exam	Total number of women of childbearing age who undergo an X-ray exam
How often must X-ray exams be repeated because the first exam was not performed properly?	Percentage of X-ray exams repeated because of wrong patient positioning on first exam	Number of X-ray exams repeated because of wrong patient positioning on first exam	Total number of X-ray exams performed
How often is equipment unavailable because of unscheduled downtime?	Percentage of time equipment is unavailable because of unscheduled downtime	Number of hours equipment is unavailable because of unscheduled downtime	Total number of hours equipment is scheduled to be available
Do uninsured patients receive the same level of service as insured patients do?	Percentage of service complaints received from uninsured patients	Number of service complaints received from uninsured patients	Total number of service complaints received from all patients
How often is the mobile mammography unit available to people living in rural areas?	Percentage of time mobile mammography unit is available in rural areas	Number of hours the mobile mammography unit is open for business in locations more than 30 miles from the hospital	Total number of hours the mobile mammography unit is open for business

Computerized databases and handwritten documents, such as those listed next, are used to collect data for the numerator, denominator, and other elements necessary to calculate a measure:

◆ *Administrative files.* The organization's billing database is an administrative file often used to gather performance data. This file typically contains information such as patient demographics, codes that identify diagnoses and procedures performed, and charges billed. Count data, such as the number of patients who have X-rays taken, can be gathered from the billing database. Other databases include those maintained by pharmacies and insurance companies.

◆ *Patient records.* Treatment results are found in patient records. Patient records are often the only source of data for outcome measures, such as the percentage of patients who reacted adversely to X-ray dyes. Gathering data from electronic patient records is usually easier and less time consuming than gathering data from paper-based records.

◆ *Miscellaneous business and clinical information.* Performance measurement data may also be available from patient and employee surveys; patient care logs maintained by clinics and EDs; and the results of special studies, such as observation reviews that evaluate compliance with patient care requirements.

Any data source has advantages and drawbacks to its use. For example, patient databases used by pharmacies and health insurance companies may lack pertinent clinical details. Providers' billing databases, designed primarily for financial and administrative uses, often lack information needed to measure quality (e.g., measures requiring a time stamp are not included in most billing databases). Patient records also may lack information needed to measure quality. For instance, patient records used by clinics often include the names of prescribed medications but may not include documentation confirming that the physician counseled the patient about the medication's side effects. To know how often counseling occurs, the physician would need to document this activity or the information would have to be collected via another source, such as observation. No data source is perfect; trade-offs must always be considered.

When planning for data collection, first look for existing information sources. Often, data are readily available and easily gathered. In some situations, however, the data needed to calculate a measure are not easy to obtain and new data sources must be developed. Let's look at the radiology department example to learn how to identify data sources for a performance measure.

The radiology manager wants to gather data to determine the percentage of results communicated to patients' doctors within 48 hours of an outpatient X-ray exam. To create this measure, the manager needs to collect two sets of data: (1) the date and time each outpatient X-ray exam is performed and (2) the date and time each outpatient exam report is telephoned, e-mailed, or faxed to the doctor. The manager also notes that a calculation is required to generate the measure. He will need to count the number of hours between completion of an outpatient X-ray exam and the report to the patient's doctor to determine whether that period is shorter than 48 hours.

The manager investigates whether the data necessary to create the measure are currently available. Ideally, they are already being collected and will only need to be retrieved to generate the measure. The manager finds that the department's X-ray technicians document the date and time of each exam in the department's electronic information system. These data will be easy to retrieve.

The date and time that exam results are reported to the patient's doctor will not be as easy to gather. The manager discovers that doctors receive outpatient X-ray exam results in two different ways. Sometimes the radiologist telephones preliminary results to the doctor and later faxes or e-mails the report to the doctor's office. At other times, the radiologist does not telephone preliminary results to the doctor and only faxes or e-mails the report. Clerical staff in the radiology department document the date and time that reports are faxed or e-mailed, but the radiologists do not record the date and time preliminary results are phoned to the doctor. To create the measure, the manager needs the radiologists to enter the date and time of these telephone communications in the department's electronic information system.

To finish designing the data collection system, the manager must make four more decisions, addressing the what, who, when, and how of data collection.

What

What refers to the population that will be measured. Will the denominator represent a **sample** of the population to be measured or the entire population? For some measures, the answer is evident. A calculation determining the percentage of a nursing home's new hires who undergo required background checks would be inaccurate if only half of the new hire population were included in the denominator, unless this half was representative of the whole. For some measures, the entire population does not need to be included in the denominator if the data are derived from a sample that is representative of the entire population. For instance, data on all prescriptions filled by the pharmacist are not necessary to determine the percentage accurately filled. A sample of filled prescriptions can provide reliable measurement data.

The Joint Commission and CMS encourage healthcare organizations to use sampling to measure performance, where appropriate. National quality measurement projects, such as those sponsored by CMS and The Joint Commission, have data specifications that must be followed by the organizations submitting data. These specifications may indicate whether samples can be used and the minimum acceptable sample size for each measure. Following are the sample size requirements for facilities that submitted measurement data in 2017 to the CMS national quality program and to The Joint Commission (CMS and Joint Commission 2016):

◆ For a monthly population of fewer than 51, review 100 percent of the population.

◆ For a monthly population of 51–254, review 51 cases from the population.

Sample
A representative portion of a larger group.

◆ For a monthly population of 255–509, review 20 percent of the initial population size.

◆ For a monthly population of 510 or more, review 102 cases from the population.

Measurement specifications in national quality projects can change. Organizations participating in these projects should comply with the most up-to-date requirements.

Who

Who refers to the data collectors. Will the manager gather all data needed for performance measurement purposes? Will employees be asked to collect some data? Will information specialists in the organization be asked to retrieve data from clinical or administrative databases? If more than one person is responsible for data collection, how will the collectors ensure they are gathering data consistently (i.e., demonstrating **interrater reliability**)?

Once identified, data collectors often need training. They must know what data are necessary to create each measure and how to gather accurate information. For example, what is the definition of "adverse reaction to X-ray dye"? What symptoms are documented when a patient reacts adversely? Where are they documented? What should the data collector do if the documentation is ambiguous? If these questions are not clearly answered, the accuracy and consistency of information gathered for measurement purposes are jeopardized.

Interrater reliability
The probability that a measurement is free from random error and yields consistent results regardless of the individuals gathering the data. (For example, a measure with high interrater reliability means that two or more people working independently will gather similar data.)

When

When refers to the frequency of data collection and reporting. How often will information be gathered? How frequently will performance measure results be reported? What are the cost implications of different data collection and reporting intervals? These decisions may be left to managers, or the organization may set the reporting frequency (e.g., monthly, quarterly) on the basis of external reporting requirements and internal priorities.

How

How refers to the process used to gather data. Several methods can be used to retrieve information for performance measures, including questionnaires, observations, electronic database queries, reviews of paper documents, and check sheets. The case study at the beginning of this chapter describes a questionnaire used to gather satisfaction data from clinic patients. Exhibit 3.12 shows a form used by data collectors to record information found in hospital patient records. The information helps to measure nurses' compliance with Joint Commission patient education standards. If nurses are using an EHR to document

Exhibit 3.12
Form Used to
Collect Data from
Hospital Patient
Records

Patient's medical record number: Date of discharge:

Nursing unit: Date of record review:

ASSESSMENT OF PATIENT'S LEARNING NEEDS	YES	NO	N/A
Does the assessment of learning needs based on the admission assessment include the following data:			
• Cultural and religious beliefs?			
• Emotional barriers?			
• Desire and motivation to learn?			
• Physical or cognitive limitations and barriers to communication?			
Is comprehension of education provided to patient and family documented?			

MEDICATION EDUCATION	YES	NO	N/A
Medication education documented in:			
• Patient education intervention			
• Nurses' notes			
Educated patient on food/drug interactions:			
• Coumadin			
• Diuretics			
• Antidiabetics			

PATIENT EDUCATION AND TRAINING	YES	NO	N/A
Is there documentation that the patient and/or family were educated about the following as appropriate:			
• Plan for care, treatment, and services?			
• Basic health and safety practices?			
• Safe and effective use of medications?			
• Nutrition interventions, modified diets, and oral health?			
• Safe and effective use of medical equipment or supplies when provided by the hospital?			
• Techniques used to help reach maximum independence?			
Is there documentation that the patient and/or family were educated about pain, including the following:			
• Understanding pain?			
• The risk of pain?			
• The importance of effective pain management?			
• The pain assessment process?			
• Methods for pain management?			

patient education activities, it may be possible to electronically download the data needed to measure compliance.

The data-gathering process must be carefully planned so the information derived will be accurate and useful. Revisit the radiology department example to learn how data are gathered for one performance measure. To evaluate the safety of department services, the radiology manager wants to know how often the pregnancy status of women of child-bearing age is confirmed before an X-ray exam. Because the department serves many patients in this age category, gathering information about the entire population would be burdensome, so the manager chooses a sample of records. Each month, a radiology clerk reviews 25 randomly selected records from this population to look for documentation of pregnancy status. Data are collected on patients seen for different exams on different days and at different times each month to ensure the results are representative of what happens for the entire population.

Using hatch marks on a check sheet, the clerk records the review findings. A **check sheet** is a data-gathering tool that presents the data in a way that enables their conversion into useful information for decision-making. When 25 records have been reviewed and the findings recorded, the clerk tabulates the results for the manager.

Exhibit 3.13 is a completed check sheet for a three-month period (each hatch mark represents one X-ray patient record). The percentage of patients asked about their pregnancy status is calculated by dividing the number of hatch marks in the first row by 25 (the total number of randomly selected films each month). The performance results for each month are as follows:

January: 88 percent of patients were asked about pregnancy status before X-ray exam
February: 76 percent of patients were asked about pregnancy status before X-ray exam
March: 92 percent of patients were asked about pregnancy status before X-ray exam

UNDERSTAND MEASURE SPECIFICATIONS

Most of the performance measures required by purchasers and external regulatory, licensing, and accreditation groups have gone through a rigorous development and validation process. These have already defined the topic and identified the data necessary to create the measure, so healthcare organizations do not need to start from scratch. Exhibit 3.14

Check sheet
A form on which data can be sorted into categories for easier analysis.

EXHIBIT 3.13
X-ray Patient Pregnancy Status Check Sheet

Status Documented?	Month: January	Month: February	Month: March
Yes	|||| |||| |||| || |||| |||| ||||		|||| |||| |||| |||
No	|||	||||		||

shows measurement specifications for one of the measures that Medicare-eligible hospitals submit to CMS. This measure is used to evaluate the quality of care provided to patients receiving treatment for a stroke.

Detailed measurement specifications for all agencies and organizations that sponsor quality measurement projects can be found on their websites.

Measure	Percentage of ischemic or hemorrhagic patients who were assessed for rehabilitation services (CMS Measure ID: CMS102v6)
Initial Patient Population	Patients age 18 and older discharged from inpatient care (nonelective admissions) with a principal diagnosis of ischemic or hemorrhagic stroke and a length of stay less than or equal to 120 days that ends during the measurement period
Denominator Statement	Initial Population
Denominator Exclusions	• Patients with comfort measures documented. • Patients discharged to another hospital. • Patients who left against medical advice. • Patients who expired. • Patients discharged to a healthcare facility for hospice care. • Patients admitted for elective carotid intervention. This exclusion is implicitly modeled by only including nonelective hospitalizations.
Numerator Statement	Ischemic or hemorrhagic patients assessed for or who received rehabilitation services
Numerator Exclusions	Not applicable
Denominator Exceptions	None
Improvement Notation	Improvement noted as an increase in rate
Guidance	The Non-elective Inpatient Encounter value set intends to capture all nonscheduled hospitalizations. This value set is a subset of the Inpatient Encounter value set, excluding concepts that specifically refer to elective hospital admissions. Nonelective admissions include emergency, urgent, and unplanned admissions.

EXHIBIT 3.14
Measurement Specifications for CMS Measure of Care Provided to Hospital Patients Treated for a Stroke

Source: Adapted from CMS (2017b).

As more healthcare facilities adopt EHRs, the data elements available for performance measurement purposes continue to expand. Yet mining these data can be challenging. Data are often stored in many different databases and may not be consistently reliable and valid. Varying naming conventions, inconsistent definitions, and varying field lengths and values for the same data element can lead to significant data collection problems, including poor data quality (Davoudi et al. 2015). For example, inconsistent data definitions occur when a patient's sex is captured as *M*, *F*, or *U* in a hospital's admit-discharge-transfer system but captured as *male*, *female*, or *other* in the same hospital's radiology department database. To prevent such inconsistencies, healthcare organizations should have an approved data dictionary that lists the descriptive name of each data element captured electronically along with a definition for the data element and its attributes (American Health Information Management Association 2016).

The purpose of the data dictionary is to standardize definitions and ensure consistency of use within an organization. For performance measurement purposes, the dictionary is useful for identifying what electronic data are available and where the data reside.

LEARNING POINT
Creating Measures

Construction of performance measures involves three main steps:

1. Identify the topic of interest.
2. Develop the measure.
3. Design the data collection system.

These steps can be time consuming but are essential to ensuring that the measures are consistent and reliable for quality management purposes. Most performance measures required by purchasers and external regulatory, licensing, and accreditation groups have gone through a rigorous development and validation process.

National Quality Forum (NQF)
A public–private partnership formed in 1999 to develop and implement a national strategy for improving healthcare quality.

Many externally mandated measures are reviewed and approved for use by the **National Quality Forum (NQF)**, a public–private partnership composed of representatives from provider organizations, regulatory and accreditation bodies, medical professional societies, healthcare purchasers, consumer groups, and other healthcare quality stakeholders. NQF was formed in 1999 to develop and implement a national strategy for improving healthcare quality. Part of this effort has focused on identifying valid and reliable performance measures to assess quality across the healthcare continuum. Subcommittees of the NQF use four criteria to assess a measurement for endorsement (NQF 2017b):

1. *Importance.* Is there a gap in performance? Is there potential for improvement?
2. *Scientific acceptability.* Is the measure reliable, valid, and precise?
3. *Usability.* Can measurement information be used to make decisions and/or take actions? Are the performance results statistically and clinically meaningful?

4. *Feasibility.* Can the measurement data be obtained within the normal flow of patient care? Can the measure be implemented by a healthcare organization without undue burden?

In 2017, about 300 NQF-endorsed measures were used by all types of public and private payers for a variety of purposes, including feedback, benchmarking, public reporting, and incentive-based payment (NQF 2017a).

MEASURES OF CLINICAL DECISION-MAKING

Many healthcare performance measures are similar to those used in other service industries. Hotels, for example, are service oriented. The measures of quality used by a hotel focus on topics such as customer satisfaction, timeliness of registration and checkout, billing accuracy, personal safety, and cleanliness of the property. One aspect of healthcare performance not found in other service industries is clinical decision-making. This is the process by which physicians and other clinicians determine which patients need what and when. For instance, when you have a migraine headache and seek treatment, your doctor decides which tests are needed, if any, and which treatment is right for you.

Healthcare organizations measure both the service aspects of performance and the quality of clinical decision-making. The same principles of measurement applicable to the service aspects of healthcare also apply to clinical decision-making.

> **⊛ LEARNING POINT**
> Evidence-Based Clinical Measures
>
> Many performance measures that healthcare organizations use for quality management purposes are similar to those found in other service industries. One aspect of healthcare not found in most service industries is the clinical decision-making process, which must be evaluated with performance measures derived from clinical practice guidelines developed by medical professional groups. These measures are referred to as *evidence-based measures*.

Process measures are used to determine whether clinicians are making the right patient management choices. Outcome measures are used to evaluate the results of those choices. Clinical decision-making measures undergo the same three-step construction process: (1) identify the topic of interest, (2) develop the measure, and (3) design the data collection system.

FACTORS SPECIFIC TO CLINICAL DECISION-MAKING

One factor particular to measures of clinical decision-making is the basis for measurement. The radiology manager in the previous case scenario established a departmental performance expectation that X-ray results are to be telephoned, e-mailed, or faxed to the ordering physician within 48 hours of an exam. He then measured how often this expectation was met.

Performance expectations related to clinical decision-making are established in a different manner. They are often found in **clinical practice guidelines** developed by medical professional organizations. Clinical practice guidelines are defined by Graham and colleagues (2011, 4) as "statements that include recommendations intended to optimize patient care that are informed by a systematic review of evidence and an assessment of the benefits and harms of alternative care options."

Guidelines are important to healthcare quality improvement because they can reduce variations in practice and change physician behavior to promote the use of interventions supported by the best evidence available. Guideline recommendations are based on current medical research and professional consensus. For instance, the American Association of Neurological Surgeons recommends against CT scans for children with mild head injuries unless the child exhibits signs that a severe injury has occurred (Kuppermann et al. 2009). These recommendations can be translated into measurable performance expectations.

Another factor unique to measures of clinical decision-making is the number of possible measurements. To evaluate the service aspects of healthcare performance, an organization can select from an almost limitless number of measures. Conceivably, each step of every patient care and business process could be measured to determine current performance. Because the resources needed to gather data for these measures would be extensive, organizations set measurement priorities.

Clinical decision-making is difficult to measure reliably and often involves uncertainty because many treatments could be effective for a patient. Measurable performance expectations can be established only for clinical decisions supported by clear and generally irrefutable research evidence or expert consensus. For this reason, measures of clinical decision-making are referred to as **evidence-based measures**. Most healthcare organizations use evidence-based measures to evaluate the quality of clinical decision-making. Some of these measures are mandated by external regulatory and accreditation groups. Exhibit 3.15 lists examples of evidence-based measures found in HEDIS, which is sponsored by NCQA (2016) and used by many state Medicaid programs for evaluating provider performance.

? DID YOU KNOW?

In 2010, Howard Brody, MD, professor of family medicine at the University of Texas Medical Branch in Galveston, called on US medical specialty societies to identify five tests and treatments that were overused in their specialty and did not provide meaningful benefit for patients. Brody's proposal was initially taken up by the National Physicians Alliance, which piloted the Five Things concept through the American Board of Internal Medicine (ABIM) Foundation. This led to the Choosing Wisely campaign, launched in April 2012 as a partnership between the ABIM Foundation and *Consumer Reports*. This initiative seeks to advance a national dialogue on avoiding wasteful or unnecessary medical tests, treatments, and procedures. Many medical specialty societies have now identified overused tests and treatments, and the number of recommendations increases each year. More information can be found on the Choosing Wisely website, www.choosingwisely.org (Wolfson, Santa, and Slass 2014).

Topic of Interest	Evidence-Based Measure
Management of low back pain	Percentage of adults 18–50 years of age with a primary diagnosis of low back pain who did not have an imaging study (plain X-ray, MRI or CT scan) within 28 days of the diagnosis
Breast cancer screening	Percentage of women 50–74 years of age who had at least one mammogram to screen for breast cancer in the past two years
Management of chronic obstructive pulmonary disease (COPD)	Percentage of adults 40 years of age and older who have a new diagnosis of COPD or newly active COPD, who received spirometry testing to confirm the diagnosis
Immunizations for Adolescents	Percentage of adolescents 13 years of age who had one dose of meningococcal vaccine and one Tdap vaccine or one tetanus, diphtheria toxoids vaccine (Td) by their 13th birthday

EXHIBIT 3.15
Examples of Evidence-Based Performance Measures

Source: Reprinted with permission from National Committee for Quality Assurance, *HEDIS® 2017 Volume 1: Narrative*. Washington, DC: NCQA. Copyright © 2016.

To promote widespread use of quality measures by the healthcare community, AHRQ (2017) sponsors the National Quality Measures Clearinghouse (NQMC), a database of evidence-based performance measures developed by governmental, accreditation, and medical professional groups around the world. To be added to the NQMC, the measures must meet inclusion criteria, including reliability and validity assessments.

BALANCED SCORECARD OF MEASURES

Originally developed as a framework for measuring private industry performance, **balanced scorecards (BSCs)** are structures healthcare organizations use to evaluate achievement of operational objectives. Many healthcare organizations use some type of BSC to measure system-level performance (McLaughlin and Olson 2017). In addition to an overall "corporate" strategic scorecard, scorecards can be set up for each business unit in an organization. Scorecard measures are typically sorted into four strategic perspectives (McLaughlin and Olson 2017):

Balanced scorecards (BSCs)
Frameworks for displaying system-level performance measures; components of structured performance management systems that align an organization's vision and mission with operational objectives.

1. Financial

2. Customer

3. Internal business process

4. Learning and growing

Kaplan and Norton (1996) suggested that a BSC include no more than five measures for each category. Examples of system-level measures in the four typical BSC categories are provided in exhibit 3.16. Some of the measures are included more than once in different categories. For instance, measures related to patient satisfaction can be reported for both the customer perspective and the internal business process perspective. Healthcare organizations are not consistent as to the kind and number of measures they report on scorecards or how they categorize them.

Exhibit 3.16
Balanced
Scorecard
Categories and
Examples of
System-Level
Measures

Category	Measures
Financial	• Volume growth by key service lines • Dollars generated from new contracts • Dollar amount of community donations (e.g., corporate gifts) • Growth in net revenues • Operating margin • Days of cash on hand • Days in accounts receivable • Debt service coverage ratio • Amortization and expense expressed as percentage of net revenue • Cost per case • Cost per discharge • Operating room supply expense per surgical case
Customer	• Percentage of patients who would recommend the facility • Number of new managed care contracts each year • Percentage of patients satisfied with services • Percentage of payers satisfied with services • Number of service complaints • Rate of employee turnover/retention rate • Percentage of physicians satisfied with services • Dollar amount of charitable donations • Average number of patients who rate hospital food as "exceeding expectations" • Percentage of patients who report their pain was adequately controlled • Dollar amount of community donations (e.g., corporate gifts)

(continued)

Category	Measures
Internal business process	• Average patient length of stay • Percentage of patients readmitted for same/similar condition • Rate of patient falls • Rate of medication errors • Number of employee occupational injuries • Call center response times • Cost per case • Percentage of occupied beds • Percentage of emergency patients seen within 15 minutes of arrival • Number of patient complaints • Percentage of claims rejected by insurance companies because of inaccuracies • Average time from provision of service to bill creation
Learning and growth	• Percentage of capital expenditures spent on key infrastructure targets • Dollar amount of employee tuition reimbursement • Number of continuing education credits per full-time employee • Percentage of clinical staff trained in teamwork • Number of new services offered • Number of new research projects • Rate of employee turnover/retention rate • Percentage of staff attending at least one formal training session • Percentage of staff with postgraduate qualifications

EXHIBIT 3.16

Balanced Scorecard Categories and Examples of System-Level Measures *(continued)*

CONCLUSION

Measurement is the starting point of all quality management activities and an integral part of the quality management cycle (see exhibit 3.1). Measurement results, usually in the form of numbers or statistics, are used by decision-makers to evaluate the performance of patient care and business processes. To be effective for quality management purposes, measures and data collection systems must be carefully developed, and measurement results must be accurate, useful, easy to interpret, and consistently reported.

Healthcare organizations use a combination of system- and activity-level measures to evaluate four dimensions of service: structure, process, outcome, and patient experience. Many healthcare organizations must gather information for performance measures required by purchasers and external regulatory, licensing, and accreditation groups. In addition, healthcare organizations select performance measures to evaluate aspects of patient care that are important to their strategic goals.

Measurement information alone does not improve quality. In chapter 4, we discuss the second step of the quality management cycle—assessment—in which data must be analyzed to determine whether performance is acceptable and to identify areas needing improvement.

FOR DISCUSSION

1. For any healthcare activity, four performance factors can be measured: structure, process, outcome, and patient experience. Identify one measure from each of these categories that could be used to evaluate the following ambulatory surgery center admission process:

   Upon arrival, the patient reports to the center's registration or admitting area. The patient completes paperwork, provides an identification card, and supplies insurance information, if insured. Money for the patient's insurance copay or self-pay deposit is collected at this time. Often, patients register on the surgery center's website before the date of admission to facilitate the registration process. An identification bracelet, including the patient's name and doctor's name, is placed around the patient's wrist. Before any procedure is performed the patient is asked to sign a consent form. If the patient is not feeling well, a family member or caregiver can help the patient complete the admission process.

2. Describe, in fundamental terms, each measure you selected to evaluate the surgery center's admission process. What are the numerator and denominator? If the measure does not require a numerator and denominator, explain why.

3. Suppose the manager of the surgery center's registration area wants to gather data to report performance results for the measures you have chosen. What data sources could be used to gather information for the measures? Why would these data sources be best for gathering reliable data?

4. Identify one structure measure, one process measure, one outcome measure, and one customer experience measure that could be used to evaluate a manager's process for hiring a new employee. The common steps in this process are as follows: Review candidate's application, schedule interview, conduct interview, collect feedback from references, prepare employment offer, submit offer to candidate, and hire candidate if offer is accepted.

5. In your opinion, what is the greatest barrier to ensuring the quality of data used for performance measurement purposes? Support your opinion with literature references.

6. Search the NQMC (www.qualitymeasures.ahrq.gov) and identify five evidence-based performance measures related to prescribing the correct medications for patients. The measures should focus on choosing the right medication for a patient's condition. List each measure, the organization or group that developed the measure, and the date the measure was published.

WEBSITES

- AHRQ Quality Measure Tools and Resources
  www.ahrq.gov/professionals/quality-patient-safety/quality-resources/index.html

- AHRQ State Snapshots (state-specific healthcare quality information)
  www.ahrq.gov/research/data/state-snapshots/index.html

- Balanced Scorecard Institute
  www.balancedscorecard.org/

- CMS Ambulatory Surgical Center Quality Reporting
  www.cms.gov/Medicare/Quality-Initiatives-Patient-Assessment-Instruments/ASC-Quality-Reporting/index.html

- CMS Electronic Clinical Quality Measures
  https://ecqi.healthit.gov/ecqms

- CMS Quality of Care Center
  www.cms.gov/Center/Special-Topic/Quality-of-Care-Center.html

- CMS Quality Payment Program (MACRA)
  https://qpp.cms.gov

- Consumer Assessment of Healthcare Providers and Systems (CAHPS) program: Surveys and Guidance
  www.cahps.ahrq.gov

- *Designing and Implementing Medicaid Disease and Care Management Programs, Section 7: Measuring Value in a Care Management Program*
  www.ahrq.gov/professionals/systems/long-term-care/resources/hcbs/medicaidmgmt/medicaidmgmt7.html

- *Encyclopedia of Measures* (2017), published by the American Hospital Association/Health Research & Educational Trust
  www.hret-hiin.org/resources/display/encyclopedia-of-measures-eom

- Glossary of Statistical Terms
  http://stats.oecd.org/glossary

- Healthcare Financial Management Association
  www.hfma.org

- Joint Commission
  www.jointcommission.org

- Leapfrog Group (hospital surveys)
  www.leapfroggroup.org

- National Committee for Quality Assurance
  http://ncqa.org

- National Quality Forum
  www.qualityforum.org

- National Quality Measures Clearinghouse
  www.qualitymeasures.ahrq.gov

- National and state performance measures of key indicators of maternal and child health, published by the US Health Resources & Services Administration
  https://mchb.tvisdata.hrsa.gov/

- Pharmacy Quality Alliance performance measures
  http://pqaalliance.org/measures/default.asp

- Sample size calculator
  www.surveysystem.com/sscalc.htm

- Toolkit for Using the AHRQ Quality Indicators
  www.ahrq.gov/professionals/systems/hospital/qitoolkit/index.html

- *Turning Point Guidebook for Performance Measurement* in public health, published by Public Health Foundation
  www.phf.org/resourcestools/Documents/PMCguidebook.pdf

REFERENCES

Agency for Healthcare Research and Quality (AHRQ). 2017. "Quality Measures Clearing-house." Accessed November 1. www.qualitymeasures.ahrq.gov.

———. 2016. "What Is Patient Experience?" Published October. www.ahrq.gov/cahps /about-cahps/patient-experience/index.html.

American Health Information Management Association. 2016. "Practice Brief: Managing a Data Dictionary (2016 Update)." Accessed July 31, 2017. http://bok.ahima.org/doc ?oid=302014#.WX_RkumQzcc.

Blumenthal, D., and J. M. McGinnis. 2015. "Measuring Vital Signs: An IOM Report on Core Metrics for Health and Health Care Progress." *Journal of the American Medical Association* 313 (19): 1901–2.

Centers for Medicare & Medicaid Services (CMS). 2017a. "About Electronic Clinical Quality Measures (eCQMs)." Accessed November 1. https://ecqi.healthit.gov/ecqms.

———. 2017b. "Assessed for Rehabilitation: eCQMs for 2018 Reporting Period." Updated October 25. https://ecqi.healthit.gov/ecqm/measures/cms102v6.

———. 2017c. "CAHPS® Hospital Survey." Accessed November 1. www.hcahpsonline.org.

———. 2017d. "Eligible Hospital / Critical Access Hospital eCQMs." Accessed November 1. https://ecqi.healthit.gov/eligible-hospital-critical-access-hospital-ecqms.

———. 2017e. "Home Health Quality Initiative: Quality Measures." Accessed November 1. www.cms.gov/Medicare/Quality-Initiatives-Patient-Assessment-Instruments/Home HealthQualityInits/HHQIQualityMeasures.html.

———. 2017f. "Quality Payment Program." Accessed November 1. https://qpp.cms.gov.

———. 2012. "Meaningful Use Regulations." Accessed November 1, 2017. www.healthit .gov/policy-researchers-implementers/meaningful-use-regulations.

Centers for Medicare & Medicaid Services (CMS) and The Joint Commission. 2016. *Specifications Manual for National Hospital Inpatient Quality Measures*, version 5.2a. Published October 20. www.jointcommission.org/specifications_manual_for_national_hospital _inpatient_quality_measures.aspx.

Connance. 2014. "2014 Connance Consumer Impact Study Shows Link Between Business Office, Patient Payment Behaviors and Patient Satisfaction." Press release. Published December 2. www.connance.com/wp-content/uploads/6-Connance_Consumer_Impact _Study_on_12-1-14_FINAL.pdf.

Davoudi, S., J. A. Dooling, B. Glondys, T. D. Jones, L. Kadlec, S. M. Overgaard, K. Ruben, and A. Wendicke. 2015. "Data Quality Management Model (2015 Update)." *Journal of AHIMA*. Published October. http://bok.ahima.org/doc?oid=107773.

Donabedian, A. 1980. *Explorations in Quality Assessment and Monitoring, Volume 1: The Definitions of Quality and Approaches in Assessment*. Chicago: Health Administration Press.

Graham, R., M. Mancher, D. M. Wolman, S. Greenfield, and E. Steinberg (eds.). 2011. *Clinical Practice Guidelines We Can Trust*. National Academies Press. Accessed November 1, 2017. http://nationalacademies.org/hmd/Reports/2011/Clinical-Practice-Guidelines-We-Can-Trust.aspx.

Illinois General Assembly, Joint Committee on Administrative Rules. 2014. "Administrative Code, Title 77: Public Health, Chapter I: Department of Public Health, Subchapter b: Hospital and Ambulatory Care Facilities, Part 205: Ambulatory Surgical Treatment Center Licensing Requirements, Section 205.620: Statistical Data." Accessed November 1, 2017. www.ilga.gov/commission/jcar/admincode/077/077002050F06200R.html.

Institute of Medicine (IOM). 2001. *Crossing the Quality Chasm: A New Health System for the 21st Century*. Washington, DC: National Academies Press.

Joint Commission. 2017. "2017 Hospital National Patient Safety Goals." Accessed November 1. www.jointcommission.org/assets/1/6/2017_NPSG_HAP_ER.pdf.

Kaplan, R., and D. P. Norton. 1996. *The Balanced Scorecard: Translating Strategy into Action*. Boston: Harvard Business School Press.

Kuppermann, N., J. F. Holmes, P. S. Dayan, J. D. Hoyle, S. M. Atabaki, R. Holubkov, F. M. Nadel, D. Monroe, R. M. Stanley, D. A. Borgialli, M. K. Badawy, J. E. Schunk, K. S. Quayle, P. Mahajan, R. Lichenstein, K. A. Lillis, M. G. Tunik, E. S. Jacobs, J. M. Callahan, M. H. Gorelick, T. F. Glass, L. K. Lee, M. C. Bachman, A. Cooper, E. C. Powell, M. J. Gerardi, K. A. Melville, J. P. Muizelaar, D. H. Wisner, S. J. Zuspan, J. M. Dean, and S. L. Wootton-Gorges. 2009. "Identification of Children at Very Low Risk of Clinically-Important Brain Injuries After Head Trauma: A Prospective Cohort Study." *Lancet* 374 (9696): 1160–70.

LaVela, S. L., and A. S. Gallan. 2014. "Evaluation and Measurement of Patient Experience." *Patient Experience Journal* 1 (1): 28–36.

McLaughlin, D. B., and J. R. Olson. 2017. *Healthcare Operations Management*, 3rd ed. Chicago: Health Administration Press.

National Committee for Quality Assurance (NCQA). 2017. "HEDIS® and Quality Compass®." Accessed November 1. www.ncqa.org/hedis-quality-measurement/what-is-hedis.

———. 2016. *HEDIS® 2017 Volume 1: Narrative*. Accessed November 1, 2017. www.ncqa.org/hedis-quality-measurement/hedis-measures/hedis-2017.

National Quality Forum (NQF). 2017a. "NQF's Work in Quality Measurement." Accessed November 1. www.qualityforum.org/about_nqf/work_in_quality_measurement.

————. 2017b. "What NQF Endorsement Means." Accessed November 1. www.quality forum.org/Measuring_Performance/ABCs/What_NQF_Endorsement_Means.aspx.

Schuster, M. A., S. E. Onorato, and D. O. Meltzer. 2017. "Measuring the Cost of Quality Measurement: A Missing Link in Quality Strategy." *Journal of the American Medical Association* 318 (13): 1219–20.

US Food and Drug Administration, Center for Devices and Radiological Health. 2014. "Clinical Laboratory Improvement Amendments (CLIA)." Accessed November 1, 2017. www.fda.gov/medicaldevices/deviceregulationandguidance/ivdregulatoryassistance/ucm124105.htm.

Wolfson, D., J. Santa, and L. Slass. 2014. "Engaging Physicians and Consumers in Conversations About Treatment Overuse and Waste: A Short History of the Choosing Wisely Campaign." *Academic Medicine* 89 (7): 990–95.

CHAPTER 4

EVALUATING PERFORMANCE

LEARNING OBJECTIVES

After reading this chapter, you will be able to

➤ identify common ways of reporting measurement data to facilitate performance assessment,

➤ apply methods of interpreting healthcare performance measurement data,

➤ describe the role of performance targets in evaluating performance,

➤ identify common techniques for establishing performance expectations, and

➤ explain how comparative performance data are used for assessment purposes.

KEY WORDS

➤ Appropriate

➤ Bar graphs

➤ Benchmarking

➤ Central tendency

- ➤ Common cause variation
- ➤ Control chart
- ➤ Dashboard
- ➤ Data analytics
- ➤ Data visualization
- ➤ Histograms
- ➤ Horizontal axis
- ➤ Judgment
- ➤ Lower control limit
- ➤ Normal distribution
- ➤ Pareto charts
- ➤ Pareto Principle
- ➤ Performance comparison
- ➤ Performance gap

- ➤ Performance targets
- ➤ Performance trends
- ➤ Pie charts
- ➤ Process variation
- ➤ Radar charts
- ➤ Scatter diagrams
- ➤ Special cause variation
- ➤ Standard deviation
- ➤ Standards
- ➤ Statistical process control (SPC)
- ➤ Tampering
- ➤ Upper control limit
- ➤ Vertical axis

Judgment
Formation of an opinion after consideration or deliberation.

Performance assessment is the evaluation stage of quality management. Measurement data have been gathered and now must be reported and analyzed. If an organization constructs measures carefully, collects accurate data, and reports results in a meaningful way, it produces information useful for decision-making.

Assessment involves judging or evaluating measurement data for the purpose of reaching a conclusion. For instance, when I weigh myself, the scale provides useful measurement data. These data allow me to reach a conclusion: Am I losing, gaining, or maintaining my weight? My weight-loss goals influence my **judgment** of the numbers displayed on the scale. I may be pleased to see I've lost three pounds since last week, but if my goal is to lose five pounds, I'll conclude that I need more exercise. A similar assessment process occurs with healthcare performance measurement data. Measurement results are compared with expectations to judge the quality of patient care and business services.

ASSESSMENT IN QUALITY MANAGEMENT

As shown in exhibit 4.1, the assessment step follows performance measurement. In this step, the organization first judges whether its performance is acceptable. If it is acceptable, the organization continues to measure performance to ensure it does not deteriorate. If its performance is not acceptable, the organization advances to the improvement step.

Second, the organization evaluates measurement results to determine whether processes are performing as expected. Finally, it assesses those results to judge the impact of improvements.

Assessing quality does not rely on data alone. Performance goals, external factors, and other conditions must be considered when evaluating measurement results, all of which are discussed at greater length later in the chapter.

The assessment phase in quality management involves **data analytics**—the examination of raw data by which to draw conclusions about that information. This phase involves three activities:

1. Displaying measurement data

2. Comparing actual performance with expectations

3. Determining whether action is needed

Data analytics
The science of examining raw data with the purpose of drawing conclusions about that information.

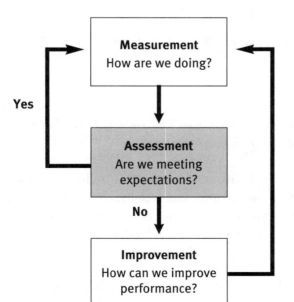

EXHIBIT 4.1
Cycle of Measurement, Assessment, and Improvement

DISPLAY DATA

The first step in analyzing performance data is deciding how the information will be presented or displayed. The data should be reported in a format from which conclusions can be easily drawn. Multiple formats can be used, such as tabulations, graphs, and statistical comparisons. Sometimes, a single data grouping will suffice for analysis purposes. To display data in an understandable format, three factors must be considered:

1. The type of data to be reported

2. The audience

3. The information's intended use

For instance, to understand how well my weight-loss diet is working, knowing the percentage of weight lost or gained at various points in time may be adequate. Alternatively, I may want to keep a daily tally of my weight so I can adjust my eating habits immediately if I am not meeting my goals. Perhaps I want to know the number of hours I exercise each week to better understand the relationship between my fitness habits and weight changes.

More important than the format in which data are displayed, however, is the accuracy and reliability of the information to help the audience answer the following questions:

◆   What is current performance?

◆   Do the data reveal a trend?

◆   Should action be taken? What kind of action?

CASE STUDY

The following case study demonstrates how data presentation influences the interpretation of performance measurement data for assessment purposes.

Continuing the radiology department case study introduced in chapter 3, the department analyzes its performance measurement results, obtained by tracking the number of outpatient X-ray exam reports it communicates to physicians within 48 hours of exam completion, to identify any trends. A line graph (also called a *run chart*) of the number of X-ray reports not communicated to patients' doctors within 48 hours of exam completion is shown in exhibit 4.2.

Although helpful, total numbers provide limited information over time. For example, the manager cannot determine whether a small or large percentage of reports are delayed. A more meaningful approach would be to graph the percentage of delayed reports—the

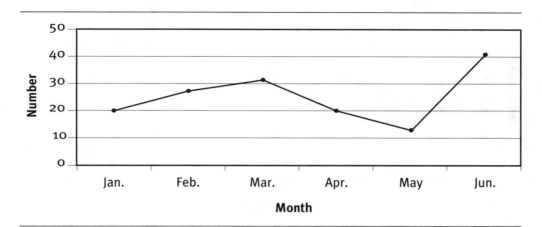

Exhibit 4.2
Line Graph
Showing Number
of Outpatient
X-ray Reports Not
Communicated to
Doctors Within 48
Hours

number of delayed X-ray reports divided by the total number of X-ray reports—as shown in exhibit 4.3.

If the radiology manager expects all outpatient X-ray reports to be communicated to patients' doctors within 48 hours, he can confirm that the performance expectation of 100 percent has not been met by simply tabulating the number of delayed reports. However, if he has set a target goal—for example, that no more than 5 percent of the reports will be delayed—he can view the data from both measurements when they are presented as a line graph that includes a target line, as shown in exhibit 4.4. With the data displayed in this manner, the radiology manager can compare actual performance each month with the performance expectations.

Reporting performance information in the right format is critical to successful quality assessment. In some cases, performance information may be displayed more effectively in a graphic format than in a tabular format. Charts and graphs can be effective media

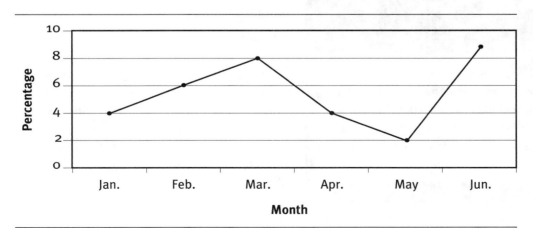

Exhibit 4.3
Line Graph
Showing
Percentage of
Outpatient X-ray
Reports Not
Communicated to
Doctors Within 48
Hours

EXHIBIT 4.4
Line Graph
Showing Target
Rate and
Percentage of
X-ray Reports Not
Communicated to
Doctors Within 48
Hours

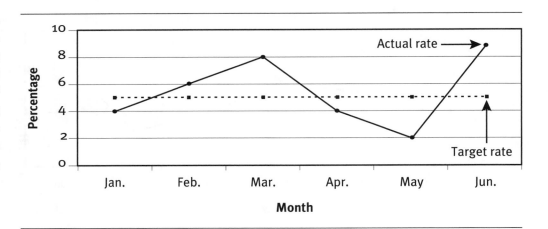

for conveying information quickly and clearly. With a swift glance, most people can glean meaningful information from pie charts and bar graphs. Graphs create a picture of the results, sometimes referred to as **data visualization**. In the rest of this section, we describe the tabular approach and common graphic display formats used by organizations to report performance data.

Data visualization
The communication of information clearly and effectively through graphical means.

SNAPSHOT REPORT FORMATS

Some performance reports provide information collected at a particular point—a snapshot of time. To create reports that represent these snapshots, data are gathered for a certain period and summarized for analysis. Common formats of snapshot reports are tabular reports, pie charts, scatter diagrams, bar graphs, histograms, Pareto charts, and radar charts.

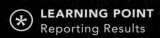

LEARNING POINT
Reporting Results

Assessment involves judging or evaluating measurement data for the purpose of reaching a conclusion. The way in which the data are presented influences their interpretation. To display data in an understandable form, three factors must be considered: the type of data to be reported, the audience, and the information's intended use.

Tabular Reports

Tabular reports, sometimes called *data tables*, are used to display numeric data gathered in one snapshot of time. Exhibit 4.5 is a tabular report showing the results of a two-month survey of patient experiences at a behavioral health clinic. A total of 47 patients completed the survey.

When considering the use of tabular reports to display performance or quality data, keep the following in mind:

◆ Tabular reports are typically used to present performance information in an easy-to-read format.

◆ Audiences may have difficulty comparing findings or identifying associations in tabular reports displaying large amounts of information. For instance, if exhibit 4.5 were to list results from 30 or more survey questions, the relationships among the lower-scoring questions would be difficult to discern. Large amounts of data are usually better displayed in a graphic design, such as the formats discussed next.

Survey Question	Mean Score $N = 47$
Overall, how would you evaluate the following:	
1. The quality of the behavioral health services you received	3.5
2. The helpfulness of the staff members	3.0
3. The courtesy shown you by the staff members	3.8
4. The staff's attention to privacy during treatment sessions	4.0
5. The professionalism of the staff members	3.9
6. The extent to which your mental health needs were addressed	3.6
7. The availability of appointments	3.5
8. The effectiveness of the medication and/or treatment you received	3.8
9. The degree to which staff members respected your confidentiality	4.1
10. Opportunities to participate in decisions about your treatment	3.9
Scale: 1 = Poor; 2 = Fair; 3 = Good; 4 = Very Good; 5 = Excellent	

EXHIBIT 4.5
Tabular Report of Results of Survey of Patient Experiences

Pie Charts

Pie charts portray the contribution of parts to a whole. For example, suppose the behavioral health clinic discussed earlier conducts a follow-up telephone survey to tally patients' most common complaints about the clinic. The results of this onetime survey can be displayed in a pie chart, as shown in exhibit 4.6.

Pie charts
Graphs in which each unit of data is represented as a pie-shaped piece of a circle. (An example of a pie chart is found in exhibit 4.6.)

EXHIBIT 4.6
Pie Chart Showing
Top Five Patient
Complaints and
Percentage of
Patients Citing
Each as Their Top
Complaint

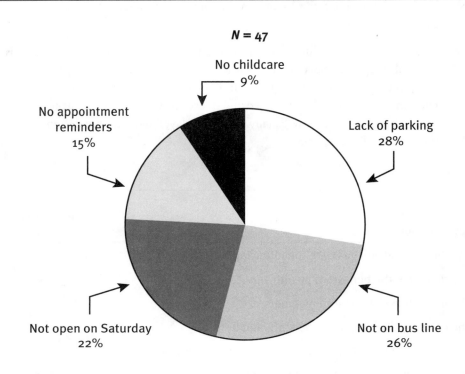

N = 47

No childcare
9%

No appointment
reminders
15%

Lack of parking
28%

Not open on Saturday
22%

Not on bus line
26%

When considering the use of pie charts, keep the following in mind:

◆ Pie charts show the data distribution from a snapshot of time.

◆ Use pie charts to illustrate the distribution or composition of a single variable. The single variable in exhibit 4.6 is patient complaints.

◆ Use pie charts only for variables with mutually exclusive values (i.e., no cases are included in more than one category). In the behavioral health clinic telephone survey, patients could pick only one complaint, which made the categories in exhibit 4.6 mutually exclusive.

◆ Avoid using pie charts for variables that have more than five categories.

Scatter diagrams
Graphs used to show
how two variables may
be related. (Examples
of scatter diagrams are
found in exhibits 4.7
and 4.8.)

Horizontal axis
The *x*-axis on a graph.

Vertical axis
The *y*-axis on a graph.

Scatter Diagrams

Scatter diagrams are tools for analyzing relationships between two variables. One variable is plotted on the **horizontal axis** (*x*-axis), and the other is plotted on the **vertical axis** (*y*-axis). The distribution of their intersecting points reveals relationship patterns, as illustrated in exhibit 4.7. If one variable increases when the other increases, the two variables are positively correlated. If one variable decreases when the other increases, they are negatively correlated. When the points appear to form a line, the variables are strongly correlated. The strength of the correlation is a measure of how likely the two variables are related to each other (Kumar 2017).

Scatter diagrams allow the user to delve beneath the surface into the cause of performance problems. For example, suppose a hospital information technology (IT) department uses computer response time as a measure of performance. The manager notices an increase in response times that has slowly developed and begins to investigate the cause. She looks at several factors and creates scatter diagrams to correlate each factor with computer response times.

The manager creates the scatter diagram shown in exhibit 4.8 to examine the relationship between computer response time (the first variable, plotted on the y-axis) and number of users connected to the computer network (the second variable, plotted on the x-axis) for 24 hours. The diagram reveals that response time increases as the number of users increases, indicating a positive cause-and-effect relationship between the two variables.

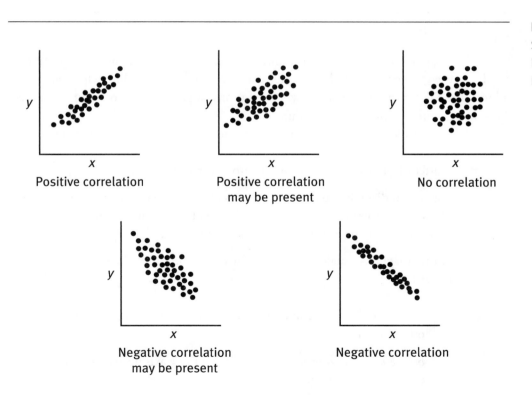

EXHIBIT 4.7
Scatter Diagram
Relationship
Patterns

EXHIBIT 4.8
Scatter Diagram
Showing
Relationship
Between Two
Variables:
Computer
Response Time
and Number of
Users Connected

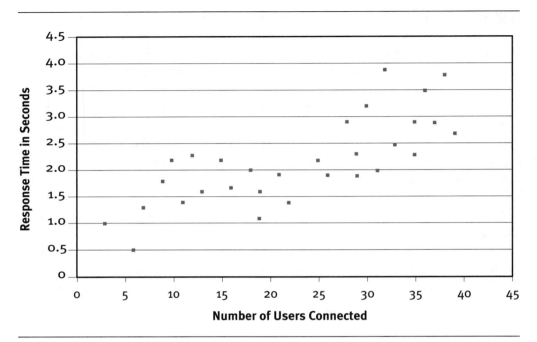

Scatter diagrams only show relationships; they do not prove that changes in one variable cause changes in the other. Scatter diagrams provide clues that help identify the culprit. The IT department manager will need to investigate further to confirm the relationship suggested by the scatter diagram.

When considering the use of scatter diagrams, keep the following in mind:

◆ Scatter diagrams show relationships from a snapshot of time.

◆ Use scatter diagrams to examine theories about cause-and-effect relationships. The scatter diagram in exhibit 4.8 helps the IT department manager narrow down what may be causing a performance problem.

◆ Scatter diagrams usually show one of five possible correlations between the two variables:

  1. *Strong positive correlation.* The value on the *y*-axis increases as the value on the *x*-axis increases.

  2. *Strong negative correlation.* The value on the *y*-axis decreases as the value on the *x*-axis increases.

3. *Possible positive correlation.* The value on the *y*-axis increases slightly as the value on the *x*-axis increases.

4. *Possible negative correlation.* The value on the *y*-axis decreases slightly as the value on the *x*-axis increases.

5. *No correlation.* No connection is evident between the two variables.

Bar Graphs

With **bar graphs**, sometimes called *bar charts*, audiences can easily compare groups of data and quickly assess their implications on performance. One axis of the chart shows the quality attribute being measured, and the other axis represents actual performance results. In Microsoft Excel, vertical bar graphs are called *column graphs* and horizontal bar graphs are called *bar graphs*.

Exhibit 4.9 is a vertical bar graph that shows average computer response times for a six-month period at each of four hospitals in a regional health system. From the graph, the hospital with the lowest average computer response time is easy to identify, and response time performance among the four hospitals is easy to compare.

Exhibit 4.10 is a horizontal bar graph displaying the number of patient falls reported in each of nine hospital units during a three-month period. One advantage of using horizontal bar graphs is that they have more room on the vertical axis to accommodate labels, which is useful when the graph contains many bars or when the label descriptors are long. The bars are arranged according to length so that units reporting the most—and the fewest—incidents are easy to identify.

Bar graphs
Graphs used to show the relative size of different categories of a variable, with each category or value of the variable represented by a bar; also called a *bar chart*. (Examples of bar graphs are found in exhibits 4.9 and 4.10.)

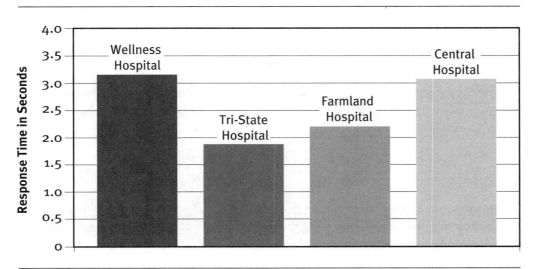

EXHIBIT 4.9
Vertical Bar Graph Comparing Computer Response Times at Four Hospitals During One Period

EXHIBIT 4.10
Horizontal Bar
Graph Showing
Number of Patient
Falls in Each
Hospital Unit,
January–March

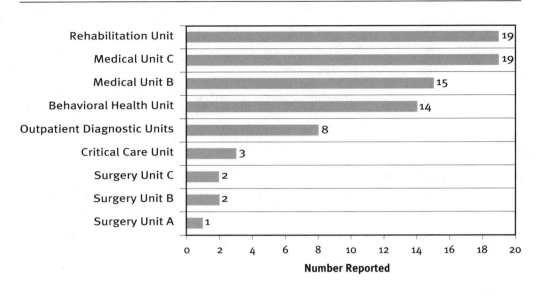

When considering the use of bar graphs, keep the following in mind:

◆ Bar graphs are an excellent way to show performance results from a snapshot of time.

◆ The height of the bar represents the frequency of incidences for that category. In exhibit 4.9, the heights of the bars represent the average computer response times at each hospital.

◆ The width of the bars within a bar graph is not relevant, but it should be consistent.

◆ Horizontal bar charts are often used when the labels along the *x*-axis are too long to fit under vertical columns or when a large number of bars are displayed.

Histograms
Bar graphs used to
show the center,
dispersion, and shape
of the distribution
of a collection of
performance data. (An
example of a histogram
is found in exhibit 4.11.)

Histograms

Histograms, sometimes referred to as *frequency distributions*, are bar charts that show a distribution of values as rankings along the *x*-axis. Exhibit 4.11 is a histogram illustrating the distribution of patient wait times in a clinic. Wait-time data were gathered for one

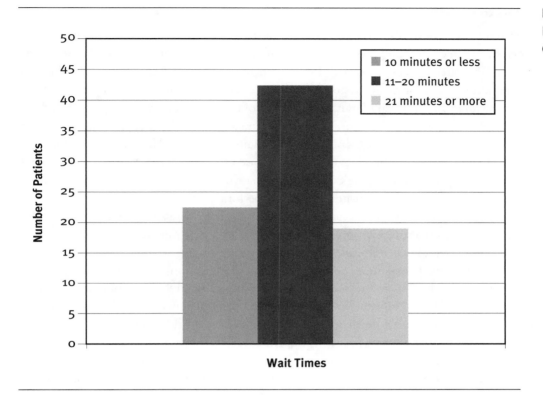

Exhibit 4.11
Histogram of
Clinic Wait Times

week, and the data were grouped into three wait-time categories. The number of patients in each category is also shown.

When considering the use of histograms, keep the following in mind:

◆ Histograms show data distribution from a snapshot of time.

◆ Use a histogram to display distributions of a variable that can be separated into rankings, such as three-month segments of a year or age ranges.

◆ As shown in exhibit 4.11, bars in a histogram should touch one another except when no cases fall into an interval along the *x*-axis.

◆ A histogram shows the **central tendency** and variability of a dataset. It can be used to quickly and easily illustrate the distribution of performance data.

Central tendency
A measure of the middle or expected center value of a dataset. The most common measures of central tendency are the arithmetic mean, the median, and the mode.

Pareto Charts

Pareto charts are similar to bar graphs, except that they sort performance data in order of decreasing frequency and include notation of other factors to highlight the **Pareto Principle**. The Pareto Principle, named after the nineteenth-century Italian economist Vilfredo Pareto, states that for many events, 80 percent of the results come from 20 percent of the inputs (Juran 1974). Joseph Juran, an originator of the science of quality, applied the Pareto Principle to quality management. Juran advised management to concentrate improvement efforts on the "vital few" sources of problems and not be distracted by those of lesser importance (Scholtes 1992). Pareto charts, then, are used to identify the 20 percent—the vital few—of the problems affecting 80 percent of performance. Organizations should resolve these problems to have the greatest impact on performance improvement.

To illustrate how a Pareto chart is used for quality assessment purposes, consider the following situation. Community Hospital starts a new practice intended to reduce problems related to patient misidentification. At the time of registration, patients scheduled for outpatient diagnostic tests now are given an identification (ID) wristband on which their name, birth date, and record number are printed. Technicians in outpatient testing areas use the ID band information to positively identify patients before performing a test. Formerly, only patients admitted to the hospital received an ID band.

Shortly after the new process is implemented, staff members in the outpatient registration area begin to complain about it. Some employees say the ink on the bands smears easily. Others say the bands are not well made and do not always fasten securely around the patient's wrist. Rather than react to random complaints, the manager of outpatient registration gathers additional information to thoroughly evaluate the situation. The manager asks employees to report ID band problems each time one occurs. At the end of 30 days, the manager tallies the data and creates a Pareto chart, shown in exhibit 4.12.

Pareto charts
Special types of bar graphs that display the most frequent problem as the first bar, the next most frequent as the next bar, and so on; also called *Pareto diagrams*. (An example of a Pareto chart is found in exhibit 4.12.)

Pareto Principle
Originally, the Pareto Principle referred to the observation that 80 percent of Italy's wealth belonged to only 20 percent of the population. The principle conveys the notion that the majority of results come from a minority of inputs (an 80/20 rule of thumb).

EXHIBIT 4.12
Pareto Chart Showing Patient ID Band Problems

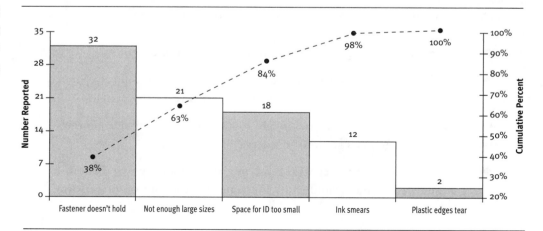

The manager concludes from these data that three main problems are triggering the complaints: the fasteners do not hold, the space provided for a patient's identifying information is too small, and the unit has too few large-sized bands on hand. A different brand of wristband—one that fastens better and has more space for the patient's identifying information—solves two of the problems. The third problem—insufficient inventory of large bands—would be solved by keeping more large bands in stock to accommodate larger patients. If these problems (20 percent of total problems, or the vital few) are resolved, complaints about ID bands should decrease by more than 80 percent.

When considering the use of Pareto charts, keep the following in mind:

◆ Pareto charts show a data distribution from a snapshot of time.

◆ Use Pareto charts to separate the few major problems (the vital few) from the many possible problems (the trivial many). Pareto charts encourage the use of data, not perception, to determine which problems are most important.

◆ Arrange performance categories or problems according to their frequency (how many), not their classification (what kind). The order should descend from left to right.

◆ The right vertical axis can be used to measure the percentage of total occurrences in each category, but in some situations, the main problems may be apparent without adding a cumulative percentage trend line.

Radar Charts

Radar charts are used to plot five to ten performance measures for an interval of time, along with performance expectations. Radar charts are sometimes called *spider charts* because of their shape. Exhibit 4.13 is a radar chart showing patient satisfaction survey results for a healthcare system. The heavy solid line represents the actual results, and the dotted line represents the expected performance or target rates. Printing these lines in different colors also can help the audience discern actual from expected performance.

When considering the use of radar charts, keep the following in mind:

◆ Radar charts show data from a snapshot of time.

◆ Radar charts show areas of relative strength and weakness and depict overall performance.

◆ In a radar chart, a point close to the center on any axis indicates a low value. A point near the edge is a high value. For example, the center point of the chart in exhibit 4.13 is 80 percent, and the edge is 100 percent.

Radar charts
Graphs used to display the differences between actual and expected performance for several measures; also called *spider charts* or *spider diagrams* because of their shape.

◆   When interpreting a radar chart, check each axis as well as the overall shape to determine overall performance.

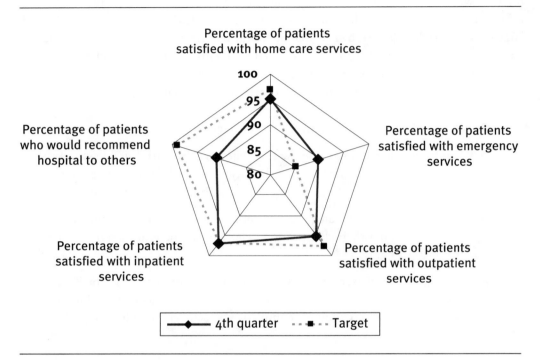

TREND REPORT FORMATS

While a report of performance from an interval of time can be helpful in some situations, decision-making often requires an understanding of performance over time. Quality is a dynamic attribute, so the ability to recognize changes in **performance trends** is important.

The volume of healthcare performance measurement data is rapidly expanding. For this reason, reports must make assessment of results as easy as possible. An audience may have difficulty absorbing information, spotting patterns, identifying aberrations, and uncovering hidden relationships from a large tabular report; graphs are usually a better choice for transforming large quantities of performance data into meaningful information. Both tabular and graph formats of performance trend reports are discussed next.

Performance trends
Patterns of gradual
change in performance;
the average or
general tendency of
performance data
to move in a certain
direction over time.

Tabular Reports

Some of the same report formats used to present snapshots of performance data can also be used to display performance trends; tabular reports are one such format. Exhibit 4.14

EXHIBIT 4.14
Tabular Report
of Home
Health Agency
Performance
Results for Four
Quarters

Performance Measure	Target	Results			
		1st Quarter	2nd Quarter	3rd Quarter	4th Quarter
Percentage of patients who report adequate pain control	≥ 90%	94%	85%	90%	92%
Percentage of patients who are admitted to an acute care hospital for at least 24 hours while a home health care patient	≤ 10%	7%	0.3%	5%	12%
Percentage of home health services delivered on the date scheduled	≥ 95%	90%	89%	92%	92%

is an excerpt from a report of system-level measures prepared for the senior leaders of a home health agency. Sometimes referred to as a **dashboard**, this type of report shows a group of performance measures; results for each period; and the performance expectation, or target, for each measure.

     Icons or color can be added to the data table to make performance problems more discernible. For example, measurement results not meeting expectations can be printed in red so the audience can easily pinpoint the results of greatest interest.

Dashboard
A set of performance measures displayed in a concise manner that allows for easy interpretation.

Line Graphs

Line graphs, sometimes called *run charts*, can be used to show changes in a performance measurement over time. The case study near the beginning of this chapter describes the radiology department manager's use of line graphs to measure the number and percentage of outpatient X-ray reports not communicated to patients' doctors within 48 hours of their exams (exhibits 4.2 and 4.3). By adding a line showing the target rate, the radiology manager was able to see how performance over time compared with expectations (see exhibit 4.4).

     One line graph can be used to report several performance measurement results. Exhibit 4.15 is a line graph showing the response rate (in seconds) to patient call lights by a hospital's nurses for 15 consecutive days. To display data effectively, line graphs should include no more than four measures. If the lines intersect, even four measures may be too many. If you are required to report many measures, consider spreading the data over more than one graph. To clarify the values along the graph lines, you might include data point markers (dots or symbols at each data point on the line). If the report identifies general

EXHIBIT 4.15

Line Graph
Showing How
Quickly Hospital
Nurses on Each
Shift Responded to
Patient Call Lights
on 15 Consecutive
Days

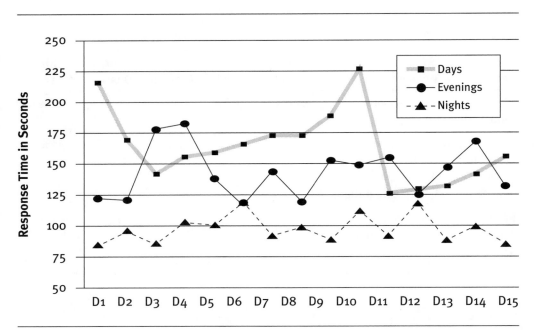

performance trends, data point markers may not be necessary. If you wish to convey exact numeric results, numbers can be added to the trend line at each data point.

Bar Graphs

Bar graphs can be used to report a snapshot of performance and also display performance data for different periods. The same three home health agency measures shown in exhibit 4.14 are reported in a horizontal bar graph in exhibit 4.16. This chart is called a *clustered bar graph* because it shows the relationship among three clusters of variables (the measurement results) for each of the four periods.

For analysis purposes, performance measurement results can be broken down into meaningful categories. For instance, on-time delivery of home health services could be reported by day of the week and the results compared from one quarter to the next. Exhibit 4.17 is a vertical bar graph showing the percentage of home health services delivered when scheduled, reported by day the service is to be provided. When the results are reported by day of the week, the home health director can see clearly where to focus improvement efforts.

Line graphs and bar graphs are the two most common ways to display performance data over time. For more than four periods, line graphs are usually the better choice. If the audience wants to see general performance trends, it may work well to use both bars and

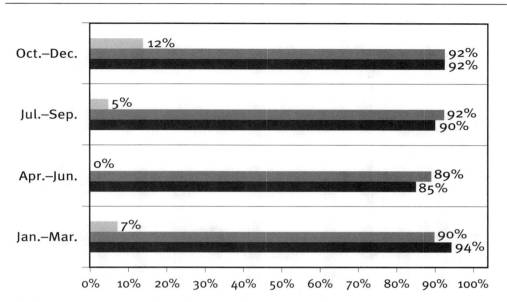

EXHIBIT 4.16

Horizontal Clustered Bar Graph Showing Home Health Agency Performance Measures

■ Percentage of home health patients admitted to hospital for at least 24 hours
■ Percentage of home health services delivered on date scheduled
■ Percentage of home health patients who report adequate pain control

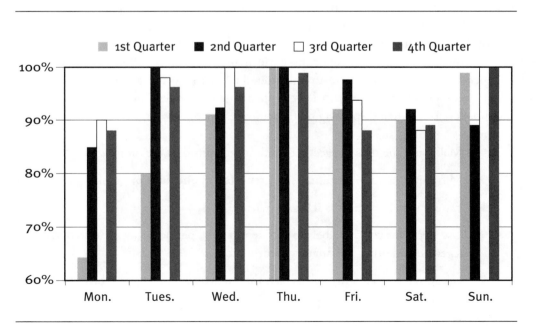

EXHIBIT 4.17

Vertical Bar Graph Showing the Percentage of Home Health Services Delivered on the Day Scheduled

EXHIBIT 4.18

Bar Graph with
Performance Trend
Line: Percentage
of Outpatient
X-ray Reports Not
Communicated to
Doctors Within 48
Hours

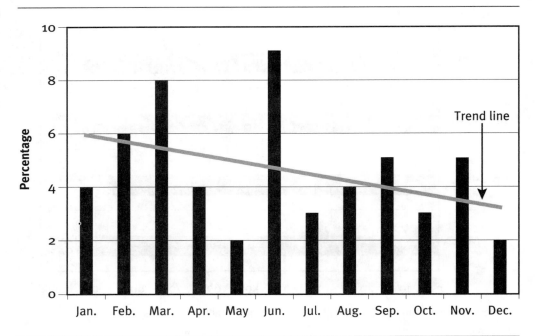

lines. For instance, exhibit 4.18 is a 12-month report of the percentage of outpatient X-ray reports not communicated to patients' doctors within 48 hours of the patients' exams. A trend line has been added to show that the overall percentages are decreasing, even though the monthly rates fluctuate.

Simplicity is the key to reporting performance measurement data, whether for a single period or for many periods. An uncluttered tabular report or graph usually conveys information more effectively than an overly data-laden one does. Several basic principles should be observed when displaying performance results:

- Make sure the data are accurate and no relevant data are omitted.

- Minimize the number of measures reported in one table or graph.

- Ensure that the report is self-explanatory.

- Use clear and concise labels for the report title, period being measured, data legends, and other explanatory information.

- Use legends or keys to explain data that may be confusing or subject to misinterpretation.

- Define abbreviations and symbols.

COMPARE RESULTS WITH EXPECTATIONS

Performance measures should be tied to a pre-defined goal or expectation. Interpretation of measurement results is meaningful only when the results are associated with goals. For instance, if I set a weight-loss goal of five pounds per month, I can compare my weight-loss performance with this goal. If I do not set a target weight, how can I interpret the numbers on my scale?

Measurement without defined performance expectations does not contribute to quality improvement. A passage from Lewis Carroll's (1999) *Alice in Wonderland* best illustrates this concept:

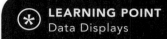

LEARNING POINT
Data Displays

Performance measurement data can be presented in many different ways. Tabular reports and bar graphs can be used to report data for a single period or for several periods. Pie charts, scatter diagrams, histograms, Pareto charts, and radar charts are typically used to report performance data from a snapshot of time. Bar and line graphs are most commonly used to display performance data over time.

"Cheshire Cat," [Alice] began. "Would you please tell me which way I ought to go from here?"

"That depends on where you want to get to," said the cat.

Without performance expectations, performance results cannot be evaluated objectively. Consider the line graph charting hand-washing compliance in exhibit 4.19. The percentage of caregivers observed washing their hands prior to patient contact shows a steady increase. Does this increase represent good performance? Without knowing the facility's performance goal, all we can say is that more people are washing their hands than before.

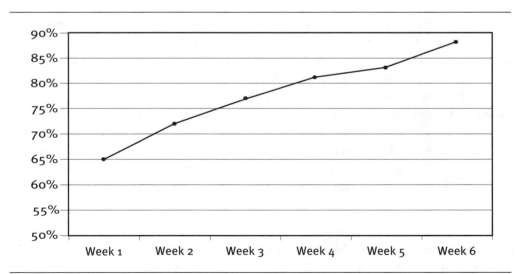

EXHIBIT 4.19
Line Graph Showing Percentage of Caregivers Observed Washing Their Hands

Alice's journey through Wonderland is similar to a healthcare organization's journey of continuous improvement. Like Alice, organizations must define their destination in terms of performance expectations. Well-defined targets have the following characteristics, known as SMART:

Specific
Measurable
Achievable
Realistic
Time-bound

SETTING EXPECTATIONS

Performance expectations should be established for every measure. These expectations are based in part on internal quality priorities, which are often influenced by the needs of stakeholders (e.g., patients, purchasers). For example, clinic patients do not like to wait a long time in the reception area, so the clinic sets an expectation for wait times to be as short as possible. Purchasers do not want to contract with a hospital that keeps patients hospitalized longer than necessary, so the hospital establishes a target for its average patient stay to be equal to or less than that of its competitors.

Government regulations and accreditation **standards** influence an organization's desired performance level. For example, the Occupational Safety and Health Administration regulations relating to employee radiation exposure state that "during any calendar quarter the dose to the whole body shall not exceed 3 rems" (US Department of Labor 1996). Radiation exposure performance expectations in radiology departments are based on these regulations.

Accreditation standards are sometimes less absolute than government regulations and give organizations leeway in setting performance expectations. For example, nursing care centers accredited by The Joint Commission (2017) are required to use at least two patient or resident identifiers when providing care, treatment, and services. The standards do not define the identifiers that can be used; they only state that the patient's or resident's room number or physical location should *not* be used. The nursing care center can select any other two patient or resident identifiers that would work best in their facility.

Except for healthcare services that must comply with absolute standards (such as standards found in government regulations), **performance targets** may be established on the basis of (1) opinion, (2) criteria, or (3) **performance comparison**.

Opinion

Performance targets may be derived from the opinion of those affected by the measure. A determination is made regarding the acceptable or desired level of performance, which

Standards
Performance expectations established by individuals or groups.

Performance targets
Desired performance.

Performance comparison
Examination of similarities or differences between one organization's performance and the performance of other organizations.

then becomes the goal. This determination is often based on people's subjective belief regarding good performance. For instance, the performance data illustrated in exhibit 4.18 show that the percentage of delayed X-ray reports is gradually declining (as evidenced by the trend line). If continued improvement of this process is a departmental goal, the following year the radiology manager will set an expectation that the percentage be lower than the current year's average rate. If maintaining the status quo is the goal, the radiology manager will set the same expectation for the following year as was achieved for the current year.

People often question why performance targets are based on opinion rather than set at 0 or 100 percent. Is less-than-perfect performance acceptable? Arguments supporting the ideal of perfection are difficult to contest, but the law of diminishing returns must be taken into consideration when setting performance goals. This law implies that larger gains are made when quality performance is low, while incremental gains diminish and become more expensive when quality is already high (Appari, Johnson, and Anthony 2013). For example, as the number of delayed X-ray reports decreases, situations that are unusually difficult to resolve may remain problematic. The manager must decide whether to direct additional efforts at achieving zero report delays or whether these efforts are better directed toward improving low performance in another area.

Criteria

Performance targets should not be established on the sole basis of opinions if relevant, professionally defined criteria are available. Professionally defined criteria are found in the standards, rules, and principles that have been developed by authoritative groups, such as clinical practice guidelines (discussed in chapter 3), consensus statements, and position papers. Physician and staff compliance with the criteria is usually considered voluntary, but organizations are encouraged to consider them when establishing expected levels of performance. For instance, the American College of Radiology (2012) recommends that imaging studies not be performed for patients with an uncomplicated headache. This recommendation may prompt the medical director of radiology to set a goal of zero imaging studies performed for this condition.

Organizations may have justifiable reasons for deviating from professionally defined criteria. In these situations, performance goals are set at less than 100 percent. For instance, the Centers for Disease Control and Prevention (2011) recommends that all healthcare practitioners and persons in training for healthcare professions be vaccinated annually against influenza, but the vaccination may not be **appropriate** for some individuals because of allergies or other contraindications. Plus, some people may choose not to follow the recommendation for personal reasons. Thus, the performance target for completion of influenza vaccinations could be set at less than 100 percent to account for such factors.

Appropriate
Suitable for a particular person, place, or condition.

Performance Comparison

Other organizations' performance is the third influence on quality targets. The use of comparative information to set performance goals is a relatively new phenomenon in healthcare. Before the mid-1980s, hospitals and other providers judged the quality of their performance primarily on the basis of internal historical trends. Organizations reviewed their current performance measurement data and compared the results with their past performance to determine whether their patient mortality rate had increased or decreased over the past year, whether patient complaints had increased or decreased, and so on. This internal attention has been replaced by a broad, externally focused type of comparison made possible by increasingly abundant, publicly available data on other organizations' achievements. Providers can use these external data to establish internal performance expectations. Exhibit 4.20 is a list of online sources of comparative performance data commonly used by healthcare organizations to set performance expectations.

The number of proprietary comparative performance databases continues to expand. For example, more than 2,500 hospitals and outpatient providers nationwide and across the world are involved in various data-sharing efforts sponsored by the National Cardiovascular Data Registry (https://cvquality.acc.org/NCDR-Home). Participants in the National Database of Nursing Quality Indicators (NDNQI) (www.pressganey.com/solutions/clinical-quality/nursing-quality) share data on structure, process, and outcome measures of nursing care at the hospital unit level. And orthopedic surgeons can submit data to FORCE-TJR, a nationwide, comprehensive database of total joint replacement surgical and patient-reported outcomes (https://forceortho.org/); in exchange, they receive quarterly reports of their results benchmarked to the national norm.

Another source of comparison data is published research. Reports on studies often provide information about performance rates. Keep in mind, however, that data from literature sources should not be blindly adopted as performance targets. For example, data from NDNQI were used by researchers to determine the prevalence of patient falls in adult medical, medical-surgical, and surgical hospital nursing units. During the study period of July 1, 2006, through September 30, 2008, a total of 315,817 falls occurred, representing a rate of 3.56 falls per 1,000 patient days (Bouldin et al. 2013). Could this fall rate be used to set a performance expectation in a hospital with similar units? The managers of the similar units would need to answer several questions to ensure a reasonably valid comparison:

◆ What is the NDNQI definition of a *patient fall*? Do we define *patient fall* the same way?

◆ How reliably did caregivers at the hospitals participating in the NDNQI report patient falls? If they did not report falls consistently, would the number of patient falls have been higher if the caregivers had reported more reliably?

◆ The researchers reported the number of patient falls per 1,000 patient days. Do we use the same reporting methodology? Do we count the number of patients who have fallen, or do we count the number of falls? (Each patient could fall more than once.)

◆ Are the patients in the hospitals participating in the NDNQI similar or dissimilar to our patient population?

◆ Does our physical environment differ from that of the hospitals participating in the NDNQI?

The term *benchmarking* is typically used to describe performance comparison activity (e.g., "We are benchmarking against other hospitals"), but it involves more than simple comparison with other organizations. **Benchmarking** uses the level of performance achieved by an exemplary or world-class organization as the standard for comparison (Sower, Duffy, and Kohlers 2007). In other words, it functions more like a scoreboard that determines whether an organization is performing above or below standard. This standard may come from an exemplary healthcare organization or from an organization outside the healthcare industry recognized for its superior performance. For example, comparison data from a hotel, a car rental company, or an airline with an excellent check-in procedure could be used to set performance goals for the patient registration process in a hospital or clinic.

> **Benchmarking**
> Learning about the best practices in other companies for the purpose of using them in your own organization.

Comparison data are not available for many aspects of healthcare services. However, any performance results from other organizations (or world-class companies) that are available should be considered when setting internal performance targets. Organizations that have achieved superior performance demonstrate the possibility that all organizations can do the same. For instance, in 2012 Maricopa Integrated Health System launched a campaign to reduce hospital-acquired infections. The campaign involved new infection prevention practices, education for the more than 4,000 staff members, and formation of the multidisciplinary Infection Prevention Champions team to investigate and recommend various other infection control strategies. As of June 2014, the system's pediatric intensive care unit had gone 457 days without a central line–associated bloodstream infection event, compared with an average interval of 79 days between events in 2011 (Maricopa Integrated Health System 2014). It is hoped that this example will stimulate other

 LEARNING POINT
Performance Goals

Performance goals are quantifiable estimates or results expected for a given period. Performance goals are set at 100 percent for aspects of healthcare that have absolute standards. In the absence of absolute standards, performance targets are based on one or more of the following factors:

• Opinion
• Criteria
• Performance comparison

EXHIBIT 4.20

Online Sources of Performance Comparison Data

Sponsor	Description of Publicly Available Data
Agency for Healthcare Research and Quality (AHRQ) (www.ahrq.gov/research/findings/nhqrdr/)	The National Healthcare Quality & Disparities Report includes national estimates of numerous performance measures, including dimensions of healthcare quality, stages of healthcare, clinical conditions, settings of care, and access to healthcare.
AHRQ Consumer Assessment of Healthcare Providers and Systems (CAHPS) (www.cahpsdatabase.ahrq.gov/cahpsidb/)	The CAHPS reporting system is an online repository for data from selected CAHPS surveys. The system contains comparative data for the CAHPS Health Plan Survey and the CAHPS Clinician & Group Survey.
American College of Surgeons Commission on Cancer (www.facs.org/quality-programs/cancer/ncdb)	The National Cancer Database (NCDB) contains information on cancer care in the United States, including tumor staging and histology characteristics, type of first-course treatment administered, disease recurrence, and survival information.
American College of Surgeons National Trauma Data Bank (NTDB) (www.facs.org/quality-programs/trauma/ntdb)	The NTDB annual adult and pediatric reports contain descriptive information about trauma patients, including demographics, injury information, and outcomes.
California Office of Statewide Health Planning and Development (www.oshpd.ca.gov/HID/#Find)	The office provides quality of care, patient safety, and outcomes data for California hospitals.
Centers for Disease Control and Prevention (CDC) (www.cdc.gov/hai/surveillance/)	The CDC provides information about national and state healthcare-associated infection rates.
Centers for Medicare & Medicaid Services (CMS) (https://data.medicare.gov)	CMS provides various performance measurement data for hospitals, nursing homes, home health agencies, and dialysis facilities.
The Commonwealth Fund (www.whynotthebest.org)	WhyNotTheBest.org is a resource for healthcare professionals interested in tracking performance on various measures of healthcare quality.
Department of Veterans Affairs (www.medicare.gov/hospitalcompare/VAData/main.html)	VA Hospital Compare contains information for consumers about the quality and safety of healthcare provided by the Veterans Health Administration.
Healthcare Cost and Utilization Project, sponsored by AHRQ (http://hcupnet.ahrq.gov)	The Healthcare Cost and Utilization Project includes health statistics and information on hospitals, including pediatric and emergency department utilization and AHRQ quality indicators.
The Joint Commission (www.qualitycheck.org)	Quality Checks are reports on the performance of accredited organizations in key areas of patient care.
The Leapfrog Group (www.leapfroggroup.org)	The Leapfrog Group conducts a hospital survey of quality and safety, focusing on hospital structures, processes of care, and outcomes.
National Committee for Quality Assurance (NCQA) (https://reportcards.ncqa.org)	NCQA provides health plan and managed behavioral healthcare organization performance measurement results for quality of care, access to care, and member satisfaction with health plans and doctors.

hospitals to work toward achieving similarly low infection rates.

STATISTICAL PROCESS CONTROL

In addition to comparing performance with pre-defined goals, healthcare organizations increasingly use **statistical process control (SPC)** to assess performance. This technique, which has traditionally been applied in industries other than healthcare, allows the user to highlight variations in performance that should be investigated. Performance variation can sometimes be a bigger problem than can consistently average performance.

> **(?) DID YOU KNOW?**
>
> In the 1860s, Florence Nightingale pioneered the systematic collection, analysis, and dissemination of comparative hospital outcomes data to understand and improve performance.

Statistical process control (SPC)
Application of statistical methods to identify and control performance.

Consider the following situation: A 450-bed urban hospital uses a centralized call center to schedule all outpatient tests, such as imaging and blood tests. Because many of its competitors offer similar outpatient services in the area, callers typically do not wait on hold for a scheduler for more than 30 to 40 seconds before hanging up. Management views a lost call as lost business.

The call center regularly measures how long callers wait on hold, and the wait time performance goal is an average of 30 seconds or less. The call center meets this performance goal each month, yet many callers hang up before a scheduler takes their call. Why? Average performance is fine; performance variation is the problem. When schedulers are busy, callers are forced to wait longer in the phone queue than they would like to. Performance appears to be acceptable when long wait times are averaged together with short wait times, but managers need a better picture of call center performance: They should apply SPC to measure variation in wait times as well as average wait time performance.

SPC concepts and methods are primarily based on the importance of reducing **process variation** to consistently achieve desired results over time. Using SPC methods, performance data are graphically displayed and analyzed to determine whether performance is in a state of statistical control. When performance reaches a state of stability and the conditions or factors present at that time remain constant, future performance is likely to stay in the same range.

Process variation
Fluctuation in process output.

The following example illustrates how SPC is used to determine whether performance is stable (in a state of statistical control) or unstable (out of statistical control). Performance stability is evaluated by determining the amount of variation.

Suppose that every day you plot on a line graph the number of minutes you take to run three miles. After a 30-day period, your daily run times vary but likely remain in a predictable range (some variation is expected in any process). At what point is your run time significantly different from the norm? To answer this question, you use data from the past 30 days to calculate the upper and lower limits of your run time norm. When you plot the current day's time on the graph, you can see whether the time lies in the normal range.

The upper and lower limits of your run time norm are derived from the statistical theory of **normal distribution**. About 68 percent of values drawn from a normal distribution are within one **standard deviation** of the mean (average), about 95 percent of the values are within two standard deviations, and about 99 percent lie within three standard deviations (Research Methods Knowledge Base 2006). If the upper and lower limits of your normal run time are set at three standard deviations from the mean, you have little chance of registering a run time outside of these parameters.

If your times remain stable (that is, they always lie in the normal range), your running performance is in a state of statistical control. The only way you can achieve better run times is to change a fundamental aspect of the process (e.g., run a different route, wear new shoes for your run). Suppose one day your run time is outside the limits of your norm. Because these limits have been statistically calculated on the basis of your past performance, you know that something unusual occurred. You will want to identify and correct the cause of the longer time.

Performance Variation

While working for Western Electric Company in the 1920s, Walter Shewhart recognized that a process can contain two types of variation: one resulting from random causes and one resulting from assignable causes (Provost and Murray 2011). W. Edwards Deming later used the expressions **common cause variation** to describe variation resulting from random causes and **special cause variation** to describe variation resulting from assignable causes (Provost and Murray 2011). Common cause variation is inherent—always present—in every process. The effect of this type of variation on performance is usually minimal and results from the regular rhythm of the process.

The different types of outpatient diagnostic tests scheduled by the hospital call center described earlier are one example of factors that can create common cause variation in a process. Each test is different, so the time required to schedule each one varies. The call center manager cannot change the fact that the tests are different; the differences are just part of the scheduling process and have to be considered when managing call wait time performance.

Special cause variation results from factors that are not inherent in the process and somehow find their way into it. They do not frequently affect the process, but when they do, their impact on performance can be huge. As an example, consider a part-time employee who works in the hospital's call center. Presume this employee is slower at scheduling test appointments than other schedulers are. Immediately, you deduce that the variation in the time callers wait on hold can be attributed to this employee's poor methods. This variation occurs infrequently (when the employee is working), has a large impact on performance (more callers on hold for longer periods), and is not a normal part of the process. To eliminate this special cause variation, the employee could receive further training or be dismissed.

You will always find some variation when you measure performance over time. During the performance assessment step, your reaction to this variation is important. Using SPC techniques, you can differentiate between common cause and special cause variation. Suppose you take an average of 29 minutes to run three miles. One day, you take 37 minutes. Does this longer time indicate a special cause variation that should be investigated and eliminated, or does it indicate a common cause variation that does not need to be investigated and eliminated?

One aspect of quality management first articulated by Shewhart (1925) is a phenomenon known as **tampering**. Tampering occurs when some action is taken in reaction to a performance result without knowing whether the result was caused by natural variation in the process (common cause) or an unusual occurrence (special cause). Process changes made in response to an instance of undesirable performance when it is just normal performance variance can damage the process further.

Tampering
Doing something in reaction to a particular performance result without knowing whether it was caused by natural variation or some unusual occurrence.

STATISTICAL PROCESS CONTROL TOOLS

Line graphs and control charts are commonly used SPC tools, in part because variations in performance data plotted on these graphs are easy to interpret. A few basic rules, discussed in detail in the following sections, should be remembered when identifying common cause variation (the process is considered stable) and special cause variation (the process is considered unstable).

Line Graph

SPC techniques can be applied to data displayed in a line graph without calculating upper and lower limits of the normal range. Only the average, or mean, of the data is calculated, and it is displayed as a center line on the graph. Ideally, the line graph has a minimum of 15 data points; some statisticians suggest a minimum of 20 data points (Woodall 2000). Performance results plotted on the graph are compared with the center line to locate significant performance shifts or trends. A shift or trend represents potentially unstable performance that needs to be investigated.

A significant shift in performance is evident when one of the following situations occurs:

◆ Seven consecutive data points appear above or below the center line on a line graph that shows fewer than 20 data points (ignore data points that fall on the center line).

◆ Eight consecutive data points appear above or below the center line on a line graph that shows 20 or more data points (ignore data points that fall on the center line).

A significant performance trend is evident when one of the following situations occurs:

◆ Seven consecutive data points move steadily upward or downward on a line graph that shows fewer than 20 data points (points may fall on or cross the center line).

◆ Eight consecutive data points move steadily upward or downward on a line graph that shows 20 or more data points (points may fall on or cross the center line).

The line graph of clinic wait time data shown in exhibit 4.21 illustrates how this SPC technique is applied during performance assessment. Starting at week 10, the wait time slightly increases. By week 16, the wait time has increased seven consecutive times—a signal that the upward trend is likely to continue. As with unusual shifts in performance, trends should be investigated.

Control Chart

A line graph that contains a mean line and upper and lower limits of the normal range (known as *control limits*) is called a statistical **control chart**. Developed by Shewhart (1925)

Control chart
A line graph that includes statistically calculated upper and lower control limits. (Examples of control charts are found in exhibits 4.22–4.25.)

EXHIBIT 4.21
Line Graph of Clinic Wait Time Data Displaying a Significant Trend

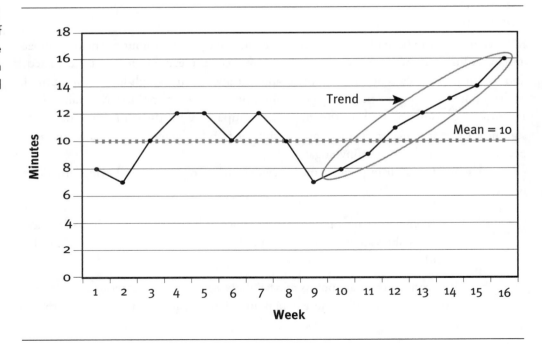

in 1924, it has become a primary tool of modern performance assessment. A set of observations (such as your run times for 30 days) is plotted on the control chart along with the mean line, called the *center line* (CL); the upper limit of the normal range, called the **upper control limit** (UCL); and the lower limit of the normal range, called the **lower control limit** (LCL). The CL almost always represents the arithmetic mean of the data. Shewhart recommended that control limits be set at plus and minus three standard deviations from the mean (Nelson 2003). In situations where performance variation must be kept to a minimum, control limits may be set at plus and minus two or even one standard deviation from the mean.

Exhibit 4.22 is a control chart showing your hypothetical three-mile run times for a 30-day period. The run times for each day are different, but these differences are normal process variation (common cause variation) because the times are within the statistically calculated UCL and LCL. Thus, according to the data in exhibit 4.22, your performance is in a state of statistical control, meaning your performance is stable and will likely remain within the control limits unless some aspect of the running process changes.

When performance data are displayed on a control chart with statistically calculated UCL and LCL, the type of variation (common cause or special cause) prompting the changes in performance is easy to determine. Exhibit 4.23 is a control chart showing performance data from a large multispecialty outpatient clinic. Each month, the clinic counts the number of insurance claims rejected because of incomplete information.

Upper control limit
The upper boundary below which data plotted on a control chart can vary without the need for change or correction.

Lower control limit
The lower boundary above which data plotted on a control chart can vary without the need for change or correction.

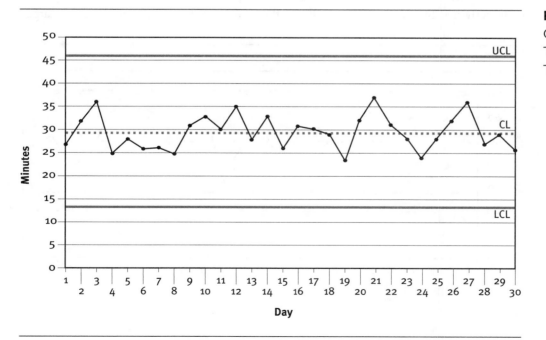

EXHIBIT 4.22
Control Chart of Three-Mile Run Times

The billing office manager has set a performance goal of no more than 60 rejections per month. Some months this target is exceeded, but the manager knows the increases result from common cause variation because the number of rejected claims is not higher than the UCL. Because performance is in a state of statistical control, the manager knows that the number of rejected claims will eventually decline and that changes to the process are not necessary. Tampering with what appears to be a stable process could make performance worse.

Exhibit 4.24 is a similar report of rejected insurance claims. As in the previous example, the performance target of no more than 60 rejections per month is exceeded in some months, but in two of these months, the number of rejections is greater than the UCL. This increase signals that an unusual occurrence—a special cause variation—took place in those months. When the manager detects that the performance target for that month has been exceeded and sees evidence of special cause variation, further investigation is needed. For example, the manager may find that two new employees were not properly trained in April. Training is provided, and the number of rejected claims declines in May. The following March, the number of rejected claims again exceeds the UCL—a signal of special cause variation. In early April, the manager investigates and discovers that in mid-March, an insurance company changed its claim submission requirements without notifying the hospital. The situation returned to normal, and as shown by the graph in exhibit 4.24, the number of insurance claim rejections in April is again in a state of statistical control.

Control charts are also useful for assessing the impact of performance improvement activities. Suppose the clinic billing office manager changes the performance target

EXHIBIT 4.23
Control Chart
of Number of
Rejected Insurance
Claims—Process
in Control

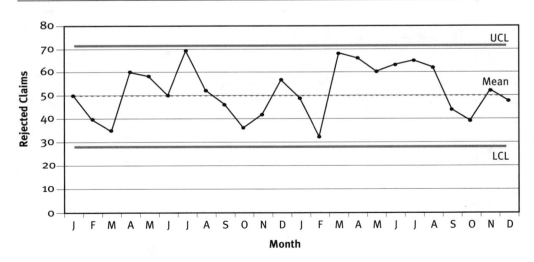

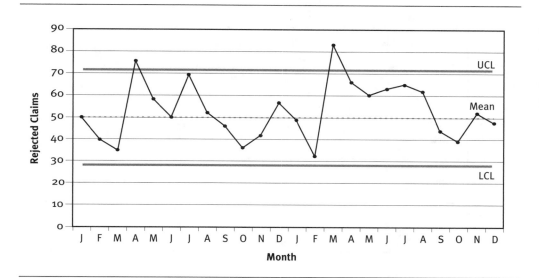

EXHIBIT 4.24
Control Chart
of Number of
Rejected Insurance
Claims—Process
Not in Control

for rejected insurance claims from no more than 60 rejections per month to no more than 40 rejections per month. To achieve this goal, employees in the billing office are trained in January to use new claims management software that is electronically linked to the clinic's new electronic health record system. In March, the manager again begins to plot the number of claim rejections each month on a control chart. The CL, UCL, and LCL are recalculated to reflect the lower target. Exhibit 4.25 shows the performance results from six months prior to the process change and the results following the process change. Not only has the number of claim rejections decreased but performance has remained in control as well. The data prove the improvement initiative was successful.

Different types of control charts (customarily denoted by letters such as *np, p, c, u, $\overline{X}$,* and *$\overline{S}$*) are appropriate for different situations (Provost and Murray 2011). Selecting the right chart requires an understanding of the type of performance measurement data that will be plotted on the chart. Additional resources on constructing and interpreting control charts appear at the end of this chapter.

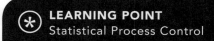

LEARNING POINT
Statistical Process Control

SPC concepts, techniques, and tools (usually line graphs and control charts) are used to distinguish between common cause and special cause variations in performance. Common cause variation is the result of normal performance fluctuations. If staff consistently follow the same procedures and all else remains unchanged, performance rates will likely exhibit only common cause variation. Unnecessary adjustments made to a process in response to common cause variation could make performance worse. If something unnatural occurs, performance rates will show signs of special cause variation. Special cause variation should be investigated, and the problem inducing atypical performance should be fixed.

EXHIBIT 4.25
Control Chart
of Number
of Rejected
Insurance Claims—
Improvement
Following Process
Change

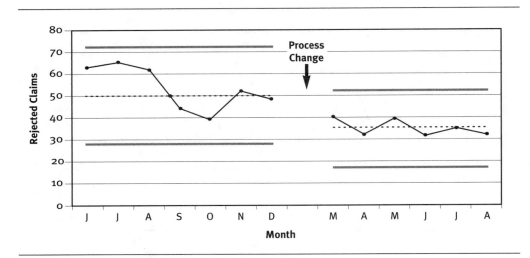

EXHIBIT 4.25
Control Chart of Number of Rejected Insurance Claims—Improvement Following Process Change

DETERMINE NEED FOR ACTION

In the final phase of performance assessment, the need for further action is decided. At this point, the measurement results have been reported and performance quality is evident. If measurement data are displayed in a control chart, the extent of performance variation is also apparent. Any of the following situations might signal the need to advance to the next step—performance improvement:

◆   Performance does not meet expectations; no signs of special cause variation are evident.

◆   Performance meets expectations; signs of special cause variation are evident.

◆   Performance does not meet expectations; signs of special cause variation are evident.

If none of the above situations exists, further investigation is unnecessary. Performance measurement should continue to ensure results do not change; sustained good performance should be celebrated with staff.

Some opportunities for improvement cannot be acted on immediately. Improvement projects are resource intensive, and an organization's leaders often need to set improvement priorities. Questions to consider when selecting topics for improvement include—but are not limited to—the following (Spath 2005):

◆   Does the issue relate to one of the organization's high-priority improvement goals?

◆   Does the issue pose a substantial risk to the safety of patients or staff?

◆   Will the organization receive substantial negative publicity or face the loss of licensure or accreditation if the concern is not addressed?

◆   If the improvement project is not executed, will staff and physician morale deteriorate or will they lose trust in leaders' commitment to ensuring high-quality patient care?

After an organization decides to advance to the performance improvement step, the people involved in the processes affecting performance investigate the **performance gap**—the problem causing the difference between actual and expected performance. Once the underlying causes are well understood, effective improvement interventions can be designed and implemented. The steps involved in performance improvement are covered in the next chapter.

Performance gap
The difference between actual and expected performance.

CONCLUSION

Performance assessment is the evaluation stage of quality management. Measurement data are reported and analyzed in this stage. The purpose of assessment is to determine whether improvement opportunities exist. Performance measurement data can be judged by comparing results with internally set performance expectations, comparing results with the achievements of other facilities, or determining whether performance is in a state of statistical control. When a gap between expected and actual performance exists or performance is unstable, further investigation is needed to determine the cause. Investigation of the cause is the starting point of performance improvement.

FOR DISCUSSION

1. The Centers for Medicare & Medicaid Services (CMS) Nursing Home Compare website (www.medicare.gov/nursinghomecompare/) allows you to compare performance at nursing homes throughout the United States. Go to this site and search for nursing homes within 50 miles of your location.

    a. Which facilities rate highest in each of the following measurement categories?

        •   Health inspections

        •   Staffing

        •   Quality measures

b. Explore the Nursing Home Compare site and review the data for each measurement category. Which performance measures in these categories are most important to consumers of nursing home services? Which performance measures are least important to consumers? Are consumers using the data on the Nursing Home Compare website to select a facility? What other factors might influence consumer choice?

2. The CMS Hospital Compare website (www.medicare.gov/hospitalcompare) allows you to compare performance at hospitals throughout the United States. Go to this site and review the data for each measurement category. Which performance measures in these categories are most important to consumers of hospital services? Which performance measures are least important to consumers? Are consumers using the data on the Hospital Compare website to select a hospital? What other factors might influence consumer choice?

3. The Joint Commission Quality Check website (www.qualitycheck.org) provides performance ratings for accredited organizations. Go to this site and look up hospitals in your area. What is different about the performance measures reported on the Quality Check website versus what is reported on the CMS Hospital Compare website? Are there any similarities? Which website provides the most detailed information about performance at the hospitals? Which website is easiest for consumers to use for performance assessment purposes?

WEBSITES

- Association for Benchmarking Health Care
  www.abhc.org

- Healthcare-Associated Infections Data Analysis and Presentation Standardization Toolkit available from the Council of State and Territorial Epidemiologists
  www.cste.org/general/custom.asp?page=HAIToolkit

- YouTube videos produced by the Institute for Healthcare Improvement:

  –   Learning About Variation by Counting Candy
      https://youtu.be/9liODQlozWQ

  –   Measurement Data and Monitoring Data: Which Is Better?
      https://youtu.be/BFHYPwV2jtk

  –   Understanding Patient Experience Data
      https://youtu.be/yW_g_G_GV6I

  –   What Do We Mean by Measurement for Judgment?
      https://youtu.be/O2dcydR97dg

STATISTICAL PROCESS CONTROL RESOURCES

Benneyan, J. C., R. C. Lloyd, and P. E. Plsek. 2003. "Statistical Process Control as a Tool for Research and Health Care Improvement." *Quality and Safety in Healthcare* 12 (6): 458–64.

Carey, R. 2003. *Improving Healthcare with Control Charts: Basic and Advanced SPC Methods and Case Studies.* Milwaukee, WI: American Society for Quality.

Kelley, D. L. 1999. *How to Use Control Charts for Healthcare.* Milwaukee, WI: American Society for Quality.

Marsteller, J. A., M. M. Huizinga, and L. A. Cooper. 2013. *Statistical Process Control: Possible Uses to Monitor and Evaluate Patient-Centered Medical Home Models.* AHRQ Publication No. 13-0031-EF. Rockville, MD: Agency for Healthcare Research and Quality. https://pcmh.ahrq.gov/page/statistical-process-controlpossible-uses-monitor-and-evaluate-patient-centered-medical-home.

MoreSteam.com. n.d. "Statistical Process Control (SPC)." www.moresteam.com/toolbox/statistical-process-control-spc.cfm.

Provost, L. P., and S. K. Murray. 2011. *The Health Care Data Guide: Learning from Data for Improvement.* San Francisco: Jossey-Bass.

Thor, J., J. Lundberg, J. Ask, J. Olsson, C. Carli, K. P. Harenstam, and M. Brommels. 2007. "Application of Statistical Process Control in Healthcare Improvement: Systematic Review." *BMJ Quality & Safety* 16 (5): 387–99.

Wheeler, D. J. 2000. *Understanding Variation: The Key to Managing Chaos*, 2nd ed. Knoxville, TN: SPC Press.

REFERENCES

American College of Radiology. 2012. "Don't Do Imaging for Uncomplicated Headache." Updated June 29, 2017. www.choosingwisely.org/clinician-lists/american-college-radiology-imaging-for-uncomplicated-headache/.

Appari, A., M. E. Johnson, and D. L. Anthony. 2013. "Meaningful Use of Electronic Health Record Systems and Process Quality of Care: Evidence from a Panel Data Analysis of U.S. Acute-Care Hospitals." *Health Services Research* 48 (2 Pt 1): 354–75.

Bouldin, E. D., E. M. Andresen, N. E. Dunton, M. Simon, T. M. Waters, M. Liu, M. J. Daniels, L. C. Mion, and R. I. Shorr. 2013. "Falls Among Adult Patients Hospitalized in the United States: Prevalence and Trends." *Journal of Patient Safety* 9 (1): 13–17.

Carroll, L. 1999. *Alice's Adventures in Wonderland*, 1st US ed. Cambridge, MA: Candlewick Press.

Centers for Disease Control and Prevention. 2011. "Immunization of Health-Care Personnel: Recommendations of the Advisory Committee on Immunization Practices (ACIP)." *Morbidity and Mortality Weekly Report*. Published November 25. www.cdc.gov/mmwr/preview/mmwrhtml/rr6007a1.htm.

Joint Commission. 2017. *National Patient Safety Goals Effective January 2017: Nursing Care Center Accreditation Program*. Accessed November 5. www.jointcommission.org/assets/1/6/NPSG_Chapter_NCC_Jan2017.pdf.

Juran, J. M. 1974. *Quality Control Handbook,* 3rd ed. New York: McGraw-Hill.

Kumar, N. 2017. "Using Data Analytics Techniques to Evaluate Performance." In *Applying Quality Management in Healthcare: A Systems Approach*, by P. L. Spath and D. L. Kelly, 126–202. Chicago: Health Administration Press.

Maricopa Integrated Health System (MIHS). 2014. "MIHS Targets Zero Hospital-Acquired Infections (HAIs)." Accessed November 5, 2017. www.mihs.org/article/mihs-targets-zero-hospital-acquired-infections-hais--.

Nelson, L. S. 2003. "When Should the Limits on a Shewhart Control Chart Be Other Than a Center Line ±3-Sigma?" *Journal of Quality Technology* 35 (4): 424–25.

Provost, L. P., and S. K. Murray. 2011. *The Health Care Data Guide: Learning from Data for Improvement*. San Francisco: Jossey-Bass.

Research Methods Knowledge Base. 2006. "Statistical Terms in Sampling." Published October 20. www.socialresearchmethods.net/kb/sampstat.php.

Scholtes, P. R. 1992. *The Team Handbook*. Madison, WI: Joiner Associates.

Shewhart, W. A. 1925. "The Application of Statistics as an Aid in Maintaining Quality of Manufactured Product." *Journal of the American Statistical Association* 20: 546–48.

Sower, V., J. A. Duffy, and G. Kohlers. 2007. *Benchmarking for Hospitals: Achieving Best-in-Class Performance Without Having to Reinvent the Wheel.* Milwaukee, WI: ASQ Press.

Spath, P. L. 2005. *Leading Your Healthcare Organization to Excellence: A Guide to Using the Baldrige Criteria.* Chicago: Health Administration Press.

US Department of Labor, Occupational Health and Safety Administration. 1996. "Occupational Safety and Health Standards — 29 CFR, Part 1910, Toxic and Hazardous Substances, Ionizing Radiation, No. 1910.1096." Accessed November 5, 2017. www.osha.gov/pls/oshaweb/owadisp.show_document?p_table=STANDARDS&p_id=10098.

Woodall, W. H. 2000. "Controversies and Contradictions in Statistical Process Control." *Journal of Quality Technology* 32 (4): 341–50.

CHAPTER 5

CONTINUOUS IMPROVEMENT

After reading this chapter, you will be able to

➤ explain the purpose of a systematic approach to improving performance,

➤ discuss common performance improvement models,

➤ recognize the similarities and differences among improvement models, and

➤ demonstrate an understanding of the steps in a performance improvement project.

➤ Analytic tools

➤ Continuous improvement

➤ Corrective action plan

➤ FADE model

➤ Improvement project

➤ Improvement team

- ➤ Kaizen event
- ➤ Lean
- ➤ Lean principles
- ➤ Lean Six Sigma
- ➤ *Muda*
- ➤ Opportunity for improvement
- ➤ Performance improvement models
- ➤ Plan-Do-Check-Act (PDCA) cycle
- ➤ Plan-Do-Study-Act (PDSA) cycle

- ➤ Process capability
- ➤ Process diagram
- ➤ Quality improvement organizations
- ➤ Rapid cycle improvement (RCI)
- ➤ Root causes
- ➤ Six Sigma
- ➤ Six Sigma quality
- ➤ Systematic

Opportunity for improvement
A problem or performance failure.

Improvement team
A group of individuals organized to work together to accomplish a specific improvement objective.

Improvement project
An initiative set up to achieve a performance improvement objective within a certain time frame.

Analytic tools
Qualitative (language) and quantitative (numeric) tools used during an improvement project; often called *quality improvement tools*.

Performance improvement is the last phase of quality management. Once an **opportunity for improvement** has been identified, action must be taken to find and fix the cause of unfavorable performance. Some performance problems can be resolved quickly, such as the two special cause variations in the rejected insurance claims example in chapter 4. Other problems require more in-depth evaluation of the complex factors affecting performance. In these situations, a team is formed to carry out an improvement project. This **improvement team** is composed of people most familiar with the processes under review. To improve performance, the team must understand the problem and the changes that will be necessary to solve it.

During an **improvement project**, all factors affecting performance are closely examined. Before changing the process, the improvement team must discover where, when, and why problems occur so that effective solutions can be implemented. To do so, the team uses **analytic tools** to scrutinize the process and select interventions that will produce successful results.

IMPROVEMENT IN QUALITY MANAGEMENT

As shown in exhibit 5.1, the improvement phase follows performance assessment. Once improvements are implemented, the quality management cycle begins again. The results of process changes are measured and analyzed to determine whether they fixed the performance problem.

Improvement projects may be launched when measurement data reveal a gap between expected and actual performance. But organizations have a finite amount of time, money,

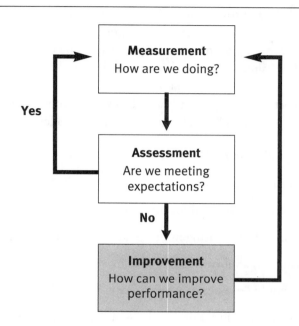

EXHIBIT 5.1
Cycle of
Measurement,
Assessment, and
Improvement

and resources to allocate to improvement projects, so they cannot work on improving all processes at once. Two factors influence the decision to initiate an improvement project: the results of performance assessment and improvement priorities. The following case study describes an improvement project initiated in response to employees' complaints that department meetings are a waste of time.

CASE STUDY

Sunrise Home Health Agency holds monthly meetings with clinical staff who visit patients in their homes. These staff members spend two hours of their busy day attending department meetings, not counting their travel time. The agency director hears staff complaining that the meetings are a waste of time. The director finds the meetings a worthwhile way to share agency news and is not sure how to make the meetings more valuable to employees. At the next meeting, the director starts a project to improve the value of staff meetings.

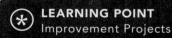

LEARNING POINT
Improvement Projects

Performance improvement projects are initiated when measurement data reveal a gap between expected and actual performance. Projects also may be initiated for other reasons. Improvement project teams include people most familiar with the process under review.

At the start of the improvement project, the director states the goal—to improve the value of staff meetings—and the discussion ground rules: All staff members' views are important, all ideas will be heard, and all opinions will be valued. The director wants to have an honest discussion and reminds everyone involved that he or she should feel comfortable voicing his or her opinions and ideas.

At the first meeting, each person is asked to voice a complaint. The director lists these concerns on a flip chart and then summarizes them as follows:

- Meeting agendas are not defined.

- Meetings usually don't start on time.

- The director rarely asks staff for input on problems.

- Problems brought up during meetings are sometimes left unresolved.

- Late afternoon is an inconvenient time for meetings.

- Meetings should be canceled when there is nothing important to discuss.

- Meetings often turn into gripe sessions and accomplish nothing.

- Meeting minutes aren't available for staff members unable to attend.

- The medical director doesn't attend all the meetings.

- Meetings last too long.

Staff members are asked to vote for their top three complaints. The following complaints receive the most votes:

- Meetings usually don't start on time.

- Late afternoon is an inconvenient time for meetings.

- Meetings often turn into gripe sessions and accomplish nothing.

To delve into the causes of these complaints, the director asks the group to answer questions about each concern. Why don't meetings start on time? Why was late afternoon originally chosen as the meeting time? Why can't the meetings be held at a different time? Why do meetings turn into gripe sessions? Answers to these questions help employees understand why they do not find staff meetings valuable. The director asks the staff members to come up with innovative, unconventional ways to eliminate these complaints.

The group reconvenes the next month to share ideas. Some are inventive. For example, two staff members suggest holding virtual meetings and provide some names of free online meeting services. As for starting meetings on time, the director acknowledges that many people (including himself) are habitually five to ten minutes late. The director suggests that meetings start at the scheduled time even if some people have not arrived. A staff member proposes that meetings be held at noon. To encourage people to attend, the agency could provide lunch. Everyone agrees that a meeting agenda will prevent the discussions from deteriorating into gripe sessions. Two employees recommend that staff be encouraged to submit agenda items.

The director lists these ideas on a flip chart, and the group selects the recommendations most likely to eliminate the top three complaints. The idea of virtual online meetings receives the most support; however, the director points out that this change requires more investigation prior to implementation. He suggests trying the second choice—holding meetings at noon and providing lunch—because it can be implemented right away. The group also decides to make two other changes: Everyone will be asked to submit a topic for the next meeting agenda. The final agenda will be distributed three days before each meeting, and all meetings will start promptly. In three months, the director will survey the staff to determine whether these changes have made a difference. He will also share information on the virtual online meeting options he will have researched.

PERFORMANCE IMPROVEMENT STEPS

Performance improvement projects should be **systematic**. Without a defined process, chaos is likely to ensue and the improvement team might not achieve desired results. A methodical improvement process has several benefits:

Systematic
Conducted using step-by-step procedures.

◆ *Performance problems are permanently solved.* The goal of performance improvement is to prevent problems from recurring, not just to clean up the mess after an undesirable event occurs.

◆ *Work–life quality improves.* Performance problems are an annoyance for everyone because they create additional work. People perform better when processes run smoothly.

◆ *Communication among employees and managers improves.* To solve problems, people from different levels of the organization and from different work groups must collaborate.

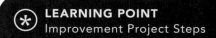

LEARNING POINT
Improvement Project Steps

Opportunities for better performance trigger improvement projects. A typical project consists of four steps:

1. Define the improvement goal.
2. Analyze current practices.
3. Design and implement improvements.
4. Measure success.

Not only does a systematic performance improvement process solve problems but also the people involved in the process acquire new habits that help the organization run more smoothly and effectively.

Over the years, several systematic **performance improvement models** have been created for use in healthcare and other industries. All these models incorporate similar steps:

1. Define the improvement goal.

2. Analyze current practices.

3. Design and implement improvements.

4. Measure success.

Performance improvement models most commonly used for healthcare improvement projects are described next.

PLAN-DO-STUDY-ACT CYCLE

Walter Shewhart, who developed the concepts and techniques of statistical process control, was one of the first quality experts to discuss a systematic model for continuous improvement. In his book *Statistical Method from the Viewpoint of Quality Control*, published in 1939, he referred to this model as the **Plan-Do-Check-Act (PDCA) cycle** (Best and Neuhauser 2006). Another renowned statistician, W. Edwards Deming, went to Japan as part of the Allied occupation after World War II to teach the Japanese industrial quality improvement methods, such as statistical process control and systematic process improvement (Best and Neuhauser 2005). Deming modified Shewhart's original model and renamed it the **Plan-Do-Study-Act (PDSA) cycle**. PDSA is the most widely recognized improvement process today (see exhibit 5.2). To ensure **continuous improvement**, the steps perpetually cycle and repeat. The following lists summarize the steps of each PDSA phase:

Plan

◆   State the objectives of the improvement project.

◆   Determine needed improvements.

◆   Design process changes to achieve the improvement objectives.

◆   Develop a plan to carry out the changes (define who, what, when, and where).

◆   Identify data that need to be collected to determine whether changes produced desired results.

Performance improvement models
Systematic approaches for conducting improvement projects.

Plan-Do-Check-Act (PDCA) cycle
The Shewhart performance improvement model.

Plan-Do-Study-Act (PDSA) cycle
The Deming performance improvement model. (An example of a PDSA improvement project is found in exhibit 5.3.)

Continuous improvement
Analyzing performance of various processes and improving them repeatedly to achieve quality objectives.

Do

- ◆ Implement the changes on a small scale.

- ◆ Document problems and unexpected events.

- ◆ Gather data to assess the changes' impact on the process.

Study

- ◆ Analyze data to determine whether the changes were effective.

- ◆ Compare results with expectations.

- ◆ Summarize lessons learned during and after implementation of the changes.

Act

- ◆ If changes were not successful, repeat the PDSA cycle.

- ◆ If changes were successful, or partially successful, implement them on a wider scale or modify them as necessary.

- ◆ Predict results.

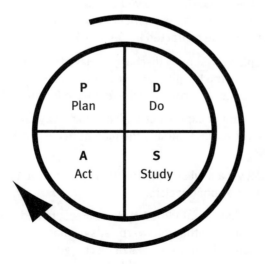

EXHIBIT 5.2
PDSA Cycle of Continuous Improvement

Source: Lean Management (2007).

Each repetition of the PDSA cycle provides greater insight into the problem. The improvement team learns from its successes and failures and uses this knowledge to plan the next process change.

A summary of a PDSA improvement project appears in exhibit 5.3. The purpose of the project is to ensure that patients discharged from the hospital know which medications they will continue taking at home, how often they must take the medications, and what

EXHIBIT 5.3
PDSA
Improvement
Project

Plan   **Objective:** To improve patient knowledge of medications to be taken after discharge from the hospital.

Plan: Pharmacists will meet with patients within 24 hours before hospital discharge to review medications, including the purpose of each medication, how to take the medication and how often, and the medication's side effects. Completion of this education session will be documented in patients' records.

Expected result: Patients will understand medications to be taken at home.

Measures: Monitor completion of medication education through review of patient records; monitor level of patient understanding of medications via follow-up call post-discharge.

Do   For two weeks, pharmacists will educate all patients in the 3-West medical unit who are about to be discharged home.

Study   Pharmacists educated 42 of the 49 patients discharged home. The 7 patients who were not educated were discharged on a Sunday. Of the 42 educated patients, 39 reported they received appropriate and adequate information about their medications. Two patients did not remember being educated. One patient could not be contacted for feedback.

Act   Modify the plan for Sunday discharges. Have the discharging nurse educate patients leaving the hospital on Sunday. Implement the modified plan in all patient care units, and consider the following for future improvements:

- Evaluate patient experience with a mail survey after the change has been in place for 30 days. Modify the plan as necessary on the basis of survey results.

- Evaluate, via a mail survey, the efficacy of instruction by nurses versus instruction by pharmacists.

- Implement a separate PDSA cycle to measure and improve compliance with the directive that follow-up calls be made to patients on four or more medications within two weeks of discharge to check their understanding of medications, compliance with dosing schedule, and side effects.

side effects they may experience. The hospital initiated the project in response to complaints from former patients and family members about inadequate medication instructions.

RAPID CYCLE IMPROVEMENT

The PDSA cycle is used in **rapid cycle improvement (RCI)** projects. Unlike a comprehensive (and often time-consuming) process analysis, an RCI project incorporates several small process changes and careful measurement of those changes to achieve an improvement goal (Varkey, Reller, and Resar 2007). This approach is an accelerated method (usually less than six weeks per improvement cycle) of collecting and analyzing data and making changes on the basis of that analysis. The first cycle is followed by a second improvement cycle to evaluate the effects of the changes on the process.

Suppose an ambulatory clinic wants to improve patient satisfaction by 20 percent during the coming year. An improvement team composed of clinic staff and physicians completes a PDSA cycle for each improvement idea. Some ideas are successful and become office practices. Ideas that fail are discarded. Over a short period, the team completes several PDSA cycles, all linked to the goal of improving patient satisfaction. This RCI process is illustrated in exhibit 5.4. Note that the four process changes are made in succession. The

> **Rapid cycle improvement (RCI)** An improvement model that supports repeated incremental improvements in a practice to optimize performance.

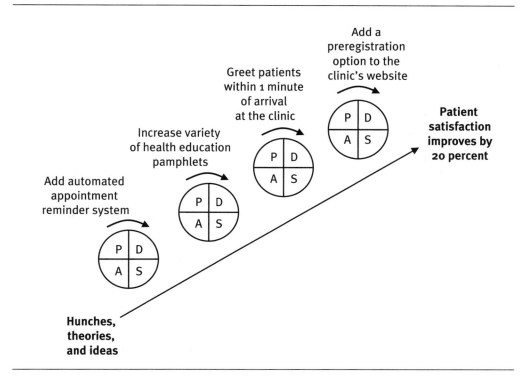

EXHIBIT 5.4
Incremental Patient Satisfaction Improvements Achieved Through Repeated PDSA Cycles

team completes one PDSA cycle change before moving on to the next one. Each adjustment brings the clinic closer to its goal.

The RCI model is used in many healthcare improvement initiatives—for example, the breakthrough projects sponsored by the Institute for Healthcare Improvement follow this model, as do the Medicare quality improvement initiatives sponsored by the Centers for Medicare & Medicaid Services and overseen at the state level by **quality improvement organizations**. RCI has been successfully applied to both the business aspects of healthcare delivery and clinical patient care processes.

Quality improvement organizations
Groups of health quality experts, clinicians, and consumers organized to improve the quality of care delivered to people with Medicare.

FOCUS-PDCA

In the early 1990s, Hospital Corporation of America, based in Nashville, Tennessee, expanded Shewhart's PDCA model by adding preliminary steps known as FOCUS (Batalden and Nolan 1992). FOCUS-PDCA, still a popular performance improvement model, involves the following steps (Hsu, Cohn, and Caban 2016):

◆ FOCUS phase

— **F**ind a process that needs improvement. Define the beginning and end of the process, and determine who will benefit from the improvement.

— **O**rganize a team of people knowledgeable about the process. This team should include employees from various levels of the organization.

— **C**larify the current process and the changes needed to achieve the improvement.

— **U**nderstand the causes of variation by measuring performance at various steps in the process.

— **S**elect actions needed to improve the process.

◆ PDCA phase

— **P**lan the change by studying the process, identifying areas needing improvement, and determining ways to measure success.

— **D**o the change on a small scale, and gather data to measure success.

— **C**heck the data to determine whether the change produced the desired improvements. Modify the change if necessary.

— **A**ct to maintain the gains. Implement the change if it is working well. Abandon the change if it is ineffective, and repeat the PDCA phase.

FADE

The **FADE model** of performance improvement is an adaptation of the original PDSA/PDCA improvement cycle. FADE was developed by Organizational Dynamics Inc. (2006), a global management consulting firm that helps all types of organizations improve quality and productivity and enhance customer satisfaction. The FADE improvement model consists of four phases (Department of Community and Family Medicine, Duke University School of Medicine 2016):

FADE model
Performance improvement model developed by Organizational Dynamics Inc.

◆ **F**ocus. Choose a problem, and write a statement to describe it.

◆ **A**nalyze. Learn more about the problem by gathering performance data.

◆ **D**evelop. Develop a solution for the problem and a plan for implementing the solution.

◆ **E**xecute. Implement the plan and monitor results. Adjust the plan as needed.

The FADE model works for all types of performance problems. The following example illustrates how the FADE model can be used to fix a computer problem:

◆ *Focus.* Occasionally my computer freezes up, and I must turn off the power and restart the computer. The most recent changes I had made to the file I was working on usually are lost and cannot be recovered. After enough recurrences, I become annoyed and decide to solve the problem permanently.

◆ *Analyze.* I review the error logs for the past six months to determine which programs are running when the computer freezes up. This log also tells me the frequency of the problem. I run a system scan to look for device driver conflicts and check the power source. My computer has been making abnormal noises lately, so I check the fan at the back of the computer and discover that it is not running smoothly. I conduct some research on the Internet and learn that an overheated computer can periodically lock up.

◆ *Develop.* I use my analysis as the basis for creating a **corrective action plan**. My computer needs a new fan. I also find that I need to update the driver for my video card. To ensure that the problem does not recur, I contact a computer repair company and arrange for an in-home service call.

Corrective action plan
A proposed solution to fix a problem or a process.

◆ *Execute.* The repairman arrives, and I watch him work so that I can fix the problem myself next time. He replaces the fan and installs updates for my video and network drivers. Three months later, the problem has yet to return. The solutions worked.

The FADE model of performance improvement is useful for focusing on a problem, analyzing the problem and its causes, developing and implementing a solution, and monitoring success.

Lean

The improvement models discussed thus far can be used to achieve any type of performance improvement objective. Some improvement models are intended for specific purposes. One such model is the **Lean** model of improvement, which is used to eliminate inefficiencies adversely affecting performance. A lean process includes only value-added steps and therefore produces little waste. The Lean model of improvement, also called *Lean manufacturing* or *Lean thinking*, originated in the Japanese automobile industry—in particular as the Toyota Production System (Womack and Jones 2003). Lean manufacturing concepts are now used in healthcare to improve efficiency and reduce errors (Nabhan, Horner, and Howell 2017).

Lean principles are applicable to an array of healthcare processes and work settings, from patient care to medical informatics to plant maintenance. Healthcare organizations eliminate waste and thus improve efficiency and quality by applying the five Lean principles of process improvement:

1. *Value.* Identify what is important to the customer and focus on it.
2. *Value stream.* Ensure all activities are necessary and add value.
3. *Flow.* Strive for continuous processing through the value stream.
4. *Pull.* Drive production with demand.
5. *Perfection.* Prevent defects and rework.

Muda, the Japanese term for waste, was coined by the late Toyota production engineer Taiichi Ohno (1988) to describe activities that add cost but no value to a process. It is estimated that 95 percent of healthcare operations contain non-value-added activities, which translates into many opportunities for efficiency improvements (Hagan 2011). The eight types of muda are listed in exhibit 5.5.

The goal of any Lean project is to create a more efficient process than is currently in place. Except for the application of Lean principles, Lean projects follow steps similar to those of other improvement projects (Zidel 2012):

1. The performance problem is stated from the process customer's viewpoint. For instance, radiology technicians are physicians' customers. If a Lean project is initiated for the process of completing X-ray exams, the performance problem

Lean
A performance improvement approach aimed at eliminating waste; also called *Lean manufacturing* or *Lean thinking*.

Lean principles
The five Lean principles are (1) value—identify what is really important to the customer and focus on that, (2) value stream—ensure all activities are necessary and add value, (3) flow—strive for continuous processing through the value stream, (4) pull—drive production with demand, and (5) perfection—prevent defects and rework.

Muda
The Japanese term for waste, a concept taken from Lean manufacturing. (Muda is anything that does not add value to the customer. Although some muda is inevitable, the goal of a Lean project is to reduce it as much as possible.)

EXHIBIT 5.5
Eight Categories
and Examples of
Waste (Muda)

Waste Category	Example
Movement	Unnecessary human movement (e.g., staff walking to various places around the work area to obtain supplies)
Waiting	People waiting for something needed to do their work (e.g., a radiologist waiting for a patient to be brought into the exam room)
Overprocessing	Doing more than is necessary to meet requirements (e.g., doing two blood tests on a patient when one would have been sufficient)
Defects	Poor quality work and rework to fix mistakes (e.g., rebilling the insurance company because the first bill contained an error)
Inventories	Inputs to the process that are waiting to be used (e.g., keeping excessive supplies on hand just in case they are needed)
Transportation	Unnecessary movement of people, supplies, equipment, and so forth (e.g., moving patients unnecessarily from one hospital unit to another)
Design	Processes that customers view as unnecessary (e.g., asking patients to handwrite a new medication list at each clinic visit)
Overproduction	Doing something that doesn't add value (e.g., performing unnecessary tests to prevent a lawsuit for malpractice)

from the technician's perspective might be "X-ray exams are delayed when ill-defined physician orders must be clarified."

2. Current work procedures are examined, and a diagram of the current process is created. The illustration of the current process is based on what is happening in the present, not recollections of what happened in the past or what should be happening. Direct observation is the preferred way to gather this information. The **process diagram** clarifies the cause of the performance problem.

3. Improvement opportunities are identified and quantified. Data are gathered to determine the frequency of the problem and the problem's impact on process customers.

4. **Root causes** of the problem are investigated. A common approach to get to the root of the problem is to ask, five times in a series, why the problem

Process diagram
A visual representation of the flow of individual steps or activities in a process.

Root causes
Primary and fundamental origins of undesirable performance.

occurs. (The Five Whys performance improvement tool is discussed in the next chapter.)

5.   A better way to work is proposed and illustrated in a process diagram. This better way is designed to alleviate the root causes identified in the previous step.

6.   An implementation plan is developed. The plan identifies the actions needed to realize the process changes and assigns plan implementation responsibilities. A deadline for completion is set.

7.   A follow-up plan is created. This plan predicts performance improvements expected to result from the implemented changes. The expected improvements are defined in measurable terms, and the means of gathering measurement data are specified.

8.   After process changes are made, results are compared with the projections made in step 7.

Kaizen event
"A focused, short-term project aimed at improving a particular process" (McLaughlin and Olson 2017, 413).

Lean projects, similar to RCI projects, are often focused on improving a particular process and are short-term. A short-term Lean project is called a **kaizen event** or blitz (McLaughlin and Olson 2017). A kaizen event usually involves a small group of people personally familiar with or interested in the process chosen for improvement. The project is typically one week long.

A Lean project often involves the creation of standardized work processes to reduce waste and continuously improve quality. The descriptions and purposes of five Lean techniques commonly used in creating standardized processes are found in exhibit 5.6.

A growing number of healthcare organizations are conducting Lean projects to improve daily operations. When these projects are successful, the organizations achieve reduced costs, improved patient satisfaction, and higher-quality performance. ThedaCare, a Wisconsin healthcare system comprising 5 hospitals and 27 physician clinics, implemented Lean in 2003. Its successes have included a 25 percent reduction in inpatient costs and significantly improved systemwide patient satisfaction (Mannon 2014). Using Lean principles, Bellevue Clinic Surgery Center in Seattle was able to reduce nonoperative patient care time by almost 50 percent, and Inova Health, an integrated system in Virginia, realized more than $6 million in labor productivity gains in its emergency departments (Toussaint and Berry 2013). A large outpatient clinic applied the Lean technique known as a *Kanban* and achieved a significant reduction in costs associated with outdated medications and medical supplies each month (Watson-Hemphill and Bradley 2016).

Lean Technique	Description	Purpose
5S methodology	A systematic process for organizing standard work that involves five phases: **S**ort, **S**traighten, **S**crub, **S**tandardize, and **S**ustain (the 5 S's).	Create an orderly and uncluttered workspace that improves efficiency, reduces errors, enhances staff morale, and presents a positive image to customers.
Kanban	*Kanban* is the Japanese word for signal or sign board, a special type of visual control used to indicate the need for movement of materials or patients. For example, a Kanban card is often used for inventory management to visually point out when an item needs to be restocked.	Make it easier for people to quickly recognize the need for movement of people or materials.
Mistake proofing	A process improvement method that involves (1) defining the mistake to be prevented, (2) determining the root cause of the mistake, and (3) developing a device or method to prevent the mistake or make it easier to identify and correct.	Improve processes to prevent mistakes or to make mistakes obvious at a glance; also called error proofing.
Value stream map	A special type of process map that illustrates the system perspective of an activity. The map includes the value-adding and non-value-adding steps and related measurements, such as the time it takes to complete a process step or the wait time between steps.	Make process waste more visible to help identify where it can be minimized and thus provide optimum value to the customer.
Visual control	A simple and nonverbal way to relay information to others. For example, color-coded patient wristbands are visual controls that communicate information about the patient's condition or allergies.	Make it easier for people to quickly recognize the current situation, understand the process, or notice when something is out of place or unusual.

EXHIBIT 5.6
Description and Purpose of Five Commonly Used Lean Techniques

To be successful, Lean projects and the accompanying Lean techniques should be part of an organization-wide commitment to continuous improvement. Leadership involvement and a supportive institutional culture, in addition to Lean quality improvement techniques, are essential to the achievement of consistent results (Mazzocato et al. 2010; Kaplan et al. 2014).

Six Sigma

Six Sigma
A disciplined methodology for process improvement that deploys a wide set of tools following rigorous data analysis to identify sources of variation in performance and ways of reducing the variation. (An example of a Six Sigma project is found in exhibit 5.7.)

Six Sigma quality
Rate of less than 3.4 defects per 1 million opportunities, which translates to a process that is 99.99966 percent defect free.

Six Sigma is a systematic, data-driven improvement approach whose goal is the near-elimination of defects from every product, process, and transaction. Six Sigma originated in the manufacturing sector at Motorola and was refined by General Electric, which has a healthcare consulting division.

Six Sigma is founded on Shewhart's statistical process control philosophies and a field of statistics known as *process capability studies* (Winton 1999). Sigma (σ) is a letter in the Greek alphabet used to denote variability. For example, let's apply Six Sigma to a hospital's process for creating billing statements. If the process is running at 3σ, almost 7 of every 100 statements are flawed in some way. The calculation from which this ratio is derived is beyond the scope of this text, but in short, the higher the sigma level at which the process is operating, the higher the amount of error-free output.

Reducing performance variability is the essence of Six Sigma. The goal of a Six Sigma project is to create processes that operate within **Six Sigma quality**, meaning the defect rate is less than 3.4 per 1 million opportunities. This rate translates into a process that is 99.99966 percent defect free. Federal Express and United Parcel Service operate between 6 and 7σ, whereas most healthcare processes operate at 3σ or lower (Swensen 2010).

Although Six Sigma projects can include a variety of structured steps, they most commonly follow the five steps of DMAIC (pronounced *dee-MAY-ick*) methodology (Barry, Smith, and Brubaker 2017):

- **D**efine the problem.
- **M**easure key aspects of the process.
- **A**nalyze the data.
- **I**mprove the system.
- **C**ontrol and sustain the improvement.

Exhibit 5.7 summarizes a Six Sigma project aimed at improving customer satisfaction with the appointment system at a hospital's imaging center.

Define the problem	The telephone appointment process at the hospital's imaging center receives low customer satisfaction scores and racks up long hold times.	**EXHIBIT 5.7** Six Sigma Project Aimed at Improving the Imaging Center Appointment Process

Measure key aspects of the process

Over the past six months, staff took an average of 2 minutes and 18 seconds to answer calls from customers wishing to schedule an imaging study. The center has received numerous customer complaints about long hold times and, as a result, lower satisfaction scores for the telephone appointment system.

Analyze the data

- The imaging center appointment desk receives more than 2,000 calls per week.
- Average customer satisfaction: 58%
- Average hold time: 2 minutes, 18 seconds
- Phone calls answered in less than 90 seconds: 55%
- Overall call abandon rate: 26%; at peak time: 49%

Improve the system

- Staffing changes were made to handle peak times.
- Shift start and end times were revised to create a 45-minute overlap between the day and evening shifts.
- Registration forms for special imaging studies were modified to make them easier for staff to complete.
- The phone menu tree and call handling were improved.
- Specifications for a future electronic scheduling system were defined.

Control and sustain the improvement

- Overall average hold time decreased to 39 seconds.
- Overall call abandon rate decreased to 11%.
- Peak-time call abandon rate decreased to 27%.
- Call volume decreased by 19% as a result of fewer callbacks.
- Further improvements are expected after installation of the electronic scheduling system. The center will continue to monitor performance during and after transition to the new system.

The following features are key characteristics of the Six Sigma improvement methodology (Barry, Smith, and Brubaker 2017):

◆ *Process variation control.* To achieve near-perfect quality, Six Sigma focuses on reducing the variations that can occur in a process. An improvement opportunity is present when a gap exists between what a process is capable of producing (**process capability**) and what the process currently produces.

◆ *Orientation toward results.* The potential impact on performance (financial, clinical, and operational) is estimated before the start of a Six Sigma project, and an evaluation is made at the end to determine whether project goals have been met.

◆ *Use of data.* Detailed information is gathered and analyzed to reveal defects in the process. Once these defects are corrected, the process operates within Six Sigma quality.

Process capability
A quantitative or qualitative description of what a process is capable of producing.

LEAN SIX SIGMA

Although common improvement models are presented separately in this chapter for discussion purposes, the models are by no means mutually exclusive. Organizations may combine elements from different models to achieve improvement goals. **Lean Six Sigma** is a popular process improvement model that combines the techniques of Lean and Six Sigma (McLaughlin and Olson 2017). By themselves, the Lean and Six Sigma models are beneficial—but when they are combined, results can be even better. Lean techniques help improve system efficiency by standardizing work, reducing inventory, and eliminating waste. The Six Sigma DMAIC approach provides a systematic framework for reducing process variations (Huang et al. 2012). For example, a value stream map—a Lean technique—can provide useful information during the design of system improvements in a Six Sigma project (De Koning et al. 2006).

The Joint Commission's Center for Transforming Healthcare has been encouraging the use of Lean and Six Sigma techniques in hospital teams throughout the country engaged in the Center's quality improvement initiatives (Chassin and Loeb 2013). Burton (2011, 148) predicts that over the next decade organizations will evolve to what he calls "adaptive and innovative Lean Six Sigma," which will improve "an organization's capability to sense, interpret, decide, act, and measure improvement activities with the integration of technology with an expanded, innovative applications tool set, and in real time." Lean Six Sigma provides facilities "with the ability to create a more resilient and flexible organization that can respond quickly, even in an unpredictable environment like healthcare" (Watson-Hemphill and Bradley 2016).

Lean Six Sigma
A process improvement model that combines the techniques of Lean and Six Sigma.

CONCLUSION

Healthcare organizations use various performance improvement models for quality management purposes. The different models share a common thread of analysis, implementation, and review. Several factors influence the selection of an approach for a project. First, the goal of the improvement project must be considered. Some improvement models work best for eliminating process inefficiencies, whereas others work best for introducing incremental improvements. The prevailing opinion of senior leaders in the organization also should be considered when selecting an improvement model.

Keep in mind that improvement does not end with the implementation of a single improvement model. Any one approach is only a means to the end of continuous improvement. Multiple improvement models should be used to tap the individual and collective power of physicians and staff members for the purpose of delivering ever-higher levels of healthcare quality.

FOR DISCUSSION

1. Many examples of improvement projects conducted by healthcare organizations can be found in the literature and on the Internet. Find an example of each type of project: PDSA, RCI, FOCUS-PDCA, FADE, Lean, Six Sigma, and Lean Six Sigma. What is similar about each project? What is different about each project?

2. Select the improvement model that would work best for the following performance problems. Explain your choices.

    • More than 25 percent of the insurance claims submitted by a clinic are rejected because of mistakes made by the clinic's billing clerks.

    • Patients experience long wait times and delays for outpatient diagnostic services.

    • A large number of hospitalized patients develop a wound infection following surgery.

    • Labor costs are too high in the radiology department.

    • Patients' overall satisfaction with the emotional support provided by nurses is lower than the satisfaction levels reported for other hospitals.

    • In a pediatric clinic, many Spanish-speaking patients are unable to communicate by phone with the receptionists and caregivers because of language barriers.

Websites

- AHRQ, Quality Improvement in Primary Care
  www.ahrq.gov/research/findings/factsheets/quality/qipc/index.html

- AHRQ, Quality improvement tools and resources for hospitals, long-term care facilities, and primary care facilities
  www.ahrq.gov/professionals/systems/index.html

- Centers for Disease Control and Prevention, Performance Management and Quality Improvement
  www.cdc.gov/stltpublichealth/Performance/index.html

- Clinical Microsystems
  http://clinicalmicrosystem.org

- Hospital Improvement Innovation Network
  www.hret-hiin.org/

- Institute for Healthcare Improvement Model for Improvement
  www.ihi.org/knowledge/Pages/HowtoImprove/

- Lean and Six Sigma resources
  www.leanhospitals.org

- National Network of Public Health Institutes: *Public Health Improvement Webinar: Kaizen! What Is the Methodology and What Can It Do for You?* (June 2014)
  https://nnphi.org/resource/public-health-improvement-webinar-kaizen-what-is-the-methodology-and-what-can-it-do-for-you/

- National Quality Center Quality Improvement Resources
  http://nationalqualitycenter.org/quality-improvement-resources

- Public Health Quality Improvement Exchange
  www.phqix.org

- Six Sigma quality resources
  www.isixsigma.com

- Society of Hospital Medicine, Quality and Innovation
  www.hospitalmedicine.org

- Virginia Mason Institute's Zero-Defect Health Care
  www.virginiamasoninstitute.org

REFERENCES

Barry, R., A. C. Smith, and C. E. Brubaker. 2017. *High-Reliability Healthcare: Improving Patient Safety and Outcomes with Six Sigma*, 2nd ed. Chicago: Health Administration Press.

Batalden, P. B., and T. W. Nolan. 1992. *Building Knowledge for Improvement: An Introductory Guide to the Use of FOCUS-PDCA*. Nashville, TN: Quality Resource Group of Hospital Corporation of America.

Best, M., and D. Neuhauser. 2006. "Walter A. Shewhart, 1924, and the Hawthorne Factory." *Quality and Safety in Healthcare* 15 (2): 142–43.

———. 2005. "W. Edwards Deming: Father of Quality Management, Patient and Composer." *Quality and Safety in Healthcare* 14 (8): 137–45.

Burton, T. T. 2011. *Accelerating Lean Six Sigma Results: How to Achieve Improvement Excellence in the New Economy*. Plantation, FL: J. Ross Publishing.

Chassin, M. R., and J. R. Loeb. 2013. "High-Reliability Health Care: Getting There from Here." *Milbank Quarterly* 91 (3): 459–90.

De Koning, H., J. P. Verver, J. van den Heuvel, S. Bisgaard, and R. J. Does. 2006. "Lean Six Sigma in Healthcare." *Journal for Healthcare Quality* 28 (2): 4–11.

Department of Community and Family Medicine, Duke University School of Medicine. 2016. "Methods of Quality Improvement." Accessed November 10, 2017. http://patientsafetyed.duhs.duke.edu/module_a/methods/methods.html.

Hagan, P. 2011. "Waste Not, Want Not: Leading the Lean Health-Care Journey at Seattle Children's Hospital." *Global Business and Organizational Excellence* 30 (3): 25–31.

Hsu, C.-D., I. Cohn, and R. Caban. 2016. "Reduction and Sustainability of Cesarean Section Surgical Site Infection: An Evidence-Based, Innovative, and Multidisciplinary Quality Improvement Intervention Bundle Program." *American Journal of Infection Control* 44 (11): 1315–20.

Huang, Y., X. Li, J. Wilck, and T. Berget. 2012. "Cost Reduction in Healthcare via Lean Six Sigma." In *Proceedings of the 2012 Industrial and Systems Engineering Research Conference,* sponsored by the Institute of Industrial Engineers, Orlando, FL, May 19–23, 1–8.

Kaplan, G. S., S. H. Patterson, J. M. Ching, and C. C. Blackmore. 2014. "Why Lean Doesn't Work for Everyone." *BMJ Quality & Safety* 23 (12): 970–73.

Lean Management. 2007. "Shewhart's PDSA Cycle." Published November 1. http://walter-a-shewart.blogspot.com.

Mannon, M. 2014. "Lean Healthcare and Quality Management: The Experience of Theda-Care." *Quality Management Journal* 21 (1): 7–10.

Mazzocato, P., C. Savage, M. Brommels, H. Aronsson, and J. Thor. 2010. "Lean Thinking in Healthcare: A Realist Review of the Literature." *BMJ Quality & Safety* 19 (5): 376–82.

McLaughlin, D. B., and J. R. Olson. 2017. *Healthcare Operations Management*, 3rd ed. Chicago: Health Administration Press.

Nabhan, C., G. Horner, and M. D. Howell. 2017. "Lean: Targeted Therapy for Care Delivery." *Journal of the National Comprehensive Cancer Network* 15 (2): 271–74.

Ohno, T. 1988. *Toyota Production System: Beyond Large-Scale Production.* New York: Productivity Press.

Organizational Dynamics Inc. 2006. "Quality Action Teams." Accessed November 10, 2017. www.orgdynamics.com/QAT.pdf.

Swensen, S. J. 2010. "Building Skyscrapers in Healthcare." In *Lessons Learned in Changing Healthcare*, edited by P. Batalden, 167–77. Toronto: Longwoods Publishing Corporation.

Toussaint, J. S., and L. L. Berry. 2013. "The Promise of Lean in Health Care." *Mayo Clinic Proceedings* 88 (1): 74–82.

Varkey, P., M. K. Reller, and R. K. Resar. 2007. "Basics of Quality Improvement in Health Care." *Mayo Clinic Proceedings* 82 (6): 735–39.

Watson-Hemphill, K., and K. N. Bradley. 2016. "Lean Six Sigma Applications in Healthcare: Making Progress Despite the Challenges." *Quality Digest.* Published April 14. www.qualitydigest.com/inside/health-care-article/041416-innovating-lean-six-sigma.html#.

Winton, D. 1999. "Process Capability Studies." Accessed November 10, 2017. http://elsmar.com/pdf_files/CPK.pdf.

Womack, J., and D. Jones. 2003. *Lean Thinking: Banish Waste and Create Wealth in Your Corporation,* 2nd ed. New York: Free Press.

Zidel, T. G. 2012. *Lean Done Right: Achieve and Maintain Reform in Your Healthcare Organization*. Chicago: Health Administration Press.

CHAPTER 6

PERFORMANCE IMPROVEMENT TOOLS

➤ Flowcharts

➤ Force field analysis

➤ Gantt charts

➤ Improvement plan

➤ Interviews

➤ Multivoting

➤ Nominal group technique

➤ Planning matrix

➤ Qualitative tools

➤ Quality storyboard

➤ Quantitative tools

➤ Questionnaires

➤ Response rate

➤ Response scales

➤ Stakeholder analysis

➤ Survey sample

➤ Surveys

➤ Workflow diagram

D uring an improvement project, various analytic tools are used to discover the causes of undesirable performance and to plan solutions. Do not confuse the performance improvement models described in chapter 5 with the analytic tools used throughout an improvement project. Think of the improvement model as the recipe—for instance, the steps you follow when baking a cake. Analytic tools are the ingredients—the materials you use while following the recipe. When baking a cake, you want to use the correct ingredients and add them to the cake mixture at the right time. The same is true for the analytic tools used during an improvement project.

QUALITATIVE IMPROVEMENT TOOLS

Analytic tools are either qualitative or quantitative. **Qualitative tools** are used to generate ideas, set priorities, maintain direction, determine problem causes, and clarify processes. **Quantitative tools** are used to measure performance, collect and display data, and monitor performance. Exhibit 6.1 is a quick reference guide to the common qualitative and quantitative analytic tools used in each step of a typical improvement project. Notice that some tools can be used in more than one step.

The quantitative tools should look familiar; they were discussed in chapter 3. Quantitative tools are typically used during the preliminary performance assessment phase of quality management to display numeric or measurement information in a manageable and useful form. They also can be used during the actual improvement project for similar

Qualitative tools
Analytic improvement tools used for generating ideas, setting priorities, maintaining direction, determining problem causes, and clarifying processes.

Quantitative tools
Analytic improvement tools used for measuring performance, collecting and displaying data, and monitoring performance.

	Qualitative Tools	Quantitative Tools
Step 1: Define the improvement goal	Affinity diagram Brainstorming Decision matrix Force field analysis Multivoting Nominal group technique Survey	Bar graph Check sheet Control chart Histogram Line graph Pareto chart Scatter diagram Survey
Step 2: Analyze current practices	Brainstorming Cause and effect diagram Five Whys Flowchart Survey Workflow diagram	Bar graph Check sheet Control chart Histogram Line graph Pareto chart Scatter diagram Survey
Step 3: Design and implement improvements	Affinity diagram Brainstorming Decision matrix Flowchart Force field analysis Nominal group technique Planning matrix Stakeholder analysis Workflow diagram	Bar graph Check sheet Control chart Histogram Line graph Pareto chart Scatter diagram Survey
Step 4: Measure success	Survey	Bar graph Check sheet Control chart Histogram Line graph Pareto chart Scatter diagram Survey

EXHIBIT 6.1
Quick Reference Guide to Analytic Improvement Tools

purposes. Qualitative tools are used to present ideas in a manageable and useful form. In other words, they give structure to a set of ideas. Qualitative tools are used throughout an improvement project. Together with quantitative tools, qualitative tools help the improvement team define the goal, understand how the process works, identify improvement opportunities, and create solutions. The qualitative tools listed in exhibit 6.1 are described in the following sections.

BRAINSTORMING

Brainstorming
An interactive decision-making technique designed to generate a large number of creative ideas.

Brainstorming is a technique used to quickly generate lots of ideas about a problem or topic. It encourages creative thinking and incites enthusiasm. The case study involving Sunrise Home Health Agency in the previous chapter described two brainstorming sessions. At the first meeting, the staff members used brainstorming to list their complaints. At the second meeting, they used the technique to generate solutions.

The most common brainstorming techniques are *structured brainstorming*, *unstructured brainstorming*, and *silent brainstorming*. In structured brainstorming, a group leader solicits ideas from group members one at a time. Participants may skip their turn if they do not have an idea to share. Structured brainstorming is advantageous in that each person has an equal chance to participate, but it is disadvantageous in that it discourages spontaneity and is restrictive.

Unstructured brainstorming is free-form; participants contribute ideas as they come to mind. Unstructured brainstorming is advantageous in that participants can build on each other's ideas in a relaxed atmosphere. It is disadvantageous in that less assertive or lower-ranking participants (such as nonleadership staff) may choose not to speak up. A few rounds of structured brainstorming followed by unstructured brainstorming may help reticent participants open up.

In silent brainstorming, participants write their ideas on small slips of paper, which are collected and posted for everyone to see. Silent brainstorming is advantageous in that everyone's ideas are captured regardless of his or her level of assertiveness or position in the organization's hierarchy. Silent brainstorming is disadvantageous in that the group does not build the synergy of an open session. Silent brainstorming is often used in combination with other brainstorming techniques.

The result of a brainstorming session is a list of ideas. A long list can be narrowed down using another qualitative tool, such as multivoting or nominal group technique.

Multivoting
A group decision-making technique used to reduce a long list of items to a manageable number by taking a series of structured votes.

MULTIVOTING

Multivoting often follows a brainstorming session. The group in the case study involving Sunrise Home Health Agency in the previous chapter used multivoting to identify its top three complaints. This technique is used to pare down a broad list of ideas and establish priorities. Which task is most important? What do we need to do first? Which solution will work best? Which improvement goals are most important?

Suppose an improvement team charged with reducing patient wait times in an outpatient clinic has identified several problems that contribute to service delays. They know they cannot fix all of these problems at once, so they use multivoting to determine which problems they should address first. The problems are listed on a flip chart in random order. Team members are given ten self-stick dots (color is irrelevant) and told to place the dots next to the problems they feel are most urgent. They are instructed to use all ten dots but to place no more than four dots on one problem. When everyone is done, the number of dots next to each problem is tallied. A few clear winners usually stand out. The problems with the highest number of dots are addressed first. Before finalizing the list of high-priority problems, the team may discuss the results to ensure everyone agrees with the selection.

> **(?) DID YOU KNOW?**
>
> The word *brainstorming* was coined by Alex Osborn, president and founder of an advertising firm in the 1930s and 1940s. He used it to help his employees generate many new ideas for the advertising business, and it was so successful that it began to be used in many different kinds of situations where ideas were needed to help solve problems. Brainstorming has developed and changed somewhat since Osborn created it, but conceptually it remains the same.

NOMINAL GROUP TECHNIQUE

Nominal group technique, a more structured form of multivoting, involves five steps. The following example illustrates the use of nominal group technique to select solutions for a performance problem.

An ambulatory surgery center forms a team to investigate why patient complaints are increasing and what is needed to fix this problem. Using nominal group technique, the team leader first states the problem and clarifies it if necessary to ensure everyone understands its nature and consequences. In the second step, each team member silently records potential solutions to the problem and does not discuss them with other team members (as in silent brainstorming). In the third step, each person shares one idea with the group, and the leader records the idea on a flip chart. The process is repeated until all solution ideas have been recorded. As in step two, the ideas are not discussed.

In the fourth step, the team clarifies the ideas listed on the flip chart. The leader may ask some team members to explain their ideas. Comments from other members are not allowed during the explanation. The goal in this step is to ensure that everyone in the group understands the suggested solutions. In the final step, the team votes on the ideas silently. Team members are asked to select five ideas they think are most effective, record

Nominal group technique
A structured form of multivoting used to identify and rank issues.

them on separate index cards, and rank them in order of importance. They mark a "5" on the card for most important, "4" for second most important, and so on.

When team members have finished ranking their ideas, the leader collects the cards and tallies the votes. Items that received one or no votes are removed from the list. Items with the highest total point values are most important to the group and should be addressed first.

The primary difference between the results of multivoting and the results of nominal group technique is that the improvement team considers the total point count for each item (adding up the values of each vote) as well as the number of votes each item received.

AFFINITY DIAGRAMS

Affinity diagrams
Charts used by improvement teams to organize ideas and issues, gain a better understanding of a problem, and brainstorm potential solutions. (An example of an affinity diagram is shown in exhibit 6.2.)

Affinity diagrams are used to organize large amounts of language data (ideas, issues, opinions) generated by brainstorming into groupings on the basis of the relationships between data items. This process helps improvement teams sift through large volumes of information and encourages new patterns of thinking. Affinity diagrams also help improvement teams identify difficult, confusing, unknown, or disorganized performance concerns.

To create an affinity diagram, team members write their ideas, issues, or opinions on separate pieces of paper or index cards and scatter them on a large table. Together, and without speaking, the team sorts related ideas into no more than eight groups. Sorting the ideas into an affinity diagram should be a creative process, so the groups should not be named until later. This categorization process takes from 10 to 20 minutes, depending on the number of ideas.

Once the ideas are sorted, the team names the groups by creating header cards and placing one at the top of each stack. The name should describe the thread or topic that ties the cards in the group together. Exhibit 6.2 is a partially completed affinity diagram created by an improvement team in a hospital's business office. The team brainstormed the problems associated with billing errors and grouped these problems into categories.

CAUSE AND EFFECT DIAGRAMS

Cause and effect diagrams
Graphic representations of the relationship between outcomes and the factors that influence them; sometimes called *Ishikawa* or *fishbone diagrams*. (Examples of cause and effect diagrams are shown in exhibits 6.3 and 6.4.)

Cause and effect diagrams are a structured brainstorming technique used to identify all possible causes of an effect (a problem or an objective). They are sometimes called *Ishikawa diagrams*—after Kaoru Ishikawa, a quality pioneer who created and first used them in the 1960s for quality control purposes (Best and Neuhauser 2008). They are also called *fishbone diagrams* because the lines connecting major cause categories resemble the backbone of a fish. Exhibit 6.3 is a cause and effect diagram created by an improvement team charged with reducing patient wait times in a clinic.

The first step in creating a cause and effect diagram is to identify the effect to be placed in the box at the right side of the diagram. The effect can be positive (an objective) or negative (a problem). The next step is to identify major factors that influence the effect.

EXHIBIT 6.2
Affinity Diagram

Training	Internal Communication	Insurance Relations
New billing clerks are not adequately trained.	Procedure charges are not consistently captured in IT system.	Insurance companies don't provide timely feedback.
Nurses don't understand the charge process for supplies.	Getting everyone together to fix charge problems is difficult.	There is no consistent procedure for confirming patient's insurance before billing.
Despite training on new IT system, some clerks still have difficulty using it.	Clerks can wait up to two weeks to be informed of billing process changes.	Insurance companies keep hospital billing clerks on hold too long.

The *four Ms*—methods, manpower, materials, and machinery—or the *four Ps*—policies, procedures, people, and plant—are commonly used as starting points. More than four factors may be identified for complex topics. The factors are placed in boxes at the end of each rib of the backbone.

Once the major factors are selected, the team identifies and categorizes the significant causes, which are usually identified through brainstorming and group members' knowledge and expertise. After the major causes are positioned on the diagram, the team digs deeper to identify the subfactors influencing the major causes. Exhibit 6.4 is a cause and effect diagram that includes the major causes and subfactors of the problem of poor fuel economy in an automobile.

Improvement teams usually create a cause and effect diagram at the beginning of an improvement project to clarify the problem. They then use quantitative tools to determine the scope of the problem. For instance, the aforementioned clinic generated lots of ideas and presumptions about potential causes of long clinic wait times (see exhibit 6.3). After completing the cause and effect diagram, the clinic will need to gather data to determine which of the presumed causes are in fact contributing to the problem. These data could be

EXHIBIT 6.3
Cause and Effect Diagram

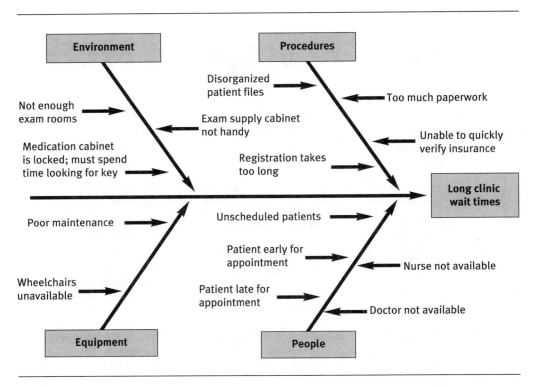

EXHIBIT 6.4
Cause and Effect Diagram with Subfactors Listed

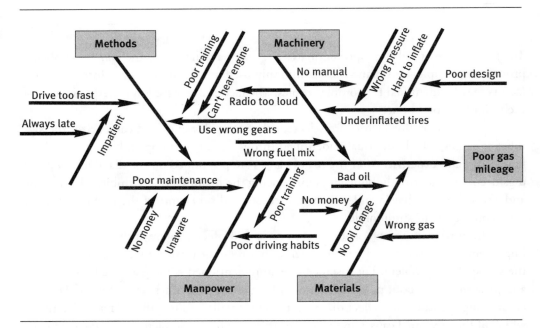

displayed in bar graphs, histograms, Pareto charts, or other graphic or tabular data reports. If the data indicate several problems, the team may use qualitative tools, such as multi-voting or a decision matrix, to prioritize them.

DECISION MATRIXES

Improvement teams can use a **decision matrix** (sometimes called a *selection matrix* or *prioritization matrix*) to systematically identify, analyze, and rate the strength of relationships between sets of information. This type of matrix is especially useful when considering a large number of decision factors and assessing each factor's relative importance. Teams frequently use this tool to select improvement priorities and evaluate alternative solutions.

   In the case study involving Sunrise Home Health Agency in the previous chapter, the director conducted a brainstorming session to solicit ideas on how to make monthly staff meetings more valuable to staff. Suppose the director had used a decision matrix (exhibit 6.5) to evaluate the suggested solutions more systematically. He would list the staff's recommendations in the first column and the criteria for evaluating each solution across the top of the remaining columns. He would then ask each staff member to score the solutions according to the ranking key. The scores are tallied, and a group average is calculated for each solution. Solutions with the highest group average are selected for implementation.

Decision matrix
A chart used to identify, analyze, and rate the strength of relationships between sets of information; it is especially useful for looking at large numbers of decision factors and assessing each factor's relative importance. (Exhibit 6.5 is an example of a decision matrix.)

EXHIBIT 6.5
Decision Matrix

Proposed Solution	Evaluation Criteria				Your Total	Group Average
	Probability of Success	Ease of Implementation	Cost-Effectiveness	Impact on Staff Satisfaction		
Hold online meetings						
Start meetings on time						
Create meeting agenda						
Allow staff to suggest agenda items						

Ranking key: 4 = excellent; 3 = very good; 2 = satisfactory; 1 = poor

Selection criteria may come from a previously prepared affinity diagram or from a brainstorming activity. Everyone involved in the improvement initiative should have a clear and common understanding of what the criteria mean. The selection criteria should be written in a way that makes a high score for each criterion represent a favorable result and a low score represent an unfavorable result. If some decision criteria are more important than others, appropriate weights can be assigned to them. The total score for each alternative is then multiplied by the weight (e.g., 1, 2, 3) assigned to it.

Five Whys
A form of analysis that delves into the causes of problems by successively asking *what* and *why* until all aspects of the situation, process, or service are reviewed and contributing factors are considered. (An example of a Five Whys analysis is shown in exhibit 6.6.)

FIVE WHYS

Before developing solutions, teams need to confirm that they have found the underlying causes of a performance problem. The **Five Whys** tool helps an improvement team dig deeper into the causes of problems by successively asking *what* and *why* until all aspects of the situation are reviewed and the underlying contributing factors are considered. Usually by the time the team has asked and answered five *why* questions, it will have reached the core problem. Teams often uncover multiple root causes during this exercise.

Exhibit 6.6 is an illustration of the Five Whys process for a problem in a nursing home involving difficulties finding equipment needed to care for the residents. The root cause is eventually discovered by asking *why* repeatedly.

EXHIBIT 6.6
The Five Whys
Process

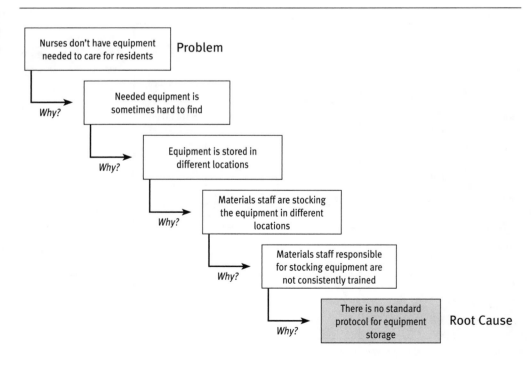

FLOWCHARTS

Flowcharts, sometimes referred to as *process diagrams* or *maps*, are used to document the flow or sequence of events in a process or to develop an optimal new process during the solution stage of improvement. They can be used to detect unexpected complexity, problem areas, redundancies, unnecessary steps, and opportunities for simplification. They also help teams agree on process steps and examine activities that most influence performance.

Standard flowchart symbols are shown in exhibit 6.7. When developing a flowchart, especially in a group environment, the goal is to illustrate the process. Do not waste time debating the best shapes to use. A flowchart that does not use these symbols can be just as useful as a chart that does. When designing a flowchart, write the process steps on index cards or sticky notes. The team can then rearrange the diagram without erasing and redrawing the chart.

After identifying the process adversely affecting performance, the improvement team defines the beginning and end of the process and the steps between these two points. It then sequences the steps in the order in which they are executed. The flowchart should illustrate the process in its current state—the way it is operating at that moment. To test for completeness, the team may validate the flowchart with people outside the team or those who execute the process. When the team is satisfied that the chart represents the process accurately, it asks questions to locate improvement opportunities:

Flowcharts
Graphic representations of a process. (Examples of flowcharts are shown in exhibits 6.8 through 6.11.)

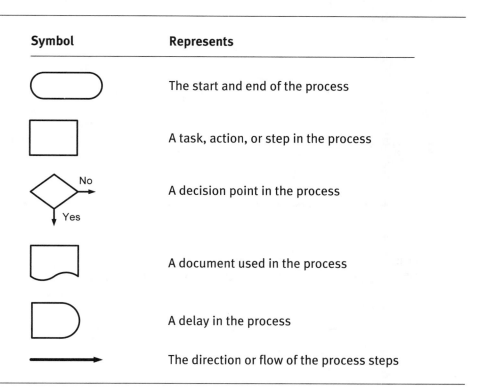

Symbol	Represents
	The start and end of the process
	A task, action, or step in the process
No / Yes	A decision point in the process
	A document used in the process
	A delay in the process
→	The direction or flow of the process steps

EXHIBIT 6.7
Standard Flowchart Symbols

- ◆ Can any steps be eliminated?

- ◆ Can any steps be combined with others?

- ◆ Can any steps be simplified?

- ◆ Can delays in the process be eliminated?

- ◆ Can rework loops be eliminated?

- ◆ Can buildup of paperwork be minimized?

- ◆ Can handoffs between people or departments be streamlined?

The improvement team may create a second flowchart that illustrates the ideal process—the best way to proceed from start to finish. While this step is not necessary, it can reveal improvement opportunities. The team can examine areas of the current process that differ from the ideal process and speculate on the reasons for the discrepancy.

Among the different types of flowcharts, high-level, detailed, deployment, and top-down charts are most commonly used. Exhibit 6.8 is a *high-level flowchart* of the steps involved in filling a prescription at a retail pharmacy. The process starts when the customer presents the prescription to the pharmacy clerk and ends when the customer receives the medication. This flowchart is considered high level because minor steps in the process have not been included.

EXHIBIT 6.8
High-Level
Flowchart of
Retail Pharmacy
Medication
Dispensing Process

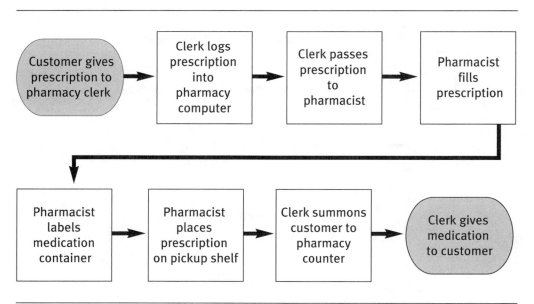

A *detailed flowchart* maps all the steps and activities that occur in the process and includes decision points, waiting periods, tasks frequently redone, and feedback loops. Exhibit 6.9 is a detailed flowchart of the patient X-ray process. This type of flowchart is particularly useful when looking for problems or inefficiencies. For example, the flowchart in exhibit 6.9 shows that delays occur when physician orders are not readily available to the X-ray technician. Delays also occur when X-rays have to be retaken for technical reasons. This flowchart was adapted from a Lean project that was implemented to reduce inefficiencies in the X-ray process.

From this flowchart, the team identified delays that could be eliminated by shifting some tasks to the radiology department's receptionists. The receptionists could confirm the availability of physician orders before patients enter the X-ray area and retrieve missing orders and escort patients to and from the dressing room, freeing up even more time for the technician. These changes would streamline the technician's job, increasing productivity.

Another type of chart, a *deployment flowchart*, shows detailed process steps and the people involved in each step. A deployment flowchart is particularly useful for mapping processes in which information or services are passed between people and groups. It also may reveal unclear responsibilities, missing information, and unshared expectations that contribute to performance problems.

Exhibit 6.10 is a deployment flowchart of an employee training process. To create this flowchart, the improvement team listed the departments involved across the top of the chart. Next, it arranged the process steps in sequence and positioned each step in the column of the department that executes the step. The process steps are connected with arrows to show where the flow lines cross from one column to the next. A handoff occurs each time the flow line crosses columns. The project team focused improvement solutions on the handoffs in the process because these transitions are prone to errors, miscommunications, and delays.

In a *top-down flowchart*, the major steps in a process are arranged sequentially across the top and the detailed steps are listed under each major step (see exhibit 6.11). Unlike a detailed flowchart, a top-down flowchart does not include decision points or other steps that might be causing inefficiencies. A top-down flowchart is useful for viewing the process in a systematic manner to better understand the activities involved and their interconnectedness.

Each type of flowchart has its strengths and weaknesses. To choose the best format for the project, the improvement team needs to understand the reason for creating the flowchart. If the team is unsure about the substeps in the process, it should create a high-level flowchart. When the team understands the process substeps and wants to better understand how the steps are carried out, it should create a detailed, deployment, or top-down flowchart. When conducting a Lean project, the team may create a value stream map instead of a flowchart. As described in chapter 5, a value stream map includes the value-adding and non-value-adding steps and related process measurements.

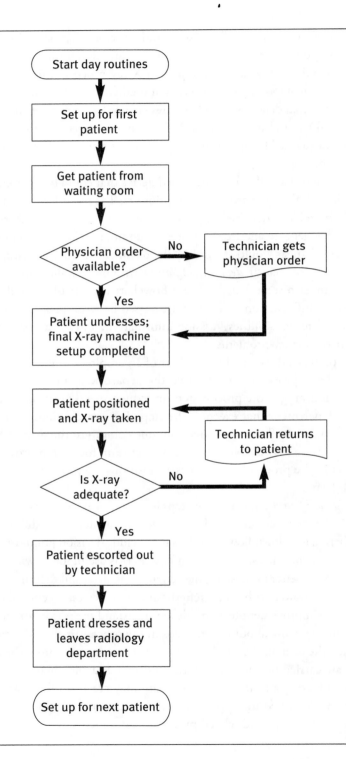

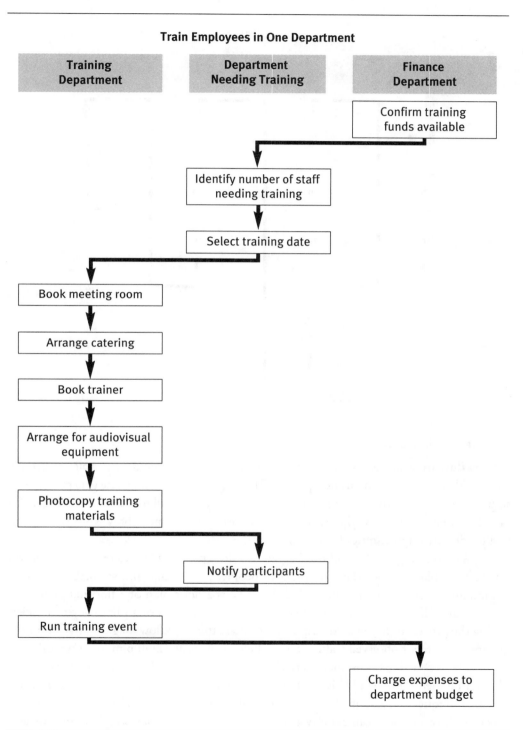

Train Employees in One Department

Training Department	Department Needing Training	Finance Department

Confirm training funds available

Identify number of staff needing training

Select training date

Book meeting room

Arrange catering

Book trainer

Arrange for audiovisual equipment

Photocopy training materials

Notify participants

Run training event

Charge expenses to department budget

EXHIBIT 6.10
Deployment Flowchart of the Employee Training Process

EXHIBIT 6.11
Top-Down
Flowchart

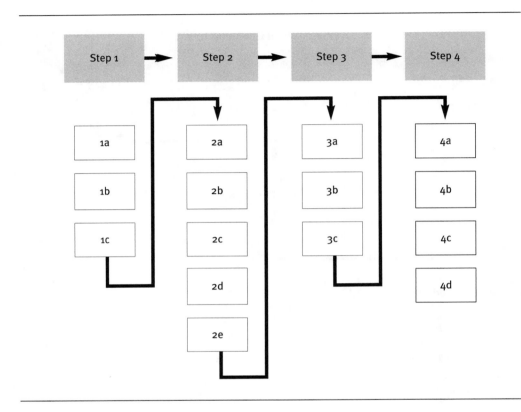

WORKFLOW DIAGRAMS

Workflow diagram
An illustration of the movement of employees or information during a process. (An example of a workflow diagram is shown in exhibit 6.12.)

A **workflow diagram** is a visual representation of the movement of people, materials, paperwork, or information during a process. The diagram can also illustrate general relationships or patterns of activity among interrelated processes (e.g., all processes occurring in the radiology department). Workflow diagrams are used to document how work is executed and to identify opportunities for improvement.

A common type of workflow diagram is a floor plan of a work site. Lines are drawn on the floor plan to trace the movement of people, paper, data, and so forth to identify redundant travel and inefficiencies. Exhibit 6.12 is a floor plan of a hospital pharmacy department. The lines on the floor plan trace the movements of a pharmacy technician during the process of filling a prescription. To create this workflow diagram, staff from the quality department observed traffic flow in the pharmacy at 12:30 p.m. on a typical day.

The technician's movements are chaotic because of the layout of the department. The central medication supply is located in the middle of the pharmacy, and medications that are infrequently prescribed line the back wall of the department. The narrow walkway between the two sections causes delay and congestion because it comfortably accommodates

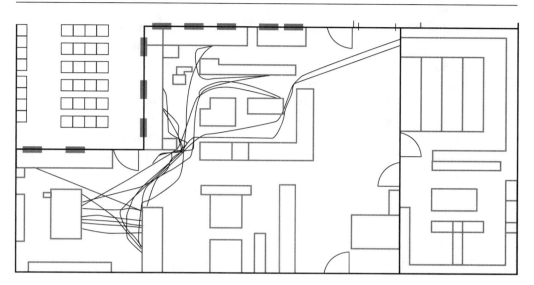

EXHIBIT 6.12
Workflow
Diagram Showing
Movement
of Pharmacy
Technician During
Peak Hours

only one person at a time. The resources needed to fill prescriptions are not easily accessible. Two printers in the lower left corner of the department, approximately 26 feet from the medication area, print prescription enclosures. The technicians must travel to this area through a narrow doorway. After studying the workflow in the pharmacy department, several changes were made to the department layout and the prescription receiving process.

SURVEYS

Surveys are instruments used to gather data or information. The case study at the beginning of chapter 3 described a survey used at the Redwood Health Center to gather satisfaction information from patients. This survey gathered quantitative (numeric rankings) and qualitative (comments) information. Researchers disagree as to whether surveys are a quantitative tool, a qualitative tool, or a combination of both. For this reason, surveys are listed as both in exhibit 6.1.

The two types of surveys are questionnaires and interviews. **Questionnaires** are usually paper or electronic instruments that the respondent completes independently. **Interviews** are conducted with the respondent face-to-face or over the phone. The interviewer is responsible for documenting the respondent's comments.

Improvement teams typically use questionnaires to gather people's perceptions of a service or process. These perceptions are not necessarily factual. For instance, suppose an improvement team at the Redwood Health Center wants to know how long patients wait in the reception area before they are escorted to an exam room. To determine the number of

Surveys
Questionnaires or interviews used to obtain information from a group of individuals about a process, product, or service.

Questionnaires
Forms containing questions to which subjects respond. (Exhibit 6.13 is an example of a questionnaire.)

Interviews
Formal discussions between two parties in which information is exchanged.

minutes patients wait, the team will need to devise a system that registers the time patients arrive at the clinic and the time they are taken to an exam room. If the center used a survey to gather wait time data, patients might over- or underestimate the time they spent in the reception area. As another example, consider the Centers for Medicare & Medicaid Services (CMS) Hospital Compare website, which publishes ratings gathered from a patient survey on hospital experiences. One survey question asks: How often did hospital staff explain about medicines before giving them to you (CMS 2017)? The majority of a hospital's patients might indicate "usually" because they remember talking to staff about their medicine, but an observational study on the subject might show that those conversations rarely included information about what the medicine was for.

Surveys can be a useful tool for gathering the opinions or perceptions of people who are not members of the improvement team. To ensure that it gathers the information necessary to complete a project, the team needs to develop questions that will elicit such data. Without adequate planning, the survey results may not yield useful information. Follow these steps when developing and administering surveys:

1. *Define the survey objectives.* Clearly define the purpose or intent of the survey. What are you trying to find out, and why do you need this information? Do not select more than five topics; otherwise, the survey will be too long. People may not respond to a request to complete a long survey. Keep the survey focused on high-priority questions that need to be answered to meet your objectives.

2. *Identify the people to be surveyed.* Whom do you need to survey to gather the information you seek? If you know what group of people you want to survey, you will be able to determine the best way to gather their responses. Will you distribute the survey at participants' work location, or will you mail it to their home? Will you bring participants together to complete the survey, or will you have them complete it on their own time?

3. *Select the survey population.* Ideally, you want to ask everyone who holds an opinion about the topic to respond to the survey. If the population is small (e.g., all employees in the health information management department), you may be able to survey everyone. If you have cost or time constraints, however, you may not be able to survey everyone, especially in a large population (e.g., all nurses who work in the hospital). You may need to settle for a sample of the population, preferably a **survey sample** that is representative of the entire population. Sampling and sample size selection are covered in chapter 3.

4. *Construct the survey.* Create a concise survey that is easy to understand and interpret. Do not include questions that might threaten the respondent. For example, if you are seeking employee feedback on an improvement plan that might involve staff cutbacks, do not ask a question such as, "Should less productive employees be laid off first?" People who feel threatened by survey

Survey sample
A subgroup of respondents derived from the target population.

questions usually give biased responses or fail to complete the survey. Do not include leading questions (i.e., questions that encourage the respondent to answer the way you want them to), and phrase items objectively. Use common rather than obscure terms, and strive for brevity and clarity.

Select the range of answers, or **response scales**, from which participants can choose. You can include a dichotomous response scale (e.g., Agree/ Disagree, True/False, Yes/No) or an interval response scale (e.g., 1 to 5, where 1 is lowest or least likely and 5 is highest or most likely). Surveys commonly include Likert scales, which offer five to seven multiple-choice alternatives (e.g., "to a very great extent," "to a great extent," "to a moderate extent," and so on) (Johnson and Morgan 2016). Other dimensions commonly used include frequency scales (how often something occurs, such as frequently–infrequently, never–always, or once per day–once per year), scales of agreement (to what degree), and scales of value (how important something is to the respondent).

> **Response scales**
> Ranges of answers from which the survey respondent can choose.

Formulate survey questions so that the answers can be graded on a continuum rather than discretely. For example, a scale that measures degrees of agreement with survey statements is a continuum. The answers on the departmental quality assessment questionnaire (exhibit 6.13) are scaled in degrees (from strongly disagree to strongly agree). In contrast, a questionnaire that asks respondents to identify sources of problems (e.g., workflow delays, waste, equipment breakdown, understaffing) must be tabulated individually. Scales usually include five to nine points, as most people have difficulty discriminating between the finer differences that would result if the scale were further divided (Johnson and Morgan 2016). A range that is too restrictive— for example, one that includes only two or three points—usually is equally ineffective and may produce meaningless results.

5. *Test the survey, and prepare the final draft.* Even well-designed surveys can pose problems. Improvement teams conduct pretests to identify and correct these problems. To conduct a pretest, prepare a few mock-ups of the survey and recruit volunteers to complete it. When they have finished, ask them for feedback. Did they find flaws or errors in the survey? Were the instructions and questions clear?

    After you correct the problems identified by your pretest volunteers, prepare a final copy of the survey for reproduction. Carefully check the final product before distribution. Errors not caught at this step can be costly, especially if you have to discard some of the survey results because of problematic questions or typographical errors.

6. *Administer the survey.* If possible, have all participants complete the survey at the same time. For example, the survey can be conducted at a department staff meeting. When such arrangements cannot be made, surveys can be

Response rate
The number of
respondents who
complete a survey out
of the number who
received the survey,
usually expressed as
a percentage; can also
apply to individual
questions.

distributed and returned by hand or internal mail. When completion of the survey is voluntary, the team should encourage a high **response rate** by using a well-designed survey, offering incentives, making personal appeals, and adopting other persuasive techniques. Low response rates are unlikely to produce valid, reliable feedback. Acceptable response rates depend on the method of survey distribution (SurveyMonkey 2008):

◆ Mail: 50 percent = adequate, 60–70 percent = good to very good

◆ Phone: 80 percent = good

EXHIBIT 6.13
Departmental
Quality
Assessment
Questionnaire

This departmental assessment survey contains 22 statements. Respond to each with the number that indicates the extent of your agreement with the statement: 1 = strongly disagree; 2 = disagree; 3 = somewhat disagree; 4 = somewhat agree; 5 = agree; 6 = strongly agree.

	Extent of Agreement
1. Work delays are uncommon in this department.	
2. Once the department starts an improvement project, it usually finishes it without undue delay.	
3. There is little waste of materials and supplies.	
4. People reuse or salvage excess materials and supplies whenever possible.	
5. Equipment is maintained and operated at peak efficiency.	
6. This department's equipment rarely requires repair.	
7. This department has sufficient personnel to accomplish its mission.	
8. The personnel turnover rate is low.	
9. Working conditions (noise, heat, light, cleanliness) are excellent.	
10. Work facilities are excellent.	
11. Department staff members are well trained.	
12. Department staff members receive the guidance and assistance they need to accomplish their work.	
13. This department's materials and supplies are well accounted for without unexplained losses.	
14. This department's materials and supplies meet quality specifications.	
15. Department staff members rarely need to shift work priorities to complete jobs.	
16. Department staff members rarely need to redo a job or task.	
17. This department's customers are satisfied with the quality of work/service.	
18. This department's customers seldom complain.	
19. This department's customers are satisfied with the quantity of work/service.	
20. This department's customers are satisfied with the timeliness of work/service.	
21. This department's customers find few errors in the work performed by staff.	
22. This department's customers find the service consistent.	

◆ E-mail: 40 percent = average, 50–60 percent = good to very good

◆ Online: 30 percent = average

◆ Face-to-face interview: 80–85 percent = good

The qualitative information gathered through questionnaires and interviews must be summarized for analysis. Often the information has to be translated into quantitative results before it can be used. Results reporting was taken into consideration when designing the departmental quality assessment survey in exhibit 6.13. Each statement corresponds to 1 of 11 quality characteristics (two statements per characteristic).

Exhibit 6.14 is a scoring tool designed to tabulate survey results. The sum of the numeric answers to each statement (two per line) is recorded in column two. The average degree of agreement for each quality characteristic is calculated by dividing the sum in column two by the number of corresponding questions (the divisor shown in column three). The average for the entire survey also can be calculated. These averages then can be reported in a data table or graph.

Statements	Sum of Responses to Statements	Divisor	Average	Quality Characteristic
1–2		2		Work flow/delays
3–4		2		Waste
5–6		2		Tools/equipment
7–8		2		Staffing
9–10		2		Facilities
11–12		2		Training
13–14		2		Supplies
15–16		2		Organization/group structure
17–18		2		Customer quality
19–20		2		Quantity
21–22		2		Reliability
All (1–22)		11		

EXHIBIT 6.14
Departmental Quality Characteristics Survey Scoring Tool

FORCE FIELD ANALYSIS

The purpose of **force field analysis** is to determine the potential support for and against (the *forces*) a particular plan or idea. Once these forces are identified, plans can be devised to strengthen support for the idea and reduce resistance against it. Teams typically use force field analysis during the solution phase of an improvement project but may also use it to prioritize their improvement goals.

Exhibit 6.15 is a force field analysis completed by an improvement project team at a children's hospital. The goal of the project is to increase parents' participation in the hospital's quality improvement efforts. To achieve this goal, the team suggested that the hospital host quarterly focus groups with the parents of former patients to solicit ways to improve parent satisfaction. The improvement team uses the force field analysis to clarify current and desired participation and identify obstacles that could impede implementation of their proposal. The vertical line at the center of the diagram represents the status quo.

Teams brainstorm to identify the driving and restraining forces and then decide which will most influence the outcome. They develop strategies to minimize the forces

EXHIBIT 6.15
Force Field Analysis for Proposed Improvement Action

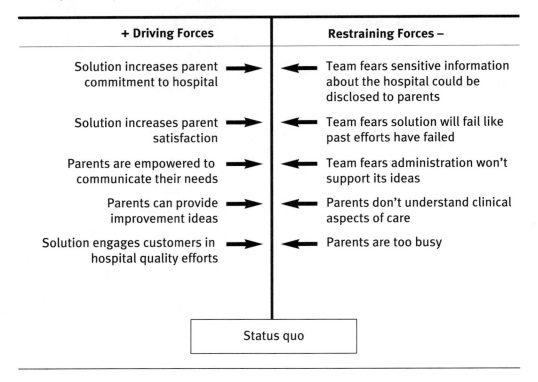

Desired situation: The hospital hosts quarterly focus group discussions with parents of former pediatric patients to solicit ideas for improving satisfaction

+ Driving Forces	Restraining Forces −
Solution increases parent commitment to hospital	Team fears sensitive information about the hospital could be disclosed to parents
Solution increases parent satisfaction	Team fears solution will fail like past efforts have failed
Parents are empowered to communicate their needs	Team fears administration won't support its ideas
Parents can provide improvement ideas	Parents don't understand clinical aspects of care
Solution engages customers in hospital quality efforts	Parents are too busy

Status quo

against, and strengthen the forces for, the desired outcome. Teams should focus on reducing or eliminating the restraining forces because they are usually more powerful than the driving forces and can prevent the change from being implemented.

STAKEHOLDER ANALYSIS

People usually resist change. If the improvement project team does not deal with this resistance, desired performance improvements may not materialize. Teams can use a **stakeholder analysis** to identify the individuals or groups that would be affected by a proposed process change. Each stakeholder is assessed to determine who would readily accept and who would resist the process changes. Stakeholders can be grouped into four main categories: allies, associates, enemies, and opponents. Not all stakeholders are equal; some have more influence on the outcome of the improvement plan than others. All of these factors are considered in a stakeholder analysis.

The Lean project team that proposed changes to the process of taking X-rays (see exhibit 6.9) used a stakeholder analysis to better understand how those affected by the change would view the new process. A stakeholder analysis matrix (exhibit 6.16) helped the team predict each group's influence on project outcomes and its level of support.

The individuals and groups that would be affected by the proposed changes to the process are listed in the first column. The team determines the specific interests these stakeholders have in the new process. The team considers such issues as

Stakeholder analysis
A tool used to identify groups and individuals who will be affected by a process change and whose participation and support are crucial to realizing successful outcomes.

- ◆ benefits to the stakeholder,

- ◆ benefits to the stakeholder's patients,

- ◆ changes the stakeholder will have to make, and

- ◆ activities that might cause conflict for the stakeholder.

These issues are recorded in the Stakeholder Incentives column.

Next, the team uses the following five-category ranking system to judge each stakeholder's support of the process change:

++	strongly in favor
+	weakly in favor
o	indifferent
−	weakly opposed
− −	strongly opposed

EXHIBIT **6.16**
Stakeholder
Analysis of
Proposed
Radiology Process
Change

Process change: Radiology receptionists will confirm the presence of a physician's order before the patient enters the X-ray area. If necessary, the receptionists will obtain the missing order from the patient's physician. Also, receptionists will escort the patient to and from the dressing room.

Stakeholder	Stakeholder Incentives	Stakeholder Support	Action(s)
Radiology receptionists	• More work for receptionists • Reception area not staffed for extra duties	−	Do time study to determine how this change will affect receptionists' workload
Radiology technicians	• Less clerical work for technicians • Could reduce opportunities to interact with patients	++	Monitor patient satisfaction surveys to determine whether reduced interactions affect radiology department satisfaction scores
Radiologists	• Increased number of X-rays performed each day	++	No action needed; group supports the changes
Physicians who order X-rays	• X-rays completed more quickly • Possible disruptions if receptionists must obtain missing orders	o	Ask radiologists to discuss the benefits of the change with physicians
Radiology manager	• Need to reevaluate staffing at reception desk • Potential to reduce overall costs and improve productivity	+	Manager is skeptical that the change will actually reduce costs or increase productivity; need to evaluate these issues closely during pilot test

++ Strongly in favor

+ Weakly in favor

o Indifferent

− Weakly opposed

− − Strongly opposed

After ranking the stakeholders, the improvement team develops strategies for gaining stakeholder support, plans for all possible barriers to success, and decides how each stakeholder should be approached about the proposed change. What kind of information does the stakeholder need? Should the team involve the stakeholder in the project? Could any other groups or individuals influence those opposed to the change? In the last column of the matrix, the team records these ideas and the actions it must take to further the project.

PLANNING MATRIX

A **planning matrix** is a diagram that shows the tasks needed to complete an activity, the people or groups responsible for completing the tasks, and an activity schedule with deadlines for task completion. A **Gantt chart** is a graphic planning matrix that displays project activities as bars measured against a horizontal time scale. Most electronic spreadsheet programs have templates for creating Gantt charts.

Exhibit 6.17 is a Gantt chart for an improvement project involving changes to the patient registration process at the Redwood Health Center. In hopes of reducing patient wait times, the team decides to implement a change to the registration process for new patients. The clinic will mail a registration form to all new patients who schedule appointments. Patients will be asked to bring the completed form on the day of their appointment. The project seems simple and straightforward, but the Gantt chart reveals that the team must complete a number of tasks to implement the change successfully.

Developing a planning matrix is especially useful in that it requires the improvement team to consider every task in the **improvement plan**. Before finalizing the planning matrix, team members should agree on the assignment of responsibility and the start and completion dates for each task.

IMPROVEMENT PROJECT REPORTS

When an improvement project is concluded, a summary of the process investigations and actions is documented. This report is used to communicate to others within the organization how process problems are being resolved and what performance gains are being achieved. Future improvement teams use project write-ups to learn from the successful and unsuccessful improvement efforts of the past.

A report that effectively conveys project results should follow the Four Cs of good communication:

- *Clear:* Use terms that committee members and staff understand and relate to.
- *Concise:* Be short and to the point.
- *Complete:* Include all relevant information.
- *Correct:* Ensure that all data are accurate. (New York State Department of Health AIDS Institute 2006, 129)

Planning matrix
A diagram that shows tasks needed to complete an activity, the persons or groups responsible for completing the tasks, and an activity schedule with deadlines for task completion.

Gantt charts
Graphic representations of a planning matrix. (Exhibit 6.17 is an example of a Gantt chart.)

Improvement plan
A plan to eliminate the cause of undesirable performance or to make good performance even better.

EXHIBIT 6.17
Gantt Chart for
Clinic Registration
Change

Task	Person Responsible	Start	End	5/15	5/30	6/15	6/30	7/15	7/30	8/15	8/30	9/15
Design a self-explanatory clinic registration form and cover letter	Clinic manager	5/15	6/1	▓	▓							
Share the form and cover letter with a sample of patients to determine whether the average patient would understand how to complete the form	Clinic manager	6/1	6/25		▓	▓						
Revise the form and cover letter as necessary and send them to printer for duplication	Clinic manager	6/30	7/15				▓	▓				
Teach the new procedure to receptionists and staff in charge of scheduling	Front-office supervisor	7/30	8/15						▓	▓		
Provide staff with registration forms, cover letters, and a supply of envelopes	Clinic manager	8/15	8/30								▓	
Alert mailroom staff to the new procedure and provide forwarding instructions for the registration forms they will receive	Front-office supervisor	8/30	9/15									▓

The content for improvement project reports varies among organizations. Common topics covered in the report are goal or aim of the project; names of team members; methods used to analyze the process and results of this investigation; improvement interventions and results; systemic changes; next steps; and lessons learned. Two potential formats for the report are a quality storyboard and an A3 report form.

QUALITY STORYBOARDS

The series of events involved in a quality improvement project can be summarized in a report called a **quality storyboard**. Storyboards were first used to plan storylines for cartoons. They were composed of a series of panels that illustrated a sequence of changes using pictures, numbers, and words. When placed together in the correct order, these panels created a story (Forsha 1995). Likewise, quality storyboards are made up of a series of words and pictures that illustrate an improvement project from start to finish. Quality storyboards typically include the following information:

Quality storyboard
A tool that visually communicates the major elements of an improvement project. (A mock-up of a quality storyboard is shown in exhibit 6.18.)

◆ Team information (names and roles)

◆ Project focus

— The opportunity for improvement

— Desired results

— Method that will be used to measure progress

◆ Analysis of current situation

— Current process steps (flowchart or workflow diagram)

— Problems identified (chart or graph)

— Quality improvement tools used to determine problem causes (diagram or chart/graph)

◆ Proposed solutions

— Actions required to resolve root problem causes (chart/graph)

— Description of stakeholders

◆ Solutions executed (timeline)

◆ Effectiveness of solutions

— Qualitative and quantitative results (charts/graphs)

— Plan for ongoing monitoring

— Next steps

— Lessons learned

Quality storyboards communicate more information and clues about intentionality through graphs and pictures than through words. Someone unfamiliar with the improvement project should be able to determine what was done and why by following the logic of the storyboard's graphical displays, data analyses, and conclusions. Storyboards can be formatted as booklets or arranged on a large poster board. Some people use presentation software such as PowerPoint to design storyboards, whereby slides are created for each panel and printed in booklet or poster format (see exhibit 6.18).

Teams usually create quality storyboards at the end of an improvement project for communication purposes, but some teams use them throughout their projects as a visual record of their progress. Quality storyboards also keep team members focused on the project goal. To create a quality storyboard for use during an improvement project, section off and label areas on a large poster board to display the team's progress for each step. Include areas for the project goal, names of team members, the work plan, activities undertaken during problem analysis and the results of those activities, the solution(s) selected, the solution(s) implemented and the results of that implementation, and other interesting or relevant information.

EXHIBIT 6.18
Quality Storyboard
Mock-Up

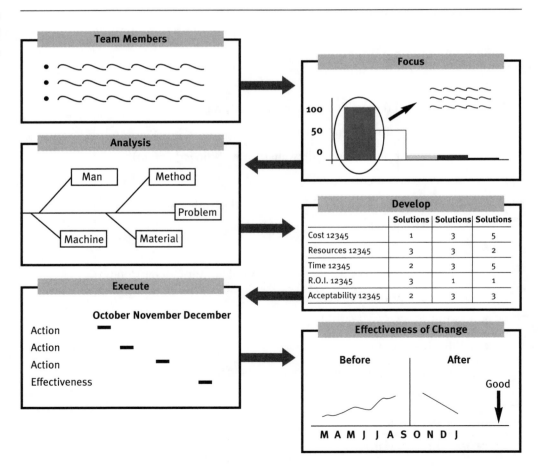

If you are using any of the analytic tools—flowcharts, cause and effect diagrams, matrixes, graphs—discussed in this chapter, include them on the storyboard as well. Performance measures, data collection forms, and graphs displaying the results are also useful inclusions. After implementing and evaluating your solution, condense the information on the storyboard and use it to communicate the improvement project story to the rest of the organization.

A3 Report Forms

The **A3 report form** was developed by Toyota to document Lean or kaizen projects. The A3 report is named after the size of the paper used for the report: standard letter size 11" × 17". "If desired, two 8.5" × 11" sheets may be used in place of the A3 sheet" (Zidel 2012, 56).

The flow of information in an A3 report often follows the Plan-Do-Study-Act improvement model cycle. One side of the form includes information about the project plan and what was found during analysis of the process. The other side of the report is used to document the do, study, and act phases of the project. An example of an A3 report template is found in exhibit 6.19. Although the A3 report was originally intended to be

A3 report form
A summary of Lean or kaizen project results presented on a one-page standard letter-sized A3 sheet of paper. (An A3 report form template is shown in exhibit 6.19.)

Exhibit 6.19
Template for an A-3 Problem-Solving Report

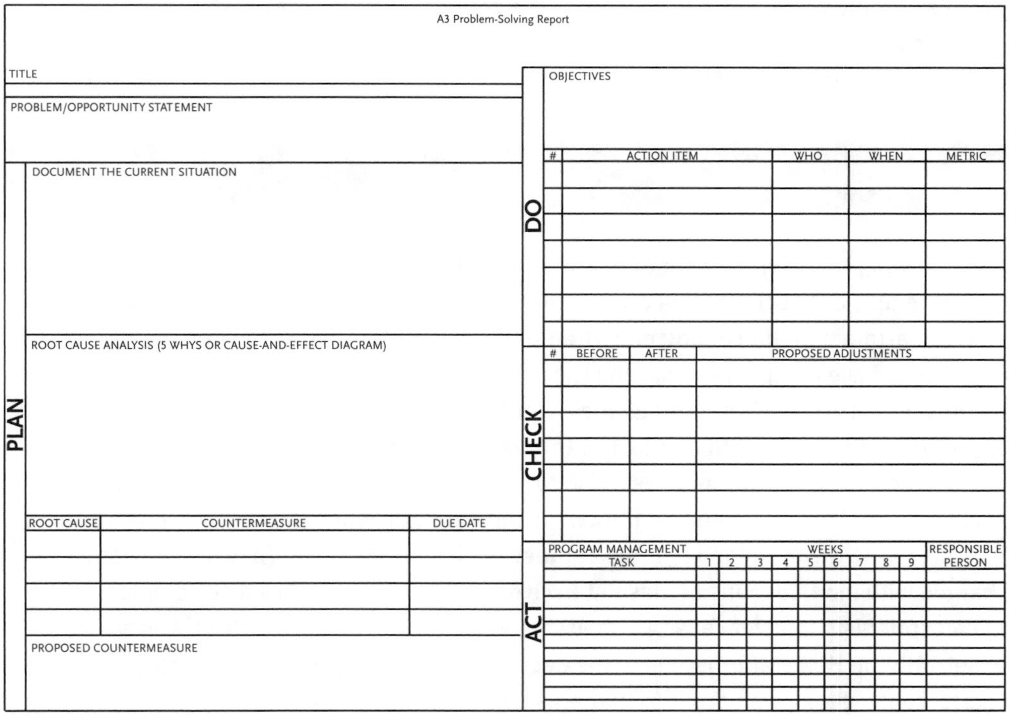

Source: Reprinted with permission from T. G. Zidel, *Lean Done Right: Achieve and Maintain Reform in Your Healthcare Organization*. Chicago: Health Administration Press. Copyright © 2012.

used to document Lean problem-solving projects, the format can be adapted as a concise report for any type of improvement project. Various other A3 report templates are available for free online.

CONCLUSION

Some quality problems can be easily solved in the course of everyday management. The solutions to more complex performance problems must be determined methodically. Several models can be used to conduct an improvement project. Although each model is different, all approaches involve analysis of current practices, implementation of solutions, and review of the solutions' effectiveness.

Teams use analytic tools throughout improvement projects to determine the causes of undesirable performance and to implement changes that result in measurable improvements. Some tools are quick and simple to use, whereas others are more complex. In most cases, experience gained from past initiatives informs a team's decisions about the tools best suited for different phases of an improvement project.

Successful project outcomes hinge on the project team's ability to address complex problems systematically and on the cooperation of professionals and departments in an organization. The third essential element, careful project management, is covered in the next chapter.

FOR DISCUSSION

Imagine you are the supervisor of the health information management (HIM) department in a large outpatient clinic. This department manages patient records. Complaints about your department are becoming more frequent and intense than in the past. Some clinic employees have complained that the HIM department takes too long to retrieve patient records. Others have expressed dismay over the rudeness of HIM staff. You decide to talk about these problems with employees throughout the clinic.

The clinic's receptionists respond to you defensively. They tell you that the HIM staff won't answer the phone and that they want some backup when they are busy with patients. You talk to the HIM staff and find their stories are just as negative. They say they are being charged with more responsibilities but have no additional help. They also complain that the receptionists transfer calls that they should be handling. The clinic's nurses are also upset with the HIM staff; they claim the department does not help them locate patient charts, causing long wait times for patients. The clinic's physicians say they cannot assume additional tasks to alleviate the situation because their days are already chaotic.

1. What improvement tool would you use to identify all possible reasons for the increase in complaints about the HIM department?

2. What improvement tool would you use to gather data to confirm the reasons for the complaints about the HIM department?

3. You hypothesize that complaints spike on certain days of the week. What improvement tool would you use to analyze this theory?

4. The HIM staff tally information about the causes of complaints. What improvement tool would you use to prioritize the problems?

5. What improvement tool would you use to define the current process for retrieving patient records?

6. You believe that cooperation between the clinic receptionists and HIM staff would improve if phone responsibilities were more clearly defined. To whom would you assign the task of defining roles and responsibilities?

7. After redesigning the record retrieval process, you want to monitor the effectiveness of your actions. What improvement tool would you use to determine whether the number of complaints has decreased?

WEBSITES

- Agency for Healthcare Research and Quality Innovations Exchange
  www.innovations.ahrq.gov

- American Society for Quality, Quality Tools
  www.asq.org/learn-about-quality/quality-tools.html

- BMJ Open Quality, quality improvement resources
  http://bmjopenquality.bmj.com/pages/about/

- Institute for Healthcare Improvement, quality improvement tools
  www.ihi.org/resources/Pages/Tools/default.aspx

- Lean Hospitals, downloadable Lean and Six Sigma project templates
  www.leanhospitals.org/downloads.php

- Minnesota Department of Public Health Quality Improvement Resources & Tools
  www.health.state.mn.us/divs/opi/qi/toolbox

- National Quality Center Quality Academy: Useful Quality Improvement Tools (tutorial)
  http://nationalqualitycenter.org/resources/nqc-quality-academy-useful-quality-improvement-tools/

- Research Methods Knowledge Base
  www.socialresearchmethods.net/kb

- Society of Hospital Medicine, quality improvement resources
  www.hospitalmedicine.org

- SurveyMonkey. 2009. "Response Rates & Surveying Techniques: Tips to Enhance Survey Respondent Participation"
  http://s3.amazonaws.com/SurveyMonkeyFiles/Response_Rates.pdf

REFERENCES

Best, M., and D. Neuhauser. 2008. "Kaoru Ishikawa: From Fishbones to World Peace." *Quality and Safety in Health Care* 17 (2): 150–52.

Centers for Medicare & Medicaid Services (CMS). 2017. "Hospital Compare." Accessed November 11. www.medicare.gov/hospitalcompare/.

Forsha, H. I. 1995. *Show Me: The Complete Guide to Storyboarding and Problem Solving.* Milwaukee, WI: ASQ Press.

Johnson, R. L., and G. B. Morgan. 2016. *Survey Scales: A Guide to Development, Analysis, and Reporting.* New York: Guilford Press.

New York State Department of Health AIDS Institute. 2006. *HIVQUAL Workbook: Guide for Quality Improvement in HIV Care.* Accessed November 11, 2017. http://nationalquality center.org/resources/hivqual-workbook-guide-for-quality-improvement-in-hiv-care-pdf/.

SurveyMonkey. 2008. "Smart Survey Design." Accessed November 11, 2017. http:// s3.amazonaws.com/SurveyMonkeyFiles/SmartSurvey.pdf.

Zidel, T. G. 2012. *Lean Done Right: Achieve and Maintain Reform in Your Healthcare Organization.* Chicago: Health Administration Press.

CHAPTER 7

IMPROVEMENT PROJECT TEAMS

LEARNING OBJECTIVES

After reading this chapter, you will be able to

➤ explain the role of improvement project participants,

➤ discuss the purpose of a team charter,

➤ recognize beneficial and disruptive team behaviors,

➤ apply leadership skills to manage team meetings effectively,

➤ describe the stages of team development, and

➤ identify strategies for preventing improvement project failures.

KEY WORDS

➤ Charter

➤ Facilitator

➤ Ground rules

➤ Independents

➤ Inputs

➤ Leadership

➤ Outputs

➤ Problem statement

➤ Process owners

➤ Sponsor

If improvement models are the recipe and if improvement tools are the ingredients, where does the improvement team fit into this analogy? When I bake a cake, I work alone; I do not need a group of people to help me. I could not work alone, however, if I had to prepare a banquet for 50 guests. I would need a team of people to help cook the meal. The more complex the process—whether cooking or improving health services quality—the greater is the need for teamwork. When improvement opportunities are identified, a group of people known as an *improvement team* is assembled. By following an improvement model and using improvement tools, the team works together to accomplish improvement goals. This team's success hinges on effective project management.

A formal team need not be assembled for every improvement opportunity. The case study at the beginning of chapter 3 describes an initiative to reduce patient wait times at the Redwood Health Center. The clinic manager did most of the work for this project. He gathered data on how long patients waited to be seen by a clinician, shared those data with other people in the clinic, and informally discussed ways of reducing wait times. An improvement team was not formed for the project. Likewise, for the improvement initiative involving patient identification wristbands at Community Hospital in chapter 4, a project team was not formed to resolve the problems people were having with the bands. After collecting information about band defects, the manager fixed the problem on her own. The case study discussing Sunrise Home Health Agency at the beginning of chapter 5 is yet another example of an informal initiative. The director and clinical staff members used regular staff meetings to revise the meeting process.

Some performance problems cannot (and should not) be solved individually or informally and require the attention of a dedicated improvement project team that includes several people familiar with the systems and processes that need to be changed. A project team should be created when the improvement goal is more likely to be achieved through the coordinated efforts of people with varying knowledge, skills, and perspectives. The greatest improvement potential lies in problems that involve different professions and departments. The team's role is to analyze and eliminate undesirable, unpredictable, or unworkable performance situations. Once the improvement project is complete, the team is disbanded.

People at all levels in the organization may be part of an improvement project team. Because projects generally take employees away from their primary work responsibilities, time spent on an improvement initiative had better produce measurable performance gains. This chapter describes ways to increase the likelihood that formal improvement projects will be successful.

PROJECT PARTICIPANTS

When the best approach to an improvement opportunity is a formal project, a team of people is chosen to fill the following roles:

◆ Sponsor

◆ Team leader

◆ Facilitator

◆ Recorder

◆ Timekeeper

◆ Team members

These roles are summarized in exhibit 7.1. Although the roles may vary, at a minimum each project has a sponsor, a team leader, and team members. Involvement of the other roles depends on the organization's resources and the scope of the project.

SPONSOR

The project **sponsor** is the individual or group that decides to initiate an improvement project. If the improvement project involves more than one department, a **leadership** representative or a quality oversight committee should sponsor the project. (The role of quality oversight committees is covered in chapter 12.) If the project affects activities in only one department or unit, the manager of that area usually serves as the sponsor.

The sponsor clearly defines the performance problem that needs to be solved by writing a **problem statement**—a description of the situation. The problem statement, sometimes called the aim statement, influences many aspects of the project, including the makeup of the team and the improvement expectations. In addition, a clearly communicated

Sponsor
An individual or a group that supports, guides, and mentors an improvement project team; serves as a link to the organization's leadership; removes barriers; and acquires the resources a team needs to achieve successful outcomes.

Leadership
An organization's senior leaders or decision makers.

Problem statement
A description of the performance problem that needs to be solved. Sometimes called the *aim statement*.

Exhibit 7.1

Roles of
Improvement
Project Participants

Project Participant	Role
Sponsor	Charters the improvement team, provides initial improvement goals, monitors team progress, and supports the team
Team leader	Coordinates project assignments and communication with external parties, removes barriers, and keeps the project on track
Facilitator	Helps manage discussions about the process during team meetings, usually by asking questions (e.g., How do we want to make this decision? What points can we agree on?)
Recorder	Captures ideas, decisions, action items, and assignments on a flip chart or whiteboard for later transcription into a written summary of the project
Timekeeper	Keeps track of time during project meetings
Team member	Participates in discussions, decision-making, and other team tasks such as gathering data, analyzing information, assisting with documentation, and sharing results

problem statement establishes project boundaries so that problem-solving activities do not escalate into larger issues or wander into unrelated topics.

The project goal should include measurable improvement expectations. For instance, the manager at Community Hospital hoped to achieve an 80 percent reduction in staff complaints about patient identification bands by making some process changes. The project sponsor sets these expectations and defines the time frame for achieving them. An explicit project goal with clearly stated, measurable expectations and time frames focuses the improvement efforts.

Once the goal is clear, the sponsor identifies people who need to be included in the project. If the sponsor already has someone in mind to serve as the team leader, that person may help the sponsor select these key people. The following questions can guide their selection:

◆ Where is the problem occurring?

◆ What tasks are involved?

◆ Who carries out these tasks?

◆ Who determines how the tasks should be done?

◆ Who provides the **inputs** to these tasks?

◆ Who uses the **outputs** of these tasks?

The people chosen for the team should possess detailed knowledge gained through experience with some part of the performance problem. They also must be willing and able to attend team meetings and make time for project work that may need to be done between meetings. Once the project is under way, the team may ask additional members to participate if critical expertise is needed or a key group is not represented. The team should be capped at five to ten members. To keep the team from expanding beyond the preferred size, some individuals may serve as consultants and attend meetings only when their expertise is needed.

In an ideal project initiation, the sponsor creates a written **charter** incorporating all the aforementioned elements: the project goal, a description of the system or process to be improved, the time frame for project completion, deliverables, measures, project scope, and team members. Exhibit 7.2 is a charter for a project aimed at improving the employee hiring process in a county-operated emergency medical service (ambulance) company.

When expectations are unclear or too broad, an improvement project can flounder. At one hospital, for example, staff members voiced concerns about the safety of the process of ordering, dispensing, and administering chemotherapy medications. An interdisciplinary team was chartered, which included representatives from the hospital's inpatient, outpatient, adult, and pediatric areas (physicians, nurses, pharmacists, and laboratory staff). Over a four-month period, the team developed a top-down flowchart of the process, which ultimately was diagrammed as 21 steps, each with multiple substeps. On review, the team realized the enormity of the project and discovered that each area had its own way of executing tasks. The charter the team developed at the outset of the project was too broad and was stalling the project. The team decided it would address only the adult outpatient population and limited the project to the medication administration phase, where most of the problems were occurring. Once the project scope and focus were better defined, the improvement initiative proceeded more quickly.

Charters keep teams focused and on track during projects. Team members may want to revisit the charter periodically to remind themselves of the project's boundaries and the objectives of the improvement effort. If the team receives new information during the project or if situations change, it may need to renegotiate its objectives or boundaries.

The sponsor supports the team throughout the project, monitoring progress and clearing obstacles that may arise. The sponsor acts as a sounding board for improvement ideas but does not become overly involved in the details of the team's work. At the end of the project, the sponsor reviews the team's improvement actions and ensures the solutions are effectively implemented.

Inputs
Products, services, or information flowing into a process.

Outputs
Products, services, or information flowing out of a process.

Charter
A written declaration of an improvement team's purpose. (An example of an improvement project charter is found in exhibit 7.2.)

EXHIBIT 7.2
Charter for
Improvement
Project

Problem Statement

- During the last fiscal year, 342 applications were received for paramedic or emergency medical technician (EMT) vacancies. In this same period, 49 applicants—14%—were hired and eventually began employment with Grant County Emergency Medical Services (EMS).
- The current hiring process for EMTs and paramedics averages 87 days with a range of 7 to 212 days from time of application.
- As of February, EMS operations are understaffed by 17% (47 vacancies for EMTs and paramedics).
- Understaffing causes an increase in EMS operational overtime, idle time during field training, and system and administrative workload.

Goal

A 5% or less vacancy rate for EMTs and paramedics

Project Scope

Individuals who apply for a paramedic or EMT position with Grant County EMS

Out-of-Project Scope

- Existing paramedic or EMT employees who are promoted or return to full-time status
- Vacancies for other positions

Measures

- Current vacancies
- Current overtime standby utilization
- Hiring process intervals (in days) and cost
- Applicants (count)
- Applicant status (percentage of overall applicants)
- Range of application date to start date

Deliverables

Within 6 months:

- Increase the hire rate of qualified applicants from 14% to 30%.
- Reduce annualized cost of EMS overtime and standby time to less than $280,000.
- Reduce cost per new hire (recruiting, advertising, and assessing) to no more than $300.

Sponsor	Robert Jones, Director, Public Safety
Team Leader	Larry McNeill, Deputy Chief, EMS Training
Team Members	• Jackie Gregory, Administrative Services • Todd O'Brien, Human Resources • Michael Fine, EMT • Gary Young, Paramedic
Team Facilitator	Sally Steward, Manager, Information Services

TEAM LEADER

The team leader organizes the project, chairs team discussions, keeps the project focused on the improvement goal, establishes the meeting schedule, and serves as a liaison between the team and the sponsor. Often, team leaders are **process owners**—supervisors, managers, or physicians in the work area most affected by the improvement project. The leader is considered a member of the team.

The team leader should be familiar with the improvement model to be used during the project and various improvement tools. She should also be skilled at managing group interactions and running a project. Some organizations assign a quality resource advisor to interdepartmental improvement projects. This person is familiar with performance improvement principles and serves as an internal consultant. The quality resource advisor helps the team understand the purpose of the project, the desired results, and team roles and responsibilities. When there is no quality advisor assigned to the project, the team leader takes on these responsibilities.

Process owners
Individuals ultimately responsible for a process, including its performance and outcomes.

> **? DID YOU KNOW?**
>
> A team leader's abilities and characteristics influence the outcome of an improvement initiative. Studies have demonstrated the importance of the following characteristics of a team leader (Turner and Müller 2005):
>
> - Problem-solving ability
> - Perspective
> - Results orientation
> - Communication skills
> - Energy and initiative
> - Negotiation skills
> - Self-confidence

FACILITATOR

The **facilitator** supports the team leader. The facilitator assists with team-building activities, keeps meeting discussions and the entire project on track, and ensures deadlines are met. The facilitator should be an objective team resource and detached from the process being improved. As a neutral party, the facilitator is particularly effective at engaging everyone on the team and helping the group reach consensus on controversial issues.

Facilitator
An individual knowledgeable about group processes and team interaction as well as performance improvement principles and techniques.

The facilitator works with the leader to plan meetings, structure tasks and assignments, and incorporate quality improvement tools into the project. The facilitator knows what data to gather, how to gather the data, and how to present the results in a meaningful graphic or tabular form.

In cases where the project is not overly complex, one person may assume the dual role of team leader and facilitator. Research suggests, however, that multifaceted healthcare improvement projects involving several departments and professions benefit from having a facilitator who is not also responsible for leading the project (Agency for Healthcare Research and Quality 2013).

RECORDER

The recorder, or notetaker, documents activities throughout the project. This position is usually assigned to one or more team members. During meetings, recorders are responsible for writing the team's ideas, decisions, and recommendations on a flip chart or whiteboard. Recorders also create meeting minutes and distribute them to team members before the next meeting. The team uses the minutes to recall previous ideas, decisions, the rationales behind the decisions, actions to be taken, the people responsible for executing those actions, and the schedule according to which those actions will be carried out.

TIMEKEEPER

The timekeeper keeps the team on track during meetings. If the time allotted for a discussion point is exceeded, the timekeeper alerts the group. The team then decides whether to accelerate the discussion, defer the item to another meeting, or end the discussion. In some cases, the leader functions as the timekeeper, or this role may be assigned to the facilitator or another team member.

TEAM MEMBERS

Team members share responsibility for achieving the improvement goal. Members participate in discussions, decision-making, and other team tasks such as data collection. Each team member should represent a program, department, or work unit significantly affected by the process to be improved or the problem to be solved. Ideally, team members should have a basic understanding of quality improvement principles, but familiarity with this topic is not a prerequisite for team membership.

Inclusion of one or two **independents**—members with little or no knowledge of the process—can also be useful. Because independents have no vested interest in the problem, they may provide a fresh and creative perspective. Some healthcare improvement projects also benefit from customer input. For example, if a hospital team is working to improve security in the maternity ward, a woman who recently delivered a baby in the facility can be included as a team member. The recent patient may be made a permanent member of the team or serve part time by attending meetings only when her input is needed.

⊛ **LEARNING POINT**
Project Participants

An improvement project involves several roles. At a minimum, each project includes a sponsor, a team leader, and team members.

Independents
Improvement team members who have little or no knowledge of the process under consideration and have no vested interest in the outcome of the project.

TEAM MEETINGS

At the first meeting, the team leader uses the project charter to introduce and explain the project goal and scope. He should discuss the charter openly to prevent misunderstandings. Any confusion or disagreement should be resolved at the first meeting.

The team leader also provides an overview of the project timeline at the first meeting. Exhibit 7.3 is a Gantt chart showing the approximate start and finish times for the steps of an improvement project.

The first meeting also is a good time to set **ground rules** for team conduct—directives stating how team members are expected to communicate in meetings, make decisions, resolve conflicts, and so forth. Critical concept 7.1 lists examples of improvement team ground rules. Teams usually adopt only a few key ground rules; however, project improvement best practices do not limit the number (Barner and Barner 2012).

Ground rules
Established guidelines for how an improvement team wants to operate; norms for behavior. (Examples of ground rules are found in critical concept 7.1.)

EXHIBIT 7.3
Gantt Chart for an Improvement Project

	March	April	May	June	July	August	September	October
Develop project charter	■							
Appoint improvement team		■						
Kick off project— first team meeting		◆						
Analyze current practices			■					
Gather performance data			■	■				
Identify improvement opportunities— second meeting					◆			
Solicit solution ideas from colleagues					■			
Finalize solutions— third meeting						◆		
Implement solutions on a trial basis						■		
Evaluate the effect of solutions— fourth meeting							◆	
Roll out successful solutions								■
Redesign ineffective solutions— fifth meeting								◆

> $\textcircled{!}$ **CRITICAL CONCEPT 7.1**
> Improvement Team Ground Rules
>
> - Participate by sharing your own opinions and experiences.
> - Contribute but do not dominate.
> - Actively listen to and consider the opinions of others.
> - Stay focused on the improvement goal.
> - Avoid side conversations.
> - Respect other people's time (e.g., arrive on time, do not leave early, return from breaks promptly).
> - Complete assignments to which you have committed.
> - Speak one at a time.
> - Leave rank at the door; all team members are equal.
> - Address conflict by dealing with the issue, not the person.
> - Turn off cell phones and other mobile devices.
> - Be a participant, not a lurker.
> - Have fun, but not at the expense of someone else's feelings.
> - Be physically and mentally present during meetings.
> - Listen, listen, listen, and respond.
> - Allow for some mistakes; acknowledge them, let go, and move on.
> - Accept conflict and its resolution as necessary catalysts for learning.
> - Be open-minded to new thoughts and different behaviors.
> - Honor confidentiality.
> - Accept diversity as a gift.
> - Begin and end all meetings on time.
> - Share in the responsibilities of the recorder.
> - Criticize ideas, not individuals.

Some organizations have a core set of ground rules for all improvement projects. From this set, teams are usually allowed to select the rules they wish to observe. If the organization has no such set of rules, the leader solicits ideas from the team members by asking them to describe acceptable team behaviors. When the list is finalized and everyone understands the ground rules, members individually acknowledge that they agree to abide by the group behaviors. Posting the rules on a large sheet of paper in the meeting room is an effective way to remind group members of the rules they agreed to follow.

IMPROVEMENT PROJECT LENGTH

The time needed to complete an improvement project varies. Some projects are elephant-sized, and some are bite-sized. Exhibit 7.4 is a timeline for completing a project involving hospital signage. At this hospital, patients occasionally have difficulty finding the outpatient testing departments. Although signs are posted to lead the way, patients may not be able to read the signs or the signs may be unclear. The director of the patient registration department brought this concern to the attention of the chief operating officer, who then sponsored a project to resolve the problem.

Not all projects are completed quickly. A project team at the University of Wisconsin Hospital and Clinics was formed for the purpose of improving the use of intravenous pumps to deliver patient medications (Tosha et al. 2006). The 22-member team included representatives from anesthesiology, biomedical engineering central supply, industrial engineering, internal medicine, nursing, and pharmacy. The team met for 46 hours over four-and-a-half months to describe the process, identify improvement opportunities, and design solutions, and then it took additional time to implement the solutions (Tosha et al. 2006).

Whether the project is long or short, the team should meet regularly; otherwise, enthusiasm for achieving the improvement goal diminishes. The project sponsor must stay informed of the progress of the initiative and intervene when progress is moving too slowly.

THE LEADER'S RESPONSIBILITIES

The team leader manages project meetings. This responsibility involves activities that ensure meetings are well run, including

- preparing the meeting agenda and distributing it at least one day in advance,

- keeping the meeting focused on the agenda,

- encouraging participation by all team members,

- fostering an environment in which team members feel safe expressing their ideas, and

- distributing the last meeting's minutes before the next meeting.

EXHIBIT 7.4
Timeline for an
Improvement
Project

Timeline	Activities
Week 1	The team meets for two hours to discuss project objectives and set ground rules. The members brainstorm reasons patients might get lost when trying to find outpatient testing departments. To determine whether these assumptions are correct, the members will gather some data over the next seven days. Some members will evaluate the current signs, and other members will interview patients and staff in the testing areas to gain their perspective.
Week 2	The team meets for two hours to review the collected data. In three locations, the signs are not at eye level, making it more difficult for people to see them. People who are having an electrocardiogram (EKG) may not recognize that they need to go to the EKG unit. Five of the interviewed patients have limited English proficiency and cannot read the signs. Several staff members confirm that lack of English proficiency is a major cause of the problem. The team comes up with three solutions: 1. Place all signs at eye level. 2. Describe outpatient departments and testing areas in terms that laypeople can understand. 3. Color code departments/testing areas (lines of the corresponding color will be painted along the wall to lead patients to the different areas). The team drafts an implementation plan for each of these solutions.
Weeks 3–7	• Team members identify signs using terminology that laypeople may not understand. New signs with patient-friendly terminology are manufactured. • Maintenance staff move existing signs to eye level and hang all new signs at eye level. • Colors are assigned to each testing area. Maintenance staff paint lines of the corresponding color along the walls leading from the registration area to the various departments. The team leader monitors the activities to ensure the solutions are implemented as expected.
Week 8	The team meets for one hour to discuss the solutions' effectiveness. Members agree to gather information to evaluate the success of the solutions. Some members will evaluate the new signs, and some members will interview staff in the testing areas to gain their perspective.
Week 9	The team meets for one hour to review data collection results. All signs are now at eye level. The director of the patient registration department reports that patients are pleased with the color coding and that no patients are having difficulty finding the outpatient departments. Staff in the testing departments report similar findings. The project is deemed a success.

The leader's responsibilities are not glamorous, but leaders keep meetings running smoothly and prevent them from becoming sloppy and unproductive. Without a leader's guidance and preparation, team members may come to meetings unprepared and fail to follow up on decisions made at prior meetings. Absent a clear agenda, meetings are likely to veer off track. When meetings deteriorate, issues are left unresolved and team members become frustrated. In their frustration, they may stop showing up for meetings. The responsibility of keeping meetings focused does not rest on the team leader alone, however. All team members must cooperate to ensure successful meeting outcomes.

To minimize disruptions, meetings should flow in an orderly manner and include the following elements:

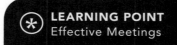

LEARNING POINT
Effective Meetings

Strong leadership is essential to a well-functioning improvement project. One of a team leader's first activities is to help the group establish ground rules and ensure the team abides by them. While team meetings are an essential part of the improvement project, meetings that lack focus, drag on, or are unproductive can be a source of frustration. Not only the leader but all team members are responsible for keeping meetings on track.

- A brief overview of the agenda, including the primary objective of the meeting

- A short update (no longer than five minutes) on work completed since the last meeting, including a synopsis of any major obstacles encountered

- A group assessment of overall progress, including a review of the improvement project timeline

- A brief discussion or time for reflection on the team's functioning as a group

- Assignment of action items to be accomplished by the next meeting

If team members talk or have questions about an issue that is not on the agenda, the leader can write the topic on a big piece of paper marked "Issues Bin" or "Parking Lot." The team can discuss these issues later or defer them to the next meeting. To keep the meeting moving, the leader may need to make arbitrary decisions about parking lot issues. If time allows, the leader can ask the group whether it wants to park the issue or discuss it.

TEAM DYNAMICS

Tension always arises between people who come together to accomplish a common goal. For instance, when my relatives plan our annual family reunion, they always disagree on the date, location, or other details. At least one contrarian in the group wants everything her way. My uncle interrupts to voice his opinions. My older sister doesn't say a word until everyone is in agreement. When she finally speaks, she complains about the decision. In the midst of this turmoil, I wonder why we bother to have reunions. In the end, though, they turn out to be lots of fun and worth the effort.

An improvement team is like a family. Each member of the team brings his values, beliefs, and personal agendas to the project. Some people show up at the first meeting thinking they already know what the problem is and how it should be fixed. Some team members are unwilling to express their opinions when a manager or leader is in the room. Some members want to be sure the improvement solutions will not require too much extra work. These people typically advocate easy-to-implement solutions even though other improvement actions might produce better results. The team leader, assisted by the facilitator, is responsible for managing this diverse group of people.

One of the team leader's greatest challenges is moving the improvement team through the stages of team development. In the 1960s, psychologist B. W. Tuckman (1965) identified four stages that all teams go through to become productive:

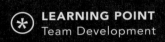

LEARNING POINT
Team Development

Improvement teams mature experientially and in stages; designating a group of individuals to function as a team is only the first step in team development. Developing a group of people into a team takes time, commitment, and energy. To achieve desired outcomes, teams must establish and focus on common goals ahead of personal needs.

1. *Forming.* The team meets and works together for the first time.

2. *Storming.* Team members "jockey" for position and struggle for control.

3. *Norming.* Team members adjust to one another and feel comfortable working together.

4. *Performing.* The team begins to function as a highly effective, problem-solving group.

Typical team characteristics and the role of the leader at each stage of development are summarized in exhibit 7.5. As mentioned earlier, if a facilitator has been assigned to the team, he will help the leader with team-building and project management responsibilities.

The rapidity of a team's progression through the four stages depends on the composition of the team, the capabilities of the team leader and members, and the tasks to be performed. But no team passes through the storming stage quickly. This stage is uncomfortable, but this discomfort and any conflict experienced are all prerequisites to successful project outcomes. When the leader is not able to help the team work through the storming phase, members are less likely to voice different perspectives. The success of the improvement project is jeopardized if team members cannot work as a cohesive group.

Stage	Team Characteristics	Role of Team Leader
Forming Members are concerned with inclusion and acceptance.	• Interactions are polite and superficial; open conflict is rare. • Groupthink (conformity of opinion) tends to dominate. • Members rely on the leader for direction. • Project goals are not clear.	The leader's role is primarily directive. She introduces the team members to the project and shares project goals and the timeline for completion. The leader helps team members become acquainted and allows time for them to get comfortable with one another while still moving the project along. Ground rules are established.
Storming Members want to be heard and begin to assert control.	• Participation increases; members want to exercise some influence on the improvement project. • Groupthink decreases; open conflict increases. • Members look more critically at the improvement process and question how and why decisions are made. • Members may challenge the team leader directly or indirectly.	The leader clarifies the team's role in achieving project goals and addresses conflicts as they surface. Ground rules are reviewed and enforced. The purpose of the improvement project is revisited. The leader engages the project sponsor in resolving conflicts that cannot be effectively handled within the team structure.
Norming Members have a good understanding of the improvement process and want to accomplish the project goals.	• Members are friendlier and more supportive of one another. • Ground rules that may have been overlooked in the beginning are now taken more seriously. • Subgroups may be formed to move the project along more quickly. • Conflict is handled openly and constructively.	The leader encourages members to spend less time on idea generation and more time on decision-making. She keeps the team on track toward improvement goals and provides time for discussion and feedback.
Performing Members are highly effective problem solvers.	• All contributions are recognized and appreciated. • Members develop a sense of cohesiveness and team identity. • Project goals are achieved. Members may look for additional improvement opportunities.	The leader takes a less directive and more supportive role as members actively take responsibility for achieving the improvement goals.

EXHIBIT 7.5

Team Characteristics and the Role of the Team Leader Through the Four Stages of Development

Improvement teams do not develop as neatly and sequentially as these stages imply. Teams can cycle from one stage to another relatively easily or become stuck in one stage. The team leader must identify where the team is along the development path and move it to the next phase with minimal fuss and resistance. Leaders with good team facilitation skills are better able to help teams progress through the stages than are leaders with poor skills in this area.

CONCLUSION

As healthcare processes become increasingly complex, teams of people working in various aspects of the delivery system must be personally involved in improving them. To achieve improvement goals, the environment must foster team interaction and open communication. Such an environment promotes the generation of new ideas and continuous improvement.

Effective teams share many characteristics, but respect for other team members is essential. Cooperation as a team requires trust among its members, focus on—and belief in—the end goal, less argument, and more exploration.

In the early stages of a team's existence, members are dependent on the initiative of the team sponsor and leader. As the team develops, it begins to take responsibility for the success of the project. It is then that each member should fully participate, suggest improvements, challenge other members when needed, and support the established ground rules.

FOR DISCUSSION

1. Of the ground rules listed in critical concept 7.1, which three are most important for a team to adopt, and why? When choosing the rules, consider your past experiences working with a team or a decision-making group.

2. Use the template in exhibit 7.2 to create a charter for an improvement project involving a healthcare process that you are familiar with. Complete as many sections of the charter as possible.

3. If you were the team leader of the group described in the following case study, how would you refocus and remotivate the team toward achieving the improvement goal?

When members were recruited for the improvement project, they were told that the team's work would be additional to their regular work responsibilities but that they had to treat team activities as a high priority. They were expected to complete team assignments on time and were required to attend meetings. Despite being aware of these clear expectations, by the third week of the project, team members started arriving late to meetings, making excuses for not having completed their assigned tasks, and neglecting to return the leader's phone calls.

WEBSITES

- Agency for Healthcare Research and Quality. *Practice Facilitation Handbook.* www.ahrq.gov/professionals/prevention-chronic-care/improve/system/pfhandbook/index.html

- Agency for Healthcare Research and Quality Primary Care Practice Facilitation learning community
www.pcmh.ahrq.gov/page/practice-facilitation

- Health Research & Educational Trust. 2013. *Leading Improvement Across the Continuum: Skills, Tools and Teams for Success.* Chicago: Health Research & Educational Trust.
www.hpoe.org/Reports-HPOE/Improvement_Continuum_October2013.pdf

- Health Resources & Services Administration, Improvement Teams
www.hrsa.gov/sites/default/files/quality/toolbox/508pdfs/improvementteams.pdf

- Institute for Patient- and Family-Centered Care, *Partnering with Patients and Families to Enhance Safety and Quality: A Mini Toolkit*
www.ihi.org/education/conferences/APACForum2012/Documents/I1_Toolkit.pdf

- National Quality Center Quality Academy: Using Teams to Improve Quality (tutorial)
http://nationalqualitycenter.org/resources/nqc-quality-academy-using-teams-to-improve-quality/

REFERENCES

Agency for Healthcare Research and Quality. 2013. *Practice Facilitation Handbook.* Published June. www.ahrq.gov/professionals/prevention-chronic-care/improve/system/pfhandbook/index.html.

Barner, R., and C. P. Barner. 2012. *Building Better Teams: 70 Tools and Techniques for Strengthening Performance Within and Across Teams.* San Francisco: Pfeiffer.

Tosha, B., T. B. Wetterneck, K. A. Skibinski, T. L. Roberts, S. M. Kleppin, M. E. Schroeder, M. Enloe, S. S. Rough, A. Schoofs Hundt, and P. Carayon. 2006. "Using FMEA to Plan Implementation of Smart IV Pump Technology." *American Journal of Health-System Pharmacy* 63 (16): 1528–38.

Tuckman, B. W. 1965. "Developmental Sequence in Small Groups." *Psychological Bulletin* 63: 384–89.

Turner, J. R., and R. Müller. 2005. "The Project Manager's Leadership Style as a Success Factor on Projects: A Literature Review." *Project Management Journal* 36 (1): 49–61.

CHAPTER 8

IMPROVING PATIENT SAFETY

LEARNING OBJECTIVES

After reading this chapter, you will be able to

➤ contrast quality management and patient safety,

➤ recognize measures of patient safety,

➤ use prospective risk analysis to improve the safety of healthcare processes,

➤ use root cause analysis to improve patient safety, and

➤ describe the patient's role in reducing adverse events.

KEY WORDS

➤ Accident

➤ Adverse event

➤ Critical failures

➤ Criticality

➤ Failure

➤ Failure mode and effects analysis (FMEA)

➤ Failure modes

➤ Faulty system design

➤ Hazard analysis

➤ Hazards

➤ High-risk activities

➤ Incident reports

➤ Incidents

➤ Medical errors

➤ Medication error

➤ Mistake proofing

➤ Near miss

➤ Patient safety

➤ Patient safety organizations (PSOs)

➤ Proactive risk assessment

➤ Reportable events

➤ Risk

➤ Risk analysis

➤ Root cause analysis (RCA)

➤ Safeguards

➤ Safety

➤ Sentinel event

➤ System

➤ Vigilant

➤ Work systems

Medical errors
Preventable adverse events or near misses during the provision of healthcare services.

Patient safety
Actions undertaken by individuals and organizations to protect healthcare recipients from being harmed by the effects of healthcare services; also defined as freedom from accidental or preventable injuries produced by medical care.

Although all healthcare professionals espouse the principle "First, do no harm," patients are occasionally harmed by caregivers' actions—or inactions. The Institute of Medicine's (IOM 2000) report *To Err Is Human: Building a Safer Health System* estimated that 44,000 to 98,000 Americans die each year as a result of preventable medical errors. IOM calculated the cost of **medical errors**, in terms of lost income, costs related to disability, and healthcare costs, at about $29 billion per year, which does not account for the incalculable emotional cost of losing a loved one. The publication caused a public outcry that led to increased attention to **patient safety**.

Despite continued efforts by healthcare organizations to improve patient safety, however, potentially avoidable safety problems still exist. A recent study by Johns Hopkins patient safety experts calculated that more than 250,000 deaths per year in the United States are due to medical errors (Makary and Daniel 2016). The *2016 National Healthcare Quality Report* revealed several opportunities for improvement (AHRQ 2017):

◆ Almost 5 percent of adult hospital patients receiving warfarin experienced an adverse drug event related to this anticoagulant.

◆ For every 1,000 live births, 1.9 percent of neonates are injured due to birth trauma.

◆ Of adult patients receiving hip joint replacement due to fracture, 9.8 percent experienced an in-hospital adverse event.

◆ More than 3 percent of hospitalized patients experience mechanical adverse events associated with central venous catheter placement.

◆ Of long-stay nursing home residents, 3.4 percent had a major injury as the result of a fall.

◆ Nearly 12 percent of adults aged 65 or older were prescribed a potentially inappropriate medication.

One of the broad quality improvement aims of every healthcare organization must be to make care safer by reducing harm caused during the delivery of care.

Safety in Healthcare

In the 2001 report *Crossing the Quality Chasm: A New Health System for the 21st Century*, IOM lists safe healthcare as one of the six dimensions of healthcare quality. Healthcare facilities have had **safety** programs in place for many years. The purpose of these programs is to provide an environment in which **hazards** are eliminated or minimized for employees, staff, patients, and visitors. Safety is promoted through several activities, including risk management, emergency preparedness, hazardous materials management, radiation safety, environmental safety and hygiene, security, and preventive maintenance. Historically, however, no organized approach has been taken to prevent medical errors that cause harm to patients.

The prevention of mistakes in healthcare is not new, but it has long been taken for granted. Error prevention was essentially entrusted to individuals: The physicians, nurses, technicians, clerical staff, and others who provide care for patients or support patient care activities were expected to do the right thing—correctly—every time. When an error occurred, the person involved usually was blamed for being careless, incompetent, or thoughtless. Organizations focused on training and hiring competent people, believing they would be less likely to make mistakes. This reliance on healthcare professionals and support staff to perform faultlessly was misguided.

Safety
The quality or condition of being safe; freedom from danger, injury, or damage.

Hazards
Events, actions, or things that can cause harm.

Faulty system design
Work system failures
that set up individuals
who work in that
system to fail.

Incidents
Events or occurrences
that could have led or
did lead to undesirable
results.

System
A set of interdependent
elements that interact
to achieve a common
aim.

Work systems
Sets of interdependent
elements, both
human and nonhuman
(e.g., equipment,
technologies), that
interact to achieve a
common aim.

Accident
An unplanned,
unexpected event,
usually with an adverse
consequence.

Vigilant
Carefully observant
or attentive; on the
lookout for possible
problems.

While the development of a competent staff is important, poor working conditions can make even the finest professionals prone to error. Investigations of mishaps, such as the Three Mile Island nuclear accident in 1979 and the space shuttle *Challenger* disaster in 1986, have found that "accidents are generally the outcome of a chain of events set in motion by **faulty system design** that either induces errors or makes them difficult to detect" (Leape et al. 1995, 35; emphasis added). Faulty system design is also a factor in most medical **incidents**. While an individual may have made a mistake, the root cause of that mistake likely lies in the design of the patient care **system**.

Healthcare professionals' decisions and actions are influenced by multiple factors, including the organizational culture, personal attitudes and qualifications, the composition of the work group, the physical resources available, and the design of **work systems** and processes. Consider the event described in critical concept 8.1. Although the radiology technician erred by not responding to what the patient was saying, this mistake was encouraged by faulty equipment and a departmental procedure that failed to account for the possibility of an equipment malfunction.

Accident research in other industries has shown that people's ability to catch and correct mistakes is not infallible (Reason 2008). Even the most explicit procedure or most exacting preventive maintenance schedule cannot eliminate the possibility of human error. Healthcare professionals watch for errors and usually catch and correct them before patients are harmed, but if faulty system design causes numerous little mistakes, healthcare professionals can easily pass over a few without noticing. According to one research study, hospital nurses encounter about one problem per hour that prevents them from continuing their tasks (Tucker and Edmondson 2003). Examples of problems include missing supplies, lack of information, and out-of-stock medications. The nurses must resolve these problems to continue with their duties. In systems that are so problem-prone, even highly competent, **vigilant** nurses are unlikely to catch every error.

 CRITICAL CONCEPT 8.1
Patient Care Event Resulting in Patient Harm

A patient tells the radiology technician that she is feeling heat from the X-ray equipment. The technician dismisses the patient's concerns and continues with the exam because the X-ray procedure states that the machine should be turned off only if the equipment's malfunction warning bulb lights up. Because the mechanical warning system failed, the patient suffers burns.

Healthcare systems that depend on perfect human performance are fatally flawed. Mistakes can be made by anyone. In general, they result from circumstances beyond the conscious control of the person who errs. To improve patient safety, systems and processes must be examined to see if changes are needed to reduce the chance that a patient will be harmed. The goal is to lessen the **risk** of errors. If an error does occur, reliable safeguards should prevent the mistake from reaching the patient. If the error does reach the patient, response mechanisms should act quickly to reduce the amount of harm to the patient.

Risk
The possibility of loss or injury.

Patient safety improvement initiatives are an important component of a healthcare organization's overall quality management effort. These initiatives focus primarily on the clinical aspects of patient care, but the same techniques used to protect patients from harm can be applied to any work activity, including billing, patient registration, plant maintenance, and housekeeping.

PREVENTING MISTAKES

Most mistakes are not intentional but occur because a process is complex. Even simple patient care processes are complex in terms of the variables involved. Consider, for example, the hospital process of obtaining a blood specimen for laboratory testing illustrated in exhibit 8.1.

The variables in this process include the method used to order the test (handwritten or electronic), the patient's location, the method used to collect the specimen, the type of vials used to store the blood, the method of laboratory analysis, the manner in which results are reported, and many more. Considering all these factors, the results are likely to be inaccurate at least some of the time.

At best, the process can be changed to make errors impossible. We encounter examples of **mistake proofing** every day. Here are just a few:

◆ Heating devices that shut off automatically so that they are not left on all day

◆ Circuit breakers that trip when circuits are overloaded

> (*) **LEARNING POINT**
> Healthcare Safety
>
> Traditionally, healthcare organizations have relied on the people providing patient care to prevent errors. However, processes that rely on perfect human performance are fatally flawed. An organized, systems improvement approach is needed to prevent errors that cause harm to patients.

Mistake proofing
Improving processes to prevent mistakes or to make mistakes obvious at a glance; also called error proofing.

EXHIBIT 8.1
High-Level Flowchart of Hospital Laboratory Testing

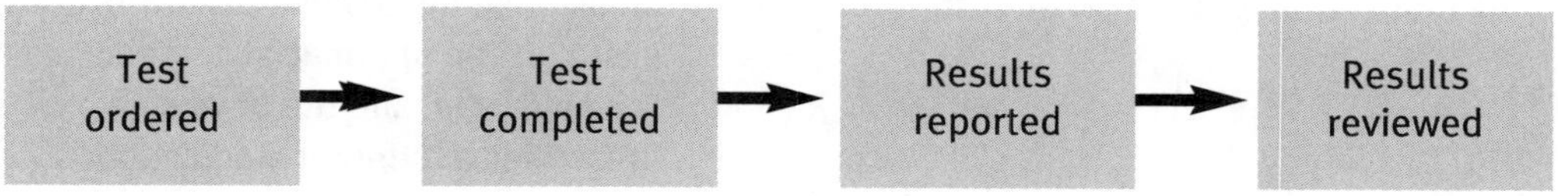

Test ordered → Test completed → Results reported → Results reviewed

◆ Computer disks that have overwrite protection

◆ Lawn mower motors that shut off when the operator lets go of the handle

◆ Containers that organize pills by day and time to prevent missed doses or accidental overdoses

    Unfortunately, elimination of all possible chances for error is not always feasible. In such cases, patient care processes should be redesigned so the chances of harmful errors are minimized. By adding **safeguards** to a process, the likelihood of causing patient harm can be greatly reduced. Exhibit 8.2 provides examples of patient care mistakes and safeguards that catch and correct the mistakes before they reach the hospitalized patient.

    High-risk activities usually incorporate several safeguards. Exhibit 8.3 is an illustration of a hospital's medication administration process and errors that could occur at

Safeguards
Physical, human, or administrative controls incorporated into a process to identify and correct errors before a patient is harmed.

High-risk activities
Tasks or processes known to be error-prone or that have the potential for causing significant patient harm should an error occur.

EXHIBIT 8.2
Mistakes and Safeguards That Prevent Patient Harm in the Hospital

Mistake	Safeguard
A surgeon starts to close a patient's surgical incision at the completion of an operation for extensive bowel repair, not knowing that a surgical sponge has been left inside the patient.	The scrub nurse conducts a sponge count and discovers one is missing. The surgeon locates the sponge inside the abdomen and removes it before closing the incision.
The phlebotomist starts to draw blood from the left arm of the patient, not knowing that the patient has just undergone a mastectomy on the left side and should not have blood drawn from that arm.	A red wristband on the patient's left arm alerts the phlebotomist that the left arm should not be used for blood draws.
A hospital dietary worker delivers an unmarked food tray to a patient room. He assumes he is delivering the tray to the correct room because it is the last tray on the cart and the patient in the room is the only patient in the nursing unit who has not yet received a meal.	A large sign indicating "nothing by mouth" is hung by the patient's bed. The dietary worker sees the sign and does not leave the food tray for the patient.
A physician prescribes a medication, not knowing that the patient is allergic to it.	The pharmacist reviews the patient's medication history and discovers the mistake. The pharmacist contacts the physician, and the physician prescribes a different medication.

various stages. Notice the reviews along the way that catch and remedy those mistakes. When these safeguards do not work as intended, mistakes can reach the patient. To further safeguard patients, healthcare organizations are adopting new error-prevention strategies and techniques, which are covered in detail in chapter 9.

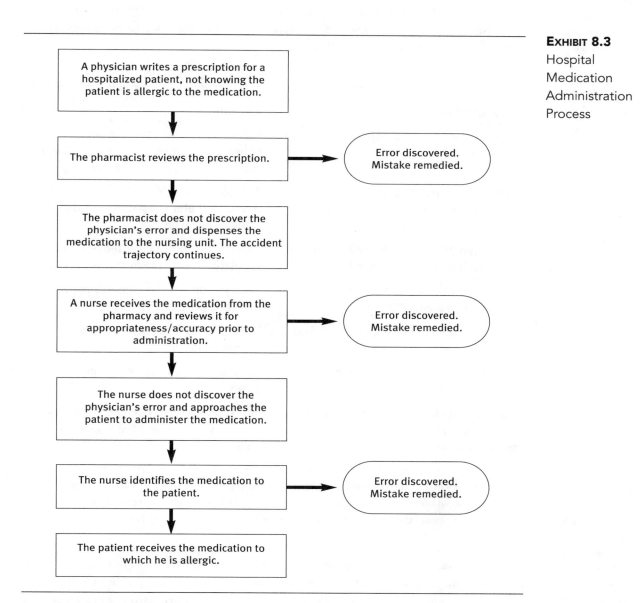

EXHIBIT 8.3
Hospital Medication Administration Process

Source: Spath (2001). Used with permission.

Adverse event

An event that results in unintended harm to the patient and is related to the care or services provided to the patient, rather than to the patient's underlying medical conditions.

MEASURING PATIENT SAFETY

The purpose of patient safety performance measurement is to discover and fix problems before an **adverse event** occurs. Measures of patient safety are like canaries in coal mines; they warn of risky situations before a mishap occurs. Patient safety measures are no different from other healthcare performance measurements. Many of the measures described in chapter 3 alert the organization to situations that are a potential safety threat to patients. Examples of patient safety topics and the system-level measures used to assess corresponding performance are shown in exhibit 8.4.

EXHIBIT 8.4
Patient Safety Topics and System-Level Measures

Topic of Interest	Measure
How often do patients develop an infection as a result of surgery?	Number of surgical cases in which patients developed an infection following surgery per 100 procedure days
How often do patients develop an infection as a result of a central venous catheter?	Average number of hospital-wide central venous catheter infections per 1,000 catheter line days
How often do patients develop pneumonia as a result of being on a ventilator?	Rate of pneumonia detected per 1,000 ventilator days in the intensive care units
How often do patients have an adverse reaction to a medication?	Average number of adverse drug events per 1,000 doses
How often do patients experience a fall?	Number of falls per 10,000 adjusted patient days*
How often do patients experience a medication error?	Number of medication errors per 1,000 doses
How often do long-stay nursing home residents who are at high risk for having a pressure ulcer actually develop one?	Percentage of high-risk long-stay nursing home residents who have a pressure ulcer

* Adjusted patient days: quantity calculated by the financial department that is based on the sum of inpatient days and financial equivalent patient days, which is determined by applying a formula to outpatient treatments, thereby accounting for inpatients and outpatients in this quantity.

Incident reports

Instruments (paper or electronic) used to document occurrences that could have led or did lead to undesirable results. (An example of an incident report is shown in exhibit 8.5.)

Incident reports, sometimes called *occurrence reports*, are paper or electronic forms used to document potential or actual patient safety concerns. Employees are asked to complete a report whenever a patient is involved in an event that has caused or has the potential to cause injury. The following are examples of **reportable events**:

◆ Error that occurs during the delivery of patient care (e.g., medication administration mistake, treatment error)

◆ Development of a condition seemingly unrelated to a patient's disease (e.g., infection, pressure ulcer)

◆ Adverse or suspected adverse reaction to a treatment, medication, or blood transfusion

◆ Serious injury or unexpected death of a patient

◆ Patient fall

◆ Malfunction of a medical device resulting in actual or potential patient injury

◆ Diagnostic or testing problem (e.g., delay in testing or reporting, **failure** to report significant abnormal results, wrong test ordered)

Reportable events
Incidents, situations, or processes that contribute to—or have the potential to contribute to—a patient injury or that degrade the provider's ability to provide safe patient care.

Failure
Compromised function or intended action.

Exhibit 8.5 is an example of a form used to report the circumstances surrounding a hospitalized patient's fall. The individual who witnessed, first discovered, or is most familiar with the incident usually completes the report. The reporter does not include his judgment on the cause of the event, only facts. The names of witnesses to the event and the employee involved in the incident (if not the reporter) are typically included in the report.

The incident reporting process is not standardized among healthcare organizations. Facilities may define reportable events differently or use different mechanisms to document events. To streamline the reporting process, some organizations have created web-based incident reporting tools and telephone hotlines.

Prompt identification of patient incidents enables an organization to immediately investigate the circumstances of the incident and, if necessary, modify the process or environment to prevent similar occurrences in the future. Incident reports are also used to identify patterns of events that indicate unsafe conditions. Various departments and committees in the organization review these reports on a regular basis. A bar graph of the types of incidents that occurred in a hospital over the course of one month is shown in exhibit 8.6.

To ensure that staff members report patient incidents, managers must strive to maintain an environment that encourages people to report mistakes, admit problems, have different opinions, and exchange ideas. Experience has shown that when employees fear reprisal, they are less likely to report patient incidents; as a result, the organization

⊛ LEARNING POINT
Improving Patient Safety

Patient safety is one component of an organization's quality management activities. The same basic cycle of measurement, assessment, and improvement used in other quality management activities applies to patient safety initiatives. The safety of patient care is measured, the measurement results are assessed, and improvements are made.

EXHIBIT 8.5
Patient Fall
Incident Report

Patient name: _____ Room #: _____ Age: _____ Gender: _____	
Admission date: _____ Date of fall: _____ Time of fall: _____	

Ask the patient:

Do you remember falling?	❑ Yes ❑ No (If the patient cannot respond, his or her family may be able to provide information.)
Were you injured?	❑ Yes (how and where?) ❑ No
What were you doing when you fell?	

Other information:

Was the nurse call light on?	❑ Yes (Include the number of minutes call light was on.) ❑ No
The activated call light belonged to:	❑ Patient ❑ Roommate
Contributing factors (specify all):	❑ Medication: ❑ Equipment: ❑ Footwear: ❑ Confusion: ❑ Urgency of bladder/bowels: ❑ Environmental issues:
Did nursing follow the risk-for-falls protocol for this patient?	❑ Yes ❑ No
Any other information from patient, family, or staff:	
Number of hours since last fall-risk assessment for this patient:	
Has this patient fallen previously during this stay?	❑ Yes ❑ No
Age:	
Injury sustained as result of fall?	❑ Yes ❑ No
Did staff witness the fall?	❑ Yes ❑ No
Was the patient identified as at risk for falls?	❑ Yes ❑ No
What fall prevention interventions were used?	
Was the patient physically restrained?	❑ Yes ❑ No

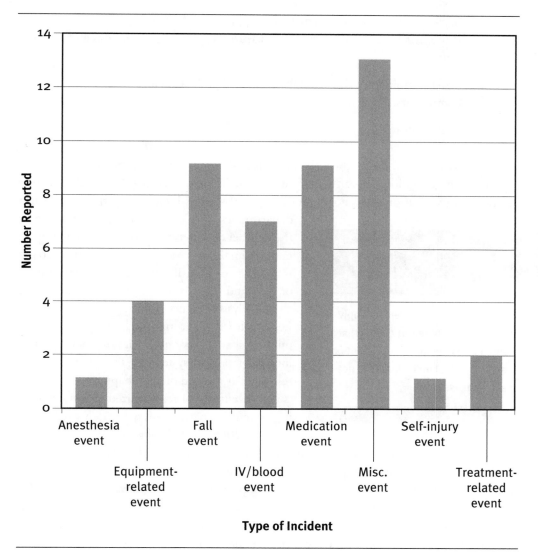

Exhibit 8.6
Bar Graph of
Patient Incidents
for Month of July

loses a valuable source of information about patient safety (Noble and Pronovost 2010). This finding is consistent with what has been discovered by officials of the NASA Aviation Safety Reporting System and the British Airways Safety Information System. These groups identified the following five practices as important to increasing the quantity and quality of employee incident reports (O'Leary and Chappell 1996):

1.   Protect people involved against disciplinary proceedings (as far as is practical).

2.   Allow confidential reporting or deidentify the reporter.

3. Separate the agency or department collecting and analyzing the reports from those that have the authority to institute disciplinary proceedings and impose sanctions.

4. Provide rapid, useful, accessible, and intelligible feedback to the reporting community.

5. Make reporting easy.

Increasingly, healthcare facilities are required to report patient incidents to entities outside the organization. More than 25 states have implemented regulations that require healthcare organizations to report certain types of serious incidents to the state health department. Some of these states publicly report the number of each type of incident. More important, maintaining state patient-incident databases is a means of identifying the underlying causes of risks and hazards in patient care because they allow analysis of events occurring at many facilities. Lessons learned through such analysis are often publicly shared. Several entities that manage state incident-reporting systems are listed in the website resources at the end of this chapter.

Eventually, a standardized national reporting system for patient safety incidents will be in place. In 2005, the federal government passed the Patient Safety and Quality Improvement Act (Patient Safety Act), which included plans to develop a national database of patient incident information. The Patient Safety Act made possible the creation of a nationwide network of **patient safety organizations (PSOs)** for the purpose of gathering and analyzing information about patient incidents from providers in all states. To qualify as a PSO, an organization must have expertise in identifying risks and hazards in the delivery of patient care, determining the underlying causes, and implementing corrective and preventive strategies.

As of this writing, the Agency for Healthcare Research and Quality (AHRQ), the federal entity responsible for administering the PSO provisions of the Patient Safety Act, has certified 83 PSOs that operate in various states, the District of Columbia, and US territories. The PSOs use common definitions and reporting formats that enable healthcare providers to collect and submit standardized information regarding patient safety events. Additional details about PSOs and the common reporting formats can be found on the AHRQ website (www.pso.ahrq.gov).

LEARNING POINT
Safety Measurement

The fundamental principles of performance measurement apply to patient safety. To encourage employees to report events that have caused or have the potential to cause injury to patients, organizations must reassure their staffs that individuals will not be disciplined for unintentional mistakes.

Patient safety organizations (PSOs)
Groups that have expertise in identifying risks and hazards in the delivery of patient care, determining the underlying causes, and implementing corrective and preventive strategies.

IMPROVING PATIENT SAFETY

Projects aimed at improving patient safety follow the same steps as any other project does:

1. Define the improvement goal.

2. Analyze current practices.

3. Design and implement improvements.

4. Measure success.

Any of the models described in chapter 5 can be used to improve patient safety. For instance, just as an ambulatory clinic can use rapid cycle improvement (RCI) to improve patient satisfaction (see exhibit 5.4), a community health center can use RCI to reduce prescription errors.

Two improvement models not described in chapter 5 are used by healthcare organizations for the explicit purpose of making patient care safer: failure mode and effects analysis and root cause analysis. These patient safety improvement models are described next.

FAILURE MODE AND EFFECTS ANALYSIS

Failure mode and effects analysis (FMEA) is a **proactive risk assessment** technique that involves a close examination of a process to determine where improvements are needed to reduce the likelihood of adverse events (Spath 2013). The technique is considered proactive because the improvement project is undertaken to prevent an adverse event. The FMEA technique promotes systematic thinking about the safety of a patient care process in terms of the following questions:

◆ What could go wrong?

◆ What will be the result if something goes wrong?

◆ What needs to be done to prevent a bad result when something does go wrong?

Risk or hazard potential is part of every process. The goal of an FMEA project is to find these hazards and make process changes to reduce the risk of error. FMEA is a formal and systematic assessment process, but individuals informally use FMEA almost every day. Here is an example:

You want to go to a music concert, expecting to buy a ticket at the door. *What could go wrong*: The concert will be sold out.

Failure mode and effects analysis (FMEA)
Systematic assessment of a process to identify the location, cause, and consequences of potential failure for the purpose of eliminating or reducing the chance of failure; also called *failure mode, effects, and criticality analysis* (FMECA) and *healthcare failure mode and effects analysis* (HFMEA). (An example of a completed FMEA is shown in exhibit 8.7.)

Proactive risk assessment
An improvement model that involves identifying and analyzing potential failures in healthcare processes or services for the purpose of reducing or eliminating risks that are a threat to patient safety.

Result: You will miss the concert, and you will be disappointed because you have waited several years for this band to come to your town.

Prevent the bad result: Buy a ticket in advance.

FMEA has been used to conduct safety system evaluations in manufacturing, aviation, computer software design, and other industries for many years. Now healthcare organizations use the technique to evaluate and improve the safety of patient care activities. Since 2002, hospitals and skilled nursing facilities accredited by The Joint Commission have been required to periodically conduct proactive risk assessments for patient safety improvement purposes. The FMEA improvement model is the most common technique used to comply with this standard (Joint Commission 2017a).

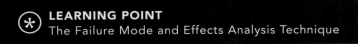

LEARNING POINT
The Failure Mode and Effects Analysis Technique

FMEA is a prospective risk-assessment technique used to reduce high-risk process failures. The probability and likelihood of detecting a failure is combined with an estimate of the impact of the failure to prioritize failures for elimination.

EXHIBIT 8.7
FMEA Steps in Relationship to PDSA Cycle

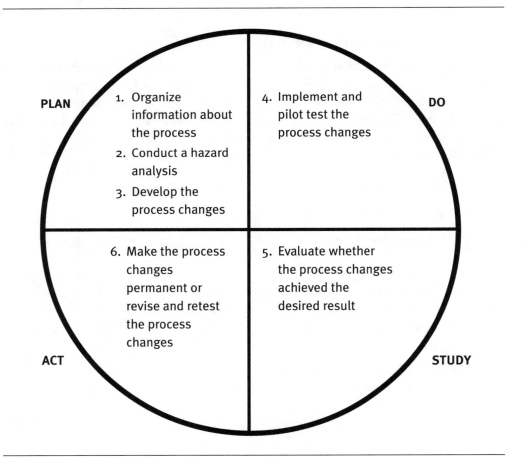

The six steps of an FMEA project are sequenced similarly to those of the Plan-Do-Study-Act improvement model (see exhibit 8.7). FMEA projects are undertaken by a team that has experience with the process under study; the team regularly carries out the activities and knows where the potential for error exists. To gain a fresh perspective, the FMEA project team may also include people who have no experience with the process.

An FMEA project begins with the development of a clear understanding of the process. The team develops a high-level flowchart to visualize each step. Next, the team conducts a **hazard analysis**, which involves a brainstorming session to develop a list of all failures that could occur at each step. The first two steps in the process of ordering outpatient laboratory tests for patients are shown in exhibit 8.8. Listed below each step are the **failure modes** or errors that could occur.

After all potential failure modes or mistakes have been identified for each step, the team determines the risk or **criticality** of each failure mode to prioritize it for elimination. Different schemes are used to calculate risk. In some FMEA models a criticality score is assigned to each potential failure on the basis of the following criteria:

◆ *Frequency*: the probability that the failure will occur

◆ *Severity*: the degree of harm the patient will experience if the failure occurs

◆ *Detection*: the likelihood that the failure will be detected before patient harm occurs

Each criterion is rated on a scale of 1 to 5, with 1 being the lowest possible rating and 5 the highest. Once the rating process is complete, a criticality score is assigned to each potential failure. This score is calculated as follows:

$$\text{Frequency} \times \text{Severity} \times \text{Detection}$$

Hazard analysis
The process of collecting and evaluating information on hazards associated with a process.

Failure modes
Different ways a process step or task could fail to provide the anticipated result.

Criticality
Ranking of potential failures according to their combined influence of severity and frequency and probability of occurrence.

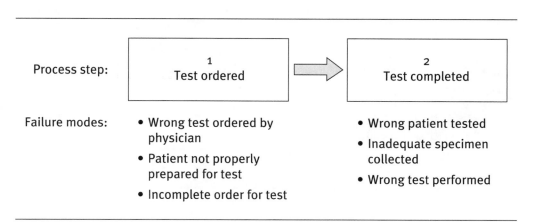

EXHIBIT 8.8
First Two Steps in Outpatient Laboratory Testing Process and Failure Modes

Critical failures
The most important process failures to prevent, according to criticality scoring results.

The potential failures with the highest criticality scores are considered the **critical failures** most in need of prevention. Exhibit 8.9 is an FMEA worksheet for the first step in the laboratory test-ordering process.

Once the critical failures are identified, the team determines what would cause these potential failures so that preventive actions can be taken. The following list provides examples of questions the team can ask about the critical failures to discover their root causes:

- Who might experience this problem? Would all the people who do the work experience it, or just some of them?
- What is the specific problem? For example, referring to the laboratory ordering process, what information is the physician likely to omit when ordering a test?
- Where might the failure occur? Where is the failure unlikely to occur?
- When would the problem likely happen (during certain times or days of the week)? When would the problem not happen?
- Why might the failure occur? Why doesn't it occur all the time?
- How many times has the problem occurred in the past? How can the process be changed to eliminate or reduce the chance this problem will occur?

The remaining steps of the FMEA project are the same as those of any improvement project. The process changes are implemented and tested to determine whether the desired results have been achieved. If the process changes reduce or eliminate the possibility that the critical failures will occur—the desired result of an FMEA project—they are incorporated into the process. Changes that do not produce the desired result are evaluated to determine why they did not work, and new process changes are developed and tested.

Exhibit 8.9
FMEA Worksheet

Step	*Potential Failure*	*Effect*	*Frequency*	*Severity*	*Detection*	*Criticality Score*
Test ordered	Wrong test ordered by physician					
	Patient not properly prepared for test					
	Incomplete order for test					

FMEA projects are usually undertaken for processes involving high-risk patient care activities prone to failure, but they can be used to reduce failure in any process. Exhibit 8.10 is a completed FMEA for the process of collecting patient demographic and insurance information in a large ambulatory health clinic for women. Members of the FMEA team included the registration area supervisor, two registration clerks, the manager of the patient accounts office, and the patient financial counselor. The clinic business manager served as team leader.

Several variations of the FMEA model described here are currently used in healthcare organizations. The Veterans Health Administration created a model called *Healthcare Failure Mode and Effects Analysis* to conduct proactive risk analyses (Stalhandske et al. 2009). Some healthcare organizations use a proactive **risk analysis** model called *failure mode, effects, and criticality analysis* (Powell et al. 2014), while other organizations use homegrown risk analysis models. All FMEA projects have similar characteristics.

ROOT CAUSE ANALYSIS

Root cause analysis (RCA) has been used for many years in other industries. NASA's (2009) use of RCA to investigate the March 2003 space shuttle *Columbia* disaster is just one example. *Columbia* was destroyed during the reentry phase of what was expected to be a routine landing, killing all seven crew members aboard. Safety improvement teams use RCA after an adverse event has occurred to determine system deficiencies that led to the event (Sanchez et al. 2017). The six steps involved in RCA follow the Plan-Do-Study-Act cycle (see exhibit 8.11).

Since 1996, organizations accredited by The Joint Commission have been required to conduct an RCA following a sentinel event. A **sentinel event** is an incident in which death or serious harm to a patient occurred. The word *sentinel* reflects the egregiousness of the injury (e.g., surgery performed on the wrong patient) and the likelihood that investigation of the event will reveal serious safety problems (Wachter 2012). The Joint Commission also encourages facilities to conduct an RCA following a near miss. A **near miss** is an incident that did not result in death or injury but could have; only by chance was the patient not harmed. An example of a near miss is the mistaken use of nonsterile rather than sterile tongue depressors by a circulating nurse in the operating room. Although no patients were harmed, this breach of care should be investigated to determine how to prevent it in the future (Cerniglia-Lowensen 2015).

Since 1996, several states have enacted regulations similar to The Joint Commission's standards. These regulations require healthcare facilities to conduct formal investigations of serious adverse events.

As with FMEA, RCA is a similar process to those that people work through almost every day. For example, a strange sound from my car (a symptom) indicates something is

Risk analysis
The process of defining, analyzing, and quantifying the hazards in a process, which typically results in a plan of action undertaken to prevent the most harmful risks or minimize their consequences.

Root cause analysis (RCA)
A structured process for identifying the underlying factors that caused an adverse event.

Sentinel event
An adverse event involving death or serious physical or psychological injury (or the risk thereof) that signals the need for immediate investigation and response.

Near miss
Any process variation that does not affect the outcome or result of an adverse event but carries a significant chance of an adverse outcome if it were to recur; also known as a *close call*.

Exhibit **8.10**
FMEA of the
Process of
Collecting Patient
Demographic
and Insurance
Information

Process Step	Potential Failure Mode	Potential Effect	Severity of Effect	Probability of Failure	Detection of Failure	Criticality Score
Verify patient's mailing address and phone number	Registration clerk does not verify address and phone number	Billing statement is sent to the wrong address; physician is unable to contact patient if necessary after patient leaves clinic	4	4	5	80
	Registration clerk enters demographic information incorrectly	Billing statement is sent to the wrong address; physician is unable to contact patient if necessary after patient leaves clinic	4	3	5	60
	Patient gives registration clerk incorrect information	Billing statement is sent to the wrong address; physician is unable to contact patient if necessary after patient leaves clinic	4	3	5	60
Verify patient's insurance information	Wrong insurance company is billed	Payment delay	5	3	3	45
	Registration clerk does not perform verification of insurance benefits	Payment delay	5	4	3	60

Rating Key

Severity rating scale:	Probability rating scale:	Detection rating scale:
1 = No effect	1 = Highly unlikely/never happened before	1 = Almost certain to be detected and corrected
2 = Minimal effect	2 = Low/relatively few failures	2 = High likelihood of being detected and corrected
3 = Moderate, short-term effect	3 = Moderate/occasional failures	3 = Moderate likelihood of being detected and corrected
4 = Significant, long-term effect	4 = High/repeated failures	4 = Low likelihood of being detected and corrected
5 = Catastrophic effect	5 = Very high/failure almost inevitable	5 = Remote likelihood of being detected and corrected

Critical Failure	Root Causes	Actions Intended to Eliminate/ Reduce Failure or Mitigate Effects	Measures of Success
Registration clerk does not verify address and phone number	Clerks are not trained and do not receive continuing education on use of address verification capabilities of registration computer system	• Provide address verification training for registration staff • Educate registration staff on importance of address verification and demonstrate correct way to document that verification was performed	• Percentage of billing statements returned because of invalid address
Registration clerk does not perform verification of insurance benefits	Management does not hold registration clerks accountable for insurance verification	• Implement policies and procedures that hold registrars accountable for verification of patient's insurance • Continue to educate registration staff on importance of insurance verification • Implement incentives for registration staff to verify insurance benefits	• Percentage of accounts for which registration clerk does not verify patient insurance benefits • Percentage of accounts with incorrect insurance identification and group numbers • Percentage of accounts billed to wrong insurance company

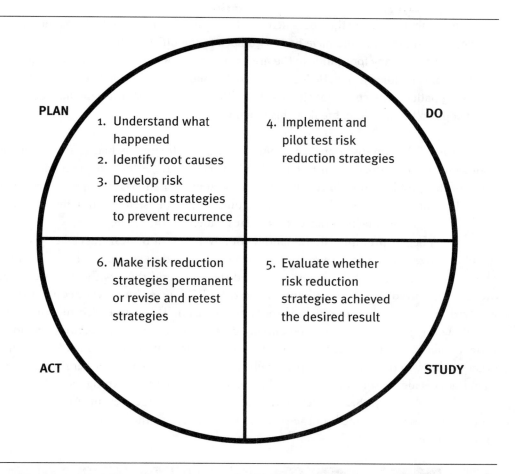

Exhibit 8.11
RCA Steps in
Relationship to
PDSA Cycle

PLAN

1. Understand what happened
2. Identify root causes
3. Develop risk reduction strategies to prevent recurrence

DO

4. Implement and pilot test risk reduction strategies

ACT

6. Make risk reduction strategies permanent or revise and retest strategies

STUDY

5. Evaluate whether risk reduction strategies achieved the desired result

wrong. Symptoms are not the cause of the problem; they are signals that something may be wrong. Turning up the radio to mask the strange sound will not fix the faulty water pump (root cause) causing the sound. My car problem will continue until the root cause is corrected. The same is true for problematic patient care processes. Delivery of the wrong medication to a nursing home resident (a symptom) signals that something is wrong with the medication administration process. If the people involved in giving medications do not find and fix the root cause of the mistake, another **medication error** is likely to occur in the future.

RCA is also a useful structured investigation process for identifying the underlying root causes of problems in nonclinical tasks. For example, a hospital conducted an RCA after the following event:

Medication error
Any preventable event that may cause or lead to inappropriate medication use or patient harm while the medication is in the control of the healthcare professional, patient, or consumer.

A housekeeper is waxing the floors near the hospital cafeteria at 1 a.m. He cannot find a wet floor sign and would have had to go back to the office to find one. He believes there will not be any foot traffic in the area at this time of night, so he does not go to the trouble of finding a sign. He leaves to take his mid-shift break while the floor dries. A young patient who could not sleep walks with his mother near the vending machine and slips on the wet floor, breaking his wrist.

The RCA team discovered the housekeeping staff frequently had to search for wet floor signs, which caused them to fall behind in their work. Although the manager was aware of this problem, no additional signs had been purchased. Making needed resources available to housekeeping staff in the future, plus reinforcing staff accountability for displaying the signs, will help to prevent a similar incident in the future.

RCA begins promptly after a sentinel or adverse event or near miss takes place. As for all improvement projects, a team of people is assembled to conduct the investigation. The team is composed of those who witnessed the event and those with expertise in the processes involved. Some consultants suggest the RCA team interview people directly involved in the event but not include them on the team. This is intended to reduce bias and allow for frank discussion of potentially difficult issues in team meetings (National Patient Safety Foundation 2015). Some organizations follow this recommendation while others include on the team people personally involved in the event. In either situation, the team leader is ideally someone who has experience using the RCA investigation technique.

Critical concept 8.2 is a description of a wrong-site surgery event. An arthroscopy should have been performed on the patient's right knee, but the procedure was done on his left knee instead.

> **(!) CRITICAL CONCEPT 8.2**
> Description of Wrong-Site Surgery Event
>
> A 62-year-old man was scheduled to undergo an arthroscopy procedure. Three weeks before the surgery, the orthopedic clinic telephoned the hospital to schedule the man's procedure. At that time, the front-office staff in the clinic mistakenly scheduled a left-knee arthroscopy instead of a right-knee arthroscopy. The surgery scheduling clerk at the hospital faxed a surgery confirmation form to the clinic. Per hospital policy, the clinic is expected to review the information on the form, verify the accuracy, and fax the signed confirmation back to the hospital. The clinic staff were busy and did not fax the confirmation back.
>
> On the day of the surgery, the patient's paperwork indicated that the surgery was to be performed on his left knee, per the original phone call from the clinic. The surgery
>
> *(continued)*

CRITICAL CONCEPT 8.2
Description of Wrong-Site Surgery Event *(continued)*

schedule, a document used to plan the day's activities in the operating area, also indicated that the patient was to have a left-knee arthroscopy. The man was taken to the preoperative holding area, where a nurse spoke with him about his upcoming procedure. Relying only on the surgery schedule, the nurse asked the patient to confirm that he was having an arthroscopy on his left knee. The man told the nurse that he had been experiencing pain in both knees and that he'd eventually need procedures on both of them. He thought he was scheduled for surgery on his right knee that day but figured that perhaps the doctor had decided to operate on his left knee instead. The nurse did not read the history and physical examination report that the patient's doctor had brought to the hospital that morning. If she had read this report, she would have noticed that it indicated the patient was to have surgery on his right knee that day.

The anesthesiologist examined the patient in the preoperative holding area. When asked about the procedure, the man was confused about which knee was to be operated on that day. The anesthesiologist wrote "knee arthroscopy" in his notes in the patient's record. The patient was taken into the operating room, where the surgeon was waiting. The surgeon spoke with the patient about the upcoming procedure on his right knee, and the patient signed a consent form indicating that surgery was to be performed on the right knee that day. The surgeon marked his initials on the man's right knee in ink to designate the surgery site.

The anesthesiologist and scrub nurse readied the room for the procedure. The patient was anesthetized and fell asleep. Thinking the man was having surgery on his left knee, the nurse placed a drape over his right knee, not noticing the surgeon's initials. The left knee was placed in the stirrup and prepped for the procedure. The nurse then asked everyone in the room to confirm that the man was the correct patient and that he was having an arthroscopy on his left knee. Everyone in the room said "yes" except the surgeon, who was busy preparing for the procedure. Distracted, he nodded his head in agreement. The nurse documented on the preoperative checklist that the patient's identity, procedure, and surgery site had been verified.

The surgeon performed the arthroscopy on the knee that had been prepped—the left one. When the patient awoke in the surgical recovery area, he asked the nurse why he felt pain in his left knee and told her the procedure should have been performed on his right knee. The nurse notified the surgeon, who immediately informed the patient and his family about the mistake.

The RCA team for the wrong-site surgery event includes the people directly involved in the procedure—the surgeon, anesthesiologist, surgical nurses, and surgery scheduling clerk—and the managers of the admission and surgical areas. The team's first task is to determine what happened by collecting and inspecting physical evidence (e.g., equipment, materials, safety devices) and reviewing documentary evidence (paper or electronic media). The team also asks the people directly and indirectly involved in the event to provide their perspectives. These discussions may occur in a team meeting, or people may be interviewed individually. Ultimately, the team develops a picture of the event and creates a high-level flowchart to illustrate the steps leading up to it (exhibit 8.12).

Next, the team looks for the root causes of the event. This step is more involved than the Five Whys tool described in chapter 6. First, the RCA team determines the causal factors. Causal factors are situations, circumstances, or conditions that collectively, with other causes, increase the likelihood of the adverse event. The team identifies several such factors for the wrong-site surgery event:

◆   The orthopedic clinic phoned the patient's surgery reservation to the hospital. According to policy, the clinic also should have confirmed the surgery reservation and provided a hard copy of it to the hospital, but it did not. Team discussion reveals that many surgeons' offices do not comply with this step.

Exhibit 8.12

High-Level Flowchart of Event

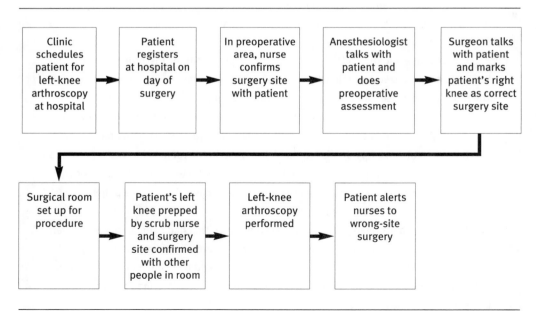

◆ The surgeon failed to provide a copy of the patient's history and physical examination to the hospital at least 72 hours before surgery, as required by policy. Without this document, the admissions and surgery scheduling clerk was unable to check the accuracy of the planned surgery before the patient's arrival.

◆ The nurse relied only on what was written on the surgical schedule to confirm the surgery site. The patient's history and physical report (which the surgeon brought to the hospital on the day of the surgery) indicated the patient was to undergo a right-knee arthroscopy, but the nurse did not read this report.

◆ The patient had a history of pain in both knees. The surgeon told him that eventually an arthroscopy would need to be performed on both knees. When the nurse and the anesthesiologist questioned the patient, he appeared confused about which knee was to be operated on that day.

◆ The surgeon correctly marked the patient's right knee as the surgery site. However, the scrub nurse placed drapes over the right knee and prepared the left knee for the procedure. The nurse had already set her mind to the fact that a left-knee arthroscopy was to be performed and did not notice the surgical-site marking on the patient's right knee.

◆ Before starting the arthroscopy, the scrub nurse asked everyone in the room to confirm the left knee as the surgery site. Everyone replied "yes" except the surgeon, who was busy at the time. He just nodded his head in agreement. According to policy, everyone in the room is supposed to stop what he or she is doing and verbally confirm the correct site.

◆ The surgeon proceeded with the left-knee arthroscopy, not noticing that he was working on the wrong knee.

Once the team is satisfied that it has identified all causal factors, it identifies the root causes. Root causes are the most fundamental reasons the event occurred. To discover the root causes, the team asks "why" questions about each causal factor. For example, why didn't the clinic provide a hard copy of the confirmed surgery reservation as required? Why didn't the nurse confirm the intended procedure by reading through the patient's history and physical report? Why didn't anyone stop to reconfirm the correct surgery site when the patient exhibited confusion about the surgery he was having? Why didn't the scrub nurse notice the surgical-site marking on the right knee before covering it with a drape? This questioning process continues until the team identifies the system problems that underlie the causal factors. System problems take many forms (Vincent 2003):

◆ Organization and management (e.g., policies and standards, organizational culture, values and priorities)

◆ Work environment (e.g., staffing levels, workload, skill mix, resource availability, managerial support)

◆ Team (e.g., communication, team leadership, level of willingness to seek help)

◆ Individual staff members (e.g., knowledge and skills, motivation and attitude)

◆ Task (e.g., availability and use of standardized procedures)

Since January 1995, The Joint Commission has been gathering information on the root causes of sentinel events. Of the 936 sentinel events reported to The Joint Commission in 2015, the most common root causes were human factors (e.g., staffing levels, staffing skill mix, staff orientation and education, competency assessment, staff and resident supervision) and inadequate communication between care providers, and inadequate leadership (Axlund 2016).

The RCA team involved in investigating the event described in critical concept 8.2 determines the following system problems to be the root causes of the wrong-site surgery:

◆ During the surgery-site verification step, members of the surgical team did not actively communicate with each other.

◆ Management does not ensure that members of the surgical team consistently comply with the standardized surgery-site verification procedures.

◆ Surgeons' offices are not held accountable for complying with the hospital's surgery scheduling processes and its requirements for history and physical exam reports.

◆ Perceived pressure for productivity (the need to start all procedures at the scheduled time) discourages members of the surgical team from interrupting the process when something unusual occurs (e.g., a patient expresses confusion about the surgery he is having).

An adverse event usually has no more than four root causes. If the team identifies more than four, questioning should continue until the fundamental reasons are apparent.

Now that the root causes of the sentinel event have been identified, the team develops solutions—a corrective action plan—to prevent such an event from occurring again. The actions "should eliminate or control system hazards or vulnerabilities that have been identified" in the RCA (Joint Commission 2017b, SE-6). A planning matrix or Gantt chart should be used to document the tasks necessary for completing the actions, the responsible individuals, and the timeline for completion (see chapter 6 for more information on these performance improvement tools).

The remaining steps of the RCA project are the same as those of any improvement project. The solutions are implemented and tested to determine whether desired results have been achieved. If the corrective actions are successful, they are made permanent. Solutions that do not achieve the desired results are evaluated to determine why they did not work, and new corrective actions are developed and tested.

FMEA and RCA are not exclusively used for improving the safety of patient care processes. Just as the FMEA improvement model can be used to conduct a prospective risk assessment of any process, the RCA model can be used to investigate the cause of any process failure.

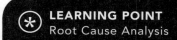

LEARNING POINT
Root Cause Analysis

RCA is an accident investigation technique undertaken to find and fix the fundamental causes of an adverse event. It is similar to any improvement method that follows the steps of the Plan-Do-Study-Act cycle.

PATIENT ENGAGEMENT IN SAFETY

A patient safety observation by authors of the IOM report *To Err Is Human* involved the role of patients in preventing medication errors (IOM 2000, 196):

> Patients themselves also could provide a major safety check in most hospitals, clinics, and practice. They should know which medications they are taking, their appearance, and their side effects, and they should notify their doctors of medication discrepancies and the occurrence of side effects.

Since that time, a growing body of research has suggested that patients and their family members can serve as additional safeguards in the healthcare system (Spath 2008; Davis, Sevdalis, and Vincent 2012; Joint Commission 2016). Following are just some of the ways patients can make their hospital experience safer:

◆ Ask caregivers to perform, or observe them performing, patient identity checks before administration of treatments.

◆ Keep a list with you of prior medical history, current treatments, and allergies, and share this list with caregivers at admission.

◆ Know how often staff should change wound dressings, and when/how/whom to ask for a dressing change.

◆ Know the type, dosage, and frequency of administration for medications; ask caregivers to explain prescribed medications to verify that they are correct; if incorrect, question the caregiver's decision to administer the medication.

◆ Observe caregivers washing their hands, or ask them to do so.

◆ Monitor the cleanliness of the equipment and the environment, and report any problems.

◆ Be informed about the usefulness of changing position in the hospital bed, and ask for position changes if they are not made as required.

◆ Request help when getting out of bed, or ask for an assistive device (e.g., cane, walker).

◆ Confirm that caregivers know what treatment the doctor has ordered for your care.

◆ Ask about equipment to understand what different sounds or noises mean; alert caregivers if you think a problem might have arisen.

In 2002, The Joint Commission joined with AHRQ, the American Medical Association, and other national groups to promote involvement of consumers in patient safety efforts. As of this writing, The Joint Commission (2017a) requires accredited organizations to foster patients' active involvement in their care to improve safety. Caregivers are required to communicate with the patient and family about all aspects of care and encourage them to report concerns about safety. If a mistake occurs and a patient is harmed, regulations in some states and The Joint Commission standards require disclosure of unanticipated outcomes of care to the patient or her representative (AHRQ Patient Safety Network 2017).

Some forward-thinking healthcare organizations are not only sharing information with patients and partnering with them for safety purposes but also including them in advisory groups and other activities to solicit safety improvement suggestions. For example, leaders at Advocate Trinity Hospital in Chicago include patients and families on leadership rounds in the nursing units to obtain their perspective and reinforce to caregivers the importance of patient and family

---

⊛ LEARNING POINT
Consumer Involvement in Patient Safety

Patients and family members can promote their safety by speaking up when they encounter a potentially unsafe or out-of-the-ordinary activity, process, or alarm. In some organizations, patients and family members are involved in internal quality management and safety improvement efforts.

input (AHRQ 2013). Many healthcare organizations have formed patient and family advisory councils to gain feedback on patient safety issues, and some organizations include community members on the patient safety committee (Health Research & Educational Trust 2015).

On occasion healthcare organizations will include the patient involved in an adverse event or the patient's family in the RCA (Zimmerman and Amori 2007). For example, the patient who experienced the wrong-site surgery event detailed in critical concept 8.2 was invited to share his perspective of what happened with the RCA team. The hope was that his input would help the team design better patient engagement strategies to lessen the chance of another similar event (Delbanco and Bell 2007). Openly soliciting the consumer perspective on healthcare quality management, including safety improvement, is gaining popularity.

CONCLUSION

For many years, healthcare organizations have relied primarily on people performing their jobs correctly to protect patients from unintended harm. Decades of research, mostly from other industries, has proven that most accidents are caused by capable but fallible people working in dysfunctional systems. Healthcare organizations are now borrowing techniques from other industries to investigate the cause of mistakes and to design safer systems.

Patient safety is only one dimension of healthcare quality, yet it receives a lot of attention from regulators, purchasers, and accreditation groups. As consumerism in healthcare grows, patients are expecting to take a more active role in safety. Consumers' involvement in safety improvement is becoming a major contributor to healthcare organizations' quality management efforts.

Patient safety includes the basic quality management components: measurement, assessment, and improvement. Two improvement models—FMEA and RCA—are often used to reduce the chance that harmful mistakes will occur.

FOR DISCUSSION

1. Go through the steps of an FMEA project for the process of taking a bath, shown in the following flowchart. Use a worksheet like the one in exhibit 8.9 to document your ideas.

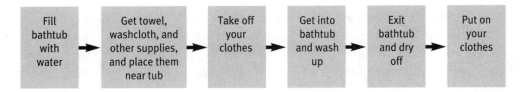

When completing the FMEA, consider your own bathing experiences and what other people may have told you about their experiences. Be creative; there are no wrong answers.

2. Read the description of the wrong-site surgery event in critical concept 8.2 and the root causes identified by the team who conducted the RCA. Conduct a literature review and Internet search for corrective actions aimed at preventing wrong-site surgeries. Which of these actions would help prevent a similar event from occurring at the hospital described in critical concept 8.2?

3. How do your healthcare providers (e.g., hospital, emergency department, personal physician, nurse practitioner, therapist, pharmacist) keep you safe from being harmed by the effects of healthcare services? What could your providers do better to keep you safe?

WEBSITES

-   Agency for Healthcare Research and Quality (AHRQ) quality and patient safety resources
    www.ahrq.gov/professionals/quality-patient-safety/index.html
-   AHRQ Patient Safety Network
    https://psnet.ahrq.gov
-   AHRQ Patient Safety Organization Program
    https://pso.ahrq.gov
-   AHRQ TeamSTEPPS: Team training for healthcare professionals
    http://teamstepps.ahrq.gov

- Always Events® Toolbox: Aspects of the patient and family experience that should always occur
  http://alwaysevents.pickerinstitute.org/?page_id=882

- American Hospital Association/Health Research & Educational Trust. *Partnering to Improve Quality and Safety: A Framework for Working with Patient and Family Advisors.*
  www.hpoe.org/resources/ahahret-guides/1828

- Consumers Advancing Patient Safety
  www.patientsafety.org

- Institute for Healthcare Improvement/National Patient Safety Foundation
  www.npsf.org

- Institute for Safe Medication Practices
  www.ismp.org

- Leapfrog Hospital Safety Grade
  www.hospitalsafetygrade.org/

- Maryland Department of Health Office of Health Care Quality
  https://health.maryland.gov/ohcq/Pages/Programs.aspx

- MedWatch: The FDA Safety Information and Adverse Event Reporting Program
  www.fda.gov/Safety/MedWatch/default.htm

- Minnesota Adverse Health Events Measurement Guide
  www.stratishealth.org/documents/MN_AE_Health_Events_Measurement_Guide.pdf

- Minnesota Department of Health, Patient Safety
  www.health.state.mn.us/patientsafety/index.html

- 100 Hospital Patient Safety Benchmarks, 2017
  www.beckershospitalreview.com/quality/100-patient-safety-benchmarks-2017.html

- Oregon Patient Safety Commission
  https://oregonpatientsafety.org

- Pennsylvania Patient Safety Authority
  http://patientsafetyauthority.org

- Safety Leaders Organization, sponsored by the Texas Medical Institute of Technology
  www.safetyleaders.org

- The Joint Commission, Sentinel Event Alerts
  www.jointcommission.org/sentinel_event.aspx

- The Joint Commission, Sentinel Event Policy and Procedures
  www.jointcommission.org/sentinel_event_policy_and_procedures/

- VA National Center for Patient Safety
  www.patientsafety.va.gov

- Vincent, C., and R. Amalberti. 2016. *Safer Healthcare: Strategies for the Real World.*
  Free e-book available at http://link.springer.com/book/10.1007/978-3-319-25559-0.

- *WebM&M*: A case-based journal and forum on patient safety
  https://psnet.ahrq.gov/webmm

- World Health Organization, Patient Safety: Education and Training
  www.who.int/patientsafety/education/en/

REFERENCES

Agency for Healthcare Research and Quality (AHRQ). 2017. *2016 National Healthcare Quality and Disparities Report.* Pub. No. 17-0001. Rockville, MD: US Department of Health and Human Services.

———. 2013. *Guide to Patient and Family Engagement in Hospital Quality and Safety.* Published June. www.ahrq.gov/professionals/systems/hospital/engagingfamilies/guide.html.

AHRQ Patient Safety Network. 2017. "Patient Safety Primers: Disclosure of Errors." Accessed November 19. http://psnet.ahrq.gov/primer.aspx?primerID=2.

Axlund, W. 2016. "Sentinel Events & Patient Safety: The Disturbing Data, Part I." *Readiness Rounds* (blog). Published March 10. www.readinessrounds.com/blog/sentinel-events-and-patient-safety.

Cerniglia-Lowensen, J. 2015. "Learning from Mistakes and Near Mistakes: Using Root Cause Analysis as a Risk Management Tool." *Journal of Radiology Nursing* 34 (1): 4–7.

Davis, R. E., N. Sevdalis, and C. A. Vincent. 2012. "Patient Involvement in Patient Safety: The Health-Care Professional's Perspective." *Journal of Patient Safety* 8 (4): 182–88.

Delbanco, T., and S. K. Bell. 2007. "Guilty, Afraid, and Alone—Struggling with Medical Error." *New England Journal of Medicine* 357 (17): 1682–83.

Health Research & Educational Trust. 2015. *Partnering to Improve Quality and Safety: A Framework for Working with Patient and Family Advisors.* Chicago: Health Research & Educational Trust.

Institute of Medicine (IOM). 2001. *Crossing the Quality Chasm: A New Health System for the 21st Century*. Washington, DC: National Academies Press.

———. 2000. *To Err Is Human: Building a Safer Health System*. Washington, DC: National Academies Press.

Joint Commission. 2017a. "Patient Safety Systems." In *2017 Comprehensive Accreditation Manual for Hospitals*. Accessed November 20. www.jointcommission.org/patient_safety_systems_chapter_for_the_hospital_program/.

———. 2017b. "Sentinel Events." In *Comprehensive Accreditation Manual for Hospitals*, Update 1. Published July. www.jointcommission.org/assets/1/6/CAMH_SE_0717.pdf.

———. 2016. *Busting the Myths About Engaging Patients and Families in Patient Safety*. Accessed November 20, 2017. www.jointcommission.org/assets/1/18/PFAC_patient_family_and_safety_white_paper.pdf.

Leape, L. L., D. W. Bates, D. J. Cullen, J. Cooper, H. J. Demonaco, T. Gallivan, R. Hallisey, J. Ives, N. Laird, G. Laffel, R. Nemeskal, L. A. Petersen, K. Porter, D. Servi, B. F. Shea, S. D. Small, B. J. Sweitzer, B. T. Thompson, and M. Vander Vliet. 1995. "Systems Analysis of Adverse Drug Events." *Journal of the American Medical Association* 274 (1): 35–43.

Makary, M. A., and M. Daniel. 2016. "Medical Error—The Third Leading Cause of Death in the US." *British Medical Journal* 353: i2139.

National Aeronautics and Space Administration (NASA). 2009. "The Columbia Accident Investigation Board." Updated September 17. https://history.nasa.gov/columbia/CAIB.html.

National Patient Safety Foundation. 2015. *RCA2: Improving Root Cause Analyses and Actions to Prevent Harm*. Boston: National Patient Safety Foundation.

Noble, D. J., and P. J. Pronovost. 2010. "Underreporting of Patient Safety Incidents Reduces Health Care's Ability to Quantify and Accurately Measure Harm Reduction." *Journal of Patient Safety* 6 (4): 247–50.

O'Leary, M., and S. L. Chappell. 1996. "Confidential Incident Reporting Systems Create Vital Awareness of Safety Problems." *International Civil Aviation Organization Journal* 51 (8): 11–13.

Powell, E. S., L. M. O'Connor, A. P. Nannicelli, L.T. Barker, R. K. Khare, N. P. Seivert, J. L. Holl, and J. A. Vozenilek. 2014. "Failure Mode Effects and Criticality Analysis: Innovative Risk Assessment to Identify Critical Areas for Improvement in Emergency Department Sepsis Resuscitation." *Diagnosis* 1 (2): 173–81.

Reason, J. T. 2008. *The Human Contribution: Unsafe Acts, Accidents and Heroic Recoveries.* Surrey, UK: Ashgate.

Sanchez, J. A., K. W. Lobdell, S. D. Moffatt-Bruce, and J. I. Fann. 2017. "Investigating the Causes of Adverse Events." *Annals of Thoracic Surgery* 103 (6): 1693–99.

Spath, P. L. 2013. "FMEA: A Proactive Resident Safety Technique." *Topics in Geriatric Medicine and Medical Direction* 35 (2): 1–4.

———. 2008. "Safety from the Patient's Point of View." In *Engaging Patients as Safety Partners: A Guide for Reducing Errors and Improving Satisfaction*, edited by P. Spath, 1–40. Chicago: Health Forum/AHA Press.

———. 2001. *The Basics of Patient Safety.* Forest Grove, OR: Brown-Spath & Associates.

Stalhandske, E., J. DeRosier, R. Wilson, and J. Murphy. 2009. "Healthcare FMEA in the Veterans Health Administration." *Patient Safety & Quality Healthcare* 6 (5): 30–33.

Tucker, A. L., and A. C. Edmondson. 2003. "Why Hospitals Don't Learn from Failures: Organizational and Psychological Dynamics That Inhibit System Change." *California Management Review* 45 (2): 55–72.

Vincent, C. 2003. "Understanding and Responding to Adverse Events." *New England Journal of Medicine* 348 (11): 1051–56.

Wachter, R. M. 2012. *Understanding Patient Safety*, 2nd ed. New York: McGraw-Hill.

Zimmerman, T. M., and G. P. Amori. 2007. "Including Patients in Root Cause and System Failure Analysis: Legal and Psychological Implications." *Journal of Healthcare Risk Management* 27 (2): 27–34.

CHAPTER 9

ACHIEVING RELIABLE QUALITY AND SAFETY

After reading this chapter, you will be able to

➤ explain the role of reliability science in the improvement of healthcare services,

➤ recognize how process reliability is measured and managed,

➤ identify strategies to increase the reliability of healthcare processes by improving the effectiveness of people and the systems in which they work, and

➤ discuss how to measure the effectiveness of improvement actions and sustain the gains.

KEY WORDS

➤ Catastrophic processes

➤ Human factors

➤ Noncatastrophic processes

➤ Reliability science

E very year, healthcare organizations throughout the United States conduct hundreds of improvement projects following the models and using the tools you studied in the preceding chapters. With all of this activity, you might think the quality of healthcare services is exemplary, with few inefficiencies and mistakes. Yet studies of healthcare performance continue to report high rates of error, overuse of services, and costly wastefulness (Agency for Healthcare Research and Quality 2016).

Why are many of the expected improvements not materializing? Does the fault lie with the improvement project models or tools? Do we need to conduct twice as many projects and involve more frontline workers? Although a lack of significant progress is caused by many factors, one element that greatly contributes to quality problems is the design of work systems. As noted by Paul Batalden, MD, director of healthcare improvement leadership development at Dartmouth Medical School in Hanover, New Hampshire, "every system is perfectly designed to get the results it gets" (McInnis 2006, 32). If we want fundamentally different results in healthcare, we must use fundamentally different improvement strategies.

Regardless of which improvement model is used for a project, at some point actions or risk reduction strategies are designed. Often these interventions focus on creating new procedures and training people to do their job correctly. Too little attention is given to the work systems that give rise to inefficiencies and human errors. Bohmer (2010) proposes that the only realistic hope for substantially improving healthcare delivery is for the core processes to be revamped.

In this chapter, we introduce the systems approach to achieving safe and reliable healthcare. These techniques are based on **reliability science**, sometimes called *human factors engineering*, which originated in the US military during World War II (Wickens et al. 2012). The concepts are commonplace in other industries and should be applied when healthcare improvement teams reach the action planning phase of a project. By thinking differently about the changes needed to improve performance, project teams can have a significant and sustainable positive impact.

Reliability science
A discipline that applies scientific know-how to a process, procedure, or health service activity so that it will perform its intended function for the required time under commonly occurring conditions.

RELIABLE PERFORMANCE

Performance reliability can be measured in various ways. The simplest way is to measure process output or outcomes. The number of actions that achieve the intended results are divided by the total number of actions taken. For instance, when you see your doctor, you expect her to have access to the results of your recently completed laboratory tests. The reliability of that process can be measured by gathering data on the occurrences of missing lab test results. If a clinic finds that 15 percent of outpatient appointments are affected by missing lab information, the process is said to have a failure rate of 15 percent and a reliability rate of 85 percent.

You may not clearly understand the concept of reliability; however, when your automobile will not start, you clearly understand the concept of failure. You also learn the cost of failure when you have to pay a mechanic to restore your automobile to a reliable condition.

Human factors scientists and engineers have studied the interactions of people, technology, and policy across multiple industries for years. Knowledge gained from these studies allows us to predict the rate of failures based on the reliability rating of the process. For instance, if the clinic's process of reporting lab results has an 85 percent reliability rating, the clinic physicians should expect missing results for one or two of every ten patients who underwent recent laboratory tests. Exhibit 9.1 shows the expected failure rates for each level of reliability (Resar 2006).

The reliability of healthcare processes varies. Studies suggest that most US healthcare organizations currently perform at the 90 percent level of reliability, meaning they have a failure rate of 1 in 10 (Nolan et al. 2004). Some hospital processes (e.g., hand hygiene, hand-off communications) fail 40 to 60 percent of the time (Bodenheimer 2008; Erasmus et al. 2010). One of the most reliable healthcare processes is giving patients compatible blood for a transfusion. Failures of this process are rare, with the reliability rate estimated to be 99.999 percent (Amalberti et al. 2005).

Human factors
"The environmental, organizational and job factors, and individual characteristics which influence behavior at work" (Clinical Human Factors Group 2016).

> ### (?) DID YOU KNOW?
>
> - You have a 1 to 2 percent chance of dying accidentally for every 10 mountains you climb in the Himalayas. The reliability rating for this high-risk activity is 80 to 90 percent. Bungee jumping has a similar risk of death.
> - Automobile travel is fairly safe, with a reliability rating of 99.99 percent. The risk of a fatal accident is low—up to 5 for every 10,000 times you ride in a car.
> - The reliability of commercial aviation is better than 99.9999 percent, with an extremely low risk of a complete engine failure leading to loss of aircraft.
>
> *Source*: Amalberti et al. (2005).

Reliability Level (%)	Expected Failure Rate
Less than 80	Unpredictable, chaotic performance
80–90	1–2 failures out of 10 opportunities
95	Up to 5 failures per 100 opportunities
99.5	Up to 5 failures per 1,000 opportunities
99.99	Up to 5 failures per 10,000 opportunities
99.999	Up to 5 failures per 100,000 opportunities
99.9999	Up to 5 failures per 1,000,000 opportunities

EXHIBIT 9.1

Process Reliability Levels and Expected Failure Rates

IMPROVING QUALITY

Reliability ratings are important for healthcare quality improvement purposes. Reliability science has demonstrated that certain process improvements are more likely to create consistent quality. When improvement actions rely mostly on people's vigilance and hard work to get things done correctly, the best level of reliability that can be achieved is 80 to 90 percent (Luria et al. 2006). On occasion, higher levels of reliability can be achieved, but they are not possible to sustain over time.

People often work in complex healthcare environments without carefully designed mistake-proofing infrastructures. For instance, hospital nurses are constantly interrupted as they carry out important patient care duties. In a review of several studies of nurse activities, the reported interruptions per hour ranged from 0.3 to 13.9 (Hopkinson and Jennings 2013). Healthcare professionals are able to cope with these situations and, most often, performance is not affected. However, people cannot be vigilant 100 percent of the time, and mistakes happen.

Exhibit 9.2 summarizes the types of actions necessary to achieve sustained reliable quality at different percentages (Amalberti et al. 2005). These actions, based on human factors and reliability science principles, should be considered in the design of actions intended to improve quality.

Not every healthcare process can be made highly reliable. Resources are insufficient, and not every process requires a high (99.5 percent or greater) level of reliability. For **noncatastrophic processes**, good outcomes depend on having at least 95 percent process reliability. For **catastrophic processes**, good outcomes depend on having 99.5 percent or better reliability. Improvement project teams should agree on the desired level of reliability and then implement actions that will achieve this level. For some healthcare processes, 80 to 90 percent reliability may be sufficient. Organizations might achieve better patient outcomes by bringing several chaotic processes to 90 percent reliability rather than concentrating on improving the reliability of just a few to 99.5 percent. This thinking coincides with the risk management concept of ALARP, which stands for "as low as reasonably practicable." Determining the extent to which workplace risks are controlled "involves weighing a risk against the trouble, time and money needed to control it" (Health and Safety Executive 2014).

The US Department of Veterans Affairs (VA) National Center for Patient Safety (2016) created an action categorization system on the basis of human factors science. These action categories are used by teams involved in root cause analyses and other patient safety improvement projects. Rather than divide improvement actions into levels of reliability, the actions are labeled as weak, intermediate, and strong. Studies at the VA have shown that when a strong action is developed and implemented, it is 2.5 times more likely to be effective at improving performance than are weak or intermediate actions (DeRosier, Taylor, and Bagian 2007). The types of actions that fall into the weak, intermediate, and strong categories are listed in exhibit 9.3.

Noncatastrophic processes
Processes that do not generally lead to patient death or severe injury within hours of a failure (e.g., hand hygiene, administration of low-risk medications).

Catastrophic processes
Processes with a high likelihood of patient death or severe injury immediately or within hours of a failure (e.g., identification of correct surgery site, administration of compatible blood for a transfusion).

Reliability Level (%)	Actions
Less than 80	Primarily rely on qualified people doing what they believe is the right thing
80–90	Implement basic failure prevention strategies, such as the following: • Standard protocols/procedures/order sheets • Personal checklists • Common equipment • Feedback on compliance • Awareness and training
95	Implement sophisticated failure prevention and basic failure identification and mitigation strategies, such as the following: • Build decision aids and reminders into the system. • Set the desired action as the default (based on scientific evidence). • Account for and take advantage of habits and patterns in the process design. • Specify process risks, and articulate actions for reducing risks. • Take advantage of scheduling. • Use redundant processes. • Operate independent backups. • Measure and provide feedback on compliance with process specifications.
99.5	Gather information to understand which failures are occurring, how often they occur, and why they occur. Then redesign the system to reduce these failures using sophisticated failure prevention, identification, and mitigation strategies: • Design the system to prevent the failure, making sure the steps in the process act independently of each other so failures can be identified and corrected. • Design procedures and relationships to make failures visible when they do occur so they may be intercepted before causing harm. • Design procedures and build capabilities for fixing failures when they are identified or mitigating the harm caused by failures when they are not detected and intercepted.
Better than 99.5	Moving beyond 99.5% requires technology and advanced system design that require significant resource investments.

EXHIBIT 9.2

Actions Necessary to Achieve Reliability Levels

Source: Adapted from Nolan et al. (2004).

EXHIBIT **9.3**
Strength of Various
Improvement
Actions

Strength of Improvement Action	Example of Action
Weak	• Double-checks • Warnings and labels • New procedure/policy • Memos • Training • Additional study/analysis
Intermediate	• Checklist/cognitive aid • Increase in staffing/decrease in workload • Redundancy • Enhanced communication (e.g., read back) • Software enhancements/modifications • Elimination of look-alikes and sound-alikes • Elimination/reduction of distractions (e.g., sterile medical environment)
Strong	• Architectural/physical plant changes • Tangible involvement and action by leadership in support of patient safety • Simplified process, with unnecessary steps removed • Standardized equipment, process, or care map • New-device usability testing before purchasing • Engineering control or interlock (forcing functions)

Source: Reprinted from National Center for Patient Safety, US Department of Veterans Affairs, "Root Cause Analysis." Retrieved from www.patientsafety.va.gov/professionals/onthejob/rca.asp. Copyright © 2016.

Improvement teams frequently favor weak interventions over higher-level actions because weak actions are lower risk and easier to create and implement. Staff training and distribution of memos telling everyone to follow procedures can be accomplished fairly easily. Unfortunately, such actions by themselves rarely have a lasting impact (Williams and Bagian 2014). Training can be made stronger by combining it with periodic competency assessments involving random observation by management. People newly trained in a procedure are more likely to follow it if they know they will be occasionally and randomly observed (Bernstein et al. 2016).

APPLYING RELIABILITY PRINCIPLES

When actions based on reliability principles are not incorporated into the design of healthcare improvement initiatives, the project goals are less likely to be achieved. Consider what happened in the following case study. An improvement team met for several weeks to design and implement actions aimed at reducing the incidence of heel pressure ulcers (skin breakdowns) among hospitalized patients.

CASE STUDY

Many patients in the hospital were developing heel ulcerations. More than 13 percent of patients aged 18 or older developed a heel ulcer within four days of admission. This rate was higher than the national average, so an improvement team was formed with representatives from nursing, physical therapy, and wound care services to reduce the incidence of heel ulcers by 50 percent within one year. The team evaluated current practices and implemented the following stepwise actions to improve the process:

1. Nurses were trained to use an assessment scoring system to identify patients at risk of heel ulcerations. A poster board showing assessment instructions was made available for five days in each nursing unit.

2. After reviewing the training material, nurses took a test to determine their proficiency in assessing a patient's heel ulcer risk. A score of 90 percent was required to pass the test.

3. Once all nurses had taken and passed the test, a new protocol was implemented that required use of the risk-assessment scoring system at the time of a patient's admission, 48 hours after admission, and whenever a significant change was seen in a patient's condition.

4. The hospital's computerized health record system was modified so nurses could add the patient's ulcer risk score into the patient's record at the required intervals.

5. Patients at moderate or high risk of a heel ulcer were started on a protocol of ulcer prevention that included application of a thin dressing or heel protectors on reddened areas and elevation of the patient's heels with pillows.

One year after the actions were completed, the incidence of hospital-acquired heel pressure ulcers had not significantly changed. An analysis of current practices found that staff nurses were not consistently completing the periodic risk assessments and that heel ulcer prevention interventions were not always employed. A lot of work had been done by the improvement team, the people who had created the training and post-training exam, and the people who had modified the computerized record system, yet no significant improvements occurred.

Everyone involved in improvement projects wants performance to improve. But good intentions are not enough to ensure good outcomes. To achieve better performance that is reliable, human factors science must be taken into consideration when making changes.

CONSIDER THE HUMAN FACTORS

Often, improvement initiatives fail because we expect people to perfectly execute their job responsibilities. Competence is important to an individual's ability to do her job—you wouldn't expect someone untrained in automobile repair to fix your car. But humans are not perfect, and there are no guarantees that mistakes will not be made. Interventions to improve performance are most successful when they address both the individuals doing the work and the way in which work gets done. For instance, the automobile mechanic must be adequately trained, have the right tools, and be provided a tolerable work environment. When healthcare improvement teams reach the action-planning phase, they must consider the human aspects that cause inconsistent performance and design systems that promote reliable quality.

Strong and effective systems make people more effective than they might be without such systems. Changes in procedures, rules, workflow, and automation; the introduction of new technology and equipment; and other system changes help to make people effective. In addition, strong and effective people make systems more effective. Rather than blaming and shaming people for not doing their job, seek to develop and enhance the competencies and skills of people in the system and ensure their needs are met. When introducing workflow changes, automation, new roles, and other interventions designed to improve performance, consider the needs of the people involved and how they will be affected. Organizations often fail in this regard by making the following mistakes (Spath 2015):

◆ Creating additional work for fewer people

◆ Removing people from roles in which they were comfortable

◆ Placing people in unfamiliar new roles as if they were interchangeable parts

◆ Not involving or consulting with the people affected by decisions but instead making assumptions about what is "good for them"

When working in complex and sometimes fast-moving healthcare environments, people can become overwhelmed with tasks, potentially causing cognitive overload—a situation in which the demands of the job exceed the individual's ability to mentally process all the information encountered regarding a situation (Ternov 2011). To ensure people are as effective as possible in their job, cognitive overload must be minimized. Critical concept 9.1 shows how to do this.

CRITICAL CONCEPT 9.1
Steps to Reduce Cognitive Overload on People

- Limit or discourage people from working when they are physically ill or under psychological duress.

- Be sure people are physically and psychologically fit for the tasks that need to be completed.

- Provide people with adequate breaks away from their job; breaks should not be optional.

- Add technologies that reduce reliance on memory, and insist that the technology be used as designed (e.g., barcoded patient identification systems, monitoring systems).

- Rotate tasks in a department when possible; when people do the same task all the time, they can become complacent and experience the effects of mental underload.

- Monitor people for excessive fatigue; a lack of adequate rest reduces productivity and efficiency.

- Place limitations on employee overtime, and provide adequate off-work intervals between shifts.

- Provide team training, including the use of simulation methods.

Source: Adapted from Kochar and Connelly (2013); Patel and Buchman (2016); Vincent and Amalberti (2016).

TEST REDESIGNED PROCESSES

Changes to processes are often implemented without a clear understanding of how the change affects other parts of the system—the people, other processes, and services. Testing the impact of redesigned processes on performance is a crucial step in all the improvement models described in chapter 5. One way to assess improvements is to test process changes, before they are implemented, on a small subset of activities or patients (usually five to ten individuals). If the changes achieve the intended goals, they can be applied to all activities or patients. Quantitative and qualitative data should be collected during the pilot phase of a process change. This information helps the project team see the impact changes will have on the people doing the work as well as on related activities and systems. It also can convince others of the value of adopting the changes organization-wide.

Testing does not end at the pilot phase. After changes have been implemented for a short time, the team must determine how well they are working.

ACHIEVE 80 TO 90 PERCENT RELIABILITY

To consistently reach 80 to 90 percent work system reliability, the improvement team must create a specific process and use staff education and vigilance to achieve standardization. The attempt at reducing heel pressure ulcers described in the case study earlier in this chapter lacked an important component: vigilance. Specific processes were designed to assess a patient's risk of a heel ulcer and to prevent one from developing, and staff was educated in these processes. But management exercised no ongoing oversight to determine if nurses were following the processes, and no actions were taken for noncompliance. Without vigilance, compliance slid, and the failure rate often exceeded 20 percent.

Standardization and vigilance are necessary to reach sustained 80 to 90 percent reliability. These contributors to quality can be instituted by creating defined protocols, requiring the use of common equipment or supplies, creating checklists that remind people what needs to be done, and following other methods for reducing process variation. Many of these techniques are the same strategies used during a Lean project to eliminate waste and improve process efficiencies (Zidel 2012).

Process standardization also improves patient safety. According to Bagian and colleagues (2011), local patient safety managers in VA facilities rated process standardization as one of the best interventions for achieving good results. Other actions rated as leading to much better results included those that improve the communication process between clinicians and those that enhance the computerized medical record through software upgrades.

If an improvement team has determined that 80 to 90 percent reliability is sufficient, it need not take further action other than periodic monitoring to ensure the failure rate does not increase. Exhibit 9.4 describes the steps that a rehabilitation facility took to reach 80 to 90 percent sustained compliance with hand-hygiene requirements. This level of reliability was the goal, so no further interventions were needed.

Additional improvement actions are necessary if a higher level of reliability is desired. They should not be taken, however, until a sustained level of 80 to 90 percent reliability has been achieved for at least six months (Baker, Crowe, and Lewis 2009). Adding improvement actions when a process is still unstable could further degrade reliability. The adverse effect of tampering was discussed in chapter 4.

Improvement Action	Measurement Results
1. Mandatory hand-hygiene and infection-control training for all patient care staff	40% compliance
2. "Clean Your Hands" posters displayed in units; weekly observation reviews by infection control team, with immediate feedback for noncompliance	Up to 60% compliance
3. Hand-hygiene process standardized using "Five Key Moments for Hand Hygiene" and staff educated in process; data gathered to better understand the causes of noncompliance so that process can be changed to prevent these failures	Up to 70% compliance
4. "Five Key Moments" posters displayed in units and patient rooms; hand-hygiene reminders included in shift change discussions and during patient bed rounds; ongoing weekly observation reviews by hand-hygiene champions, with nonconfrontational feedback for noncompliance; continued evaluation of causes of noncompliance and changes made to prevent failures	Sustained 80–90% compliance

EXHIBIT 9.4
Rehabilitation
Facility Hand-
Hygiene
Improvement
Project

ACHIEVE 95 PERCENT RELIABILITY

Moving a work system from 80 to 90 percent reliability to 95 percent requires stronger interventions than have been adopted thus far. Some actions, such as building decision aids into the system, may be as straightforward as creating paper checklist reminders for people to use. Decision aids can also take the form of more sophisticated computerized feedback that alerts people to unusual clinical situations requiring attention.

Intermediate and strong actions needed to improve the reliability of a process to 95 percent are listed in exhibits 9.2 and 9.3. Often, a number of advanced failure prevention and failure identification and mitigation strategies are needed. For instance, the inpatient psychiatric unit at Sinai Hospital of Baltimore (2017) reduced the incidence of patient elopements (unauthorized absence without permission) from four attempted and actual elopements in 2013 to none in 2016. To achieve this improvement, the unit implemented several interventions throughout 2015 and 2016:

◆ Provide staff education to improve awareness and increase staff vigilance

◆ Add more security cameras in the unit

◆ Keep patients in hospital garments for 24 hours after arrival in the unit

◆ Limit the number of outside staff with access to the locked unit

◆ Escort ancillary hospital staff pushing carts (food and linen) to the unit exit door

◆ Dress patients at risk for elopement in green gowns and green socks

◆ Place black-out tape over the five-second flashing green light on the exit door badge scanner

◆ Install safety signs to direct patients to the day area and away from high-risk elopement areas

◆ Add a "panic button" to the staff communication devices to allow for immediate and simultaneous elopement alerts

Exhibit 9.5 shows intermediate and strong actions taken by a hospital to improve the reliability of the intravenous (IV) medication and solution administration process. These actions resulted in sustained 95 percent reliability for many of the process steps. Of course, the interventions differ in their power to effect changes. Some, such as automated functions that prevent IV pumps from being incorrectly programmed, are very strong in preventing failures. Other interventions, such as labels on the IV bags, are less likely to reduce failures. An important step in any improvement project is to closely monitor the effectiveness and impact of action plans and make adjustments as needed.

ACHIEVE 99.5 PERCENT OR BETTER RELIABILITY

Some healthcare processes should function at 99.5 percent reliability or better because failures within them are likely catastrophic for patients. To achieve 99.5 percent performance or greater requires identifying failures, determining how often they occur, and understanding why they occur.

Specifically, getting to 99.5 percent reliability requires three essential steps. First, process failures must be closely monitored. Second, targeted interventions must be designed and tested until the desired level of reliability is achieved and maintained. For example, a large ambulatory health center in the South implemented several process changes to ensure patients with diabetes have regular body mass index (BMI) measurements (Baker, Crowe, and Lewis 2009). In addition to educating staff on the importance of obtaining a BMI at every patient visit, BMI was made a data element on the clinic's standardized flow sheet that serves as the front page of the record. A care manager reviews patient records the day before a visit to determine if BMI is entered into the electronic record, and job descriptions for all patient care staff were updated to include the task of ensuring BMI documentation

Type of Action	Intervention
Standardization is pervasive	• Reduce the variety of IV solutions available as floor stock to those most frequently used • Use only standard concentrations of IV solutions • Make only one kind of IV medication pump in each class available in the hospital • Develop and implement standard IV physician orders
Decision aids and reminders are built into the system	• Label all IV solutions that do not come from the pharmacy with a tag displaying the nurse's name, date, name of solution, and rate of administration • Place on each IV bag a drug-specific label containing flow rate calculations • Program standard IV orders into the computerized order entry system
The desired action is the default	• Use IV pumps with forcing functions to prevent programming errors
Habits and patterns are studied and used in the design	• Change the arrangement of the medication access control device so only one injection is available per drawer
Process risks are specified, and actions for reducing risks are articulated	• Include discussion of risks and interventions in the annual staff competency assessment process to reduce these risks
Scheduling is used to advantage	• At change of shift, double-check all potentially hazardous IVs (medications, pump settings, and IV tubing) for failure
Redundant processes are in place	• Place on each IV bag a drug-specific label containing flow rate calculations
Independent backup is in place	• Have two nurses independently double-check all IV medications, pump settings, and IV tubing before administration and before patient transfer to another location
Compliance is measured and results are shared	• Gather data on compliance with the new process and the number of incidents involving IV medication and IV solutions; regularly evaluate results and share with everyone involved in the process

Exhibit 9.5

Examples of Interventions That Improved Reliability of Administration of IV Medications and Solutions

at every visit. After experiencing negative reactions from some patients when asked to be weighed, the clinic revised its diabetic education materials with input from patients. The percentage of patients with diabetes with a completed BMI improved from less than 20 percent to 100 percent.

Third, once sustained reliability (99.5 percent or better) is achieved, performance must be regularly reviewed and feedback provided to the people doing the work. Every failure should be examined, and the information obtained should be used to redesign the process or create ways for staff to better identify and correct failures quickly or to lessen the effects of the failures.

In some situations, the healthcare organization may seek to improve reliability to 99.9 percent or better. Achieving such a high level of reliability requires more than human labor. Technology and possibly architectural changes are needed. Anesthesia administration, once thought to cause 1 to 2 deaths in every 10,000 patients receiving anesthesia, is now considered to be one of the most reliable processes occurring in healthcare delivery (Stoelting 2017). A host of changes to anesthesia administration, based on an understanding of human factors principles, were initiated throughout the United States in the 1970s. Reaching the current high level of reliability required the adoption of important safety technology (pulse oximetry, capnography, audible physiologic alarms, electronic health records) as well as improvements in the culture of safety. Overall, the combined effect of all the initiatives has been a 10- to 20-fold reduction in mortality and catastrophic morbidity for healthy patients undergoing routine anesthesia (Stoelting 2017).

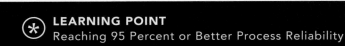

LEARNING POINT
Reaching 95 Percent or Better Process Reliability

Reaching 95 percent or better process reliability involves four main steps:

1. Agree on a measure for assessing reliability.
2. Measure how often accuracy is achieved according to the agreed-on measure, thereby establishing a baseline against which to compare results of the initiative.
3. Establish reliability goals for the measure.
4. Make stepwise improvements and measure success.

Source: Dlugacz and Spath (2011).

MONITORING PERFORMANCE

Designing process changes on the basis of reliability science is the starting point to achieving consistently high quality. The next step is to make the changes. Once the improvement team has developed action plans, leadership oversight will ensure the actions are implemented as intended. Researchers studying the implementation of corrective measures following root cause analyses found that healthcare organizations never fully implemented up to 55 percent of the proposed actions (Peerally et al. 2016).

The organization's progress in implementing action plans must be tracked and leaders kept informed of outstanding and completed action items. Exhibit 9.6 is an excerpt from a monthly report on the status of improvement actions provided to hospital leaders. When

Date of Report: _____

Current Status	Project Description	Actions	Responsible Party	Actions to Date
Needs attention	Reduce delays in start times for interventional radiology procedures	1. Revise the patient scheduling procedure	1. Imaging director	1. Done
		2. Publish an article about new policy in medical staff newsletter	2. Medical staff services office	2. Done
		3. Revise the scheduling software to accommodate new policy	3. Imaging director and software vendor	3. Vendor has repeatedly canceled on-site visit for software upgrade
		4. Conduct monitoring by radiology department for compliance with new policy	4. Imaging director	4. Radiology department unable to start new procedure due to software upgrade delay
In progress	Improve timeliness of electrocardiogram (EKG) interpretations	1. Standardize the EKG interpretation process	1. Vice president of medical affairs	1. Done
		2. Modify transmission process at off-site locations	2. Diagnostic center managers	2. Done
		3. Obtain software upgrade to enable results tracking	3. Managers of noninvasive cardiology and information technology departments	3. Funds for software in next year's capital budget

EXHIBIT 9.6
Improvement
Action Tracking
Log

delays are unacceptable, senior leaders often need to intervene to clear away implementation barriers. In chapter 12, we discuss the leadership structure necessary to support quality management activities, including the role of the organization's governing board and quality oversight groups in monitoring performance.

MEASURE EFFECTIVENESS

Improvement goals are set at the start of an improvement project. Clearly documented goals help frame the improvement initiative. The project goals guide decisions about what needs to be changed in the process and how best to accomplish the changes. Once action plans

Consider the following questions when developing measures to evaluate the success of improvement actions:

1. How will you know the action has been effective in improving performance?

2. What will you evaluate to determine if the process is more reliable?

3. Do you have any data that can be used for before-and-after comparisons?

4. How often will you measure performance (by shift, daily, weekly, biweekly, monthly, other)?

5. How will data be gathered, and by whom?

6. How long will you continue to measure performance?

7. How often will performance results be reported, and to whom?

8. Once measurement data substantiate that performance goals are met, how often will you measure to ensure improved performance is sustained?

Source: Adapted from Bagian et al. (2011).

have been implemented, evaluate whether goals have been achieved. Regardless of what improvement model is used to execute the project, it will include a step in which the effectiveness of action plans is measured.

Action plan effectiveness can be determined using process or outcome measures. Recall from chapter 3 that process measures are data describing how services are delivered, and outcome measures are data describing the results of healthcare services. Exhibit 9.7 is a description of an improvement project undertaken in a multiclinic primary care organization to improve the use of preventive care screenings. Several actions were taken, and three measures were used to evaluate the success of the actions.

Chapter 3 discusses data collection systems for gathering performance measurement information. Similar data collection systems must be enacted to measure the effectiveness of action plans. Useful and accurate performance information is needed to judge the success of action plans.

A question that often arises during discussions of how to measure the success of improvement actions is, How long must we continue to gather and report measurement data? Ideally, all of the following criteria should be met to conclude that successful corrective action plan implementation has been achieved (Minnesota Department of Health 2015):

◆ Data for the process measure were monitored over time.

◆ The goal was attained (process and outcome).

◆ You are confident that the change is permanent.

◆ The event is not repeated (if improvements were made to prevent another adverse event).

Improvement Project Goal: Increase rates of preventive care screening services

Improvement Actions:

1. Telephone patients to remind them to come to the clinic for needed preventive care screening.
2. Design a preventive care services summary in patient electronic records to document needed preventive screening, date of patient contact, and date of completion.
3. Educate staff in preventive service requirements and how to use the summary in patient records.
4. Change the workflow to include having medical assistants or nurses prepare paperwork for preventive screenings before a patient's visit and give to the provider at the time of the visit.

How Effectiveness of Actions Will Be Measured:

Measure	Data Collection Method	Goal
Percentage of patients needing preventive screenings who are contacted by phone	Quarterly query of database of patients needing screenings to determine if patient was contacted	Sustained 95 percent
Percentage of patients needing preventive screenings who receive them as required	Quarterly query of preventive care services summary database	Sustained 95 percent
Number of patients who refuse preventive screenings after discussion with provider	Quarterly query of preventive care services summary database	No more than 5 percent per quarter

EXHIBIT 9.7

Improvement Project Measures of Action Plan Effectiveness

REALIZING SUSTAINED IMPROVEMENTS

Once the desired level of reliable quality has been reached, the problems affecting undesirable performance must stay fixed. "I thought we solved that problem already" is an utterance often heard in healthcare organizations. Financial and human resources are constantly expended on improvement projects and system redesign, yet familiar problems may creep back in to disrupt the performance of key processes. Managers trying to improve performance sometimes make mistakes that could have been avoided with forethought.

CHANGE BEHAVIORS

When process improvements come undone, the cause often can be traced back to the attitudes or behaviors of the people doing the work—behaviors that should have been modified but were not. Process improvement efforts tend to focus on standardizing and error-proofing work steps and sometimes overlook the human part of the process. For instance, nurses in a hospital that implemented a barcoded patient identification system to reduce medication errors found the process too cumbersome and began to take shortcuts (Koppel et al. 2008). The nurses made duplicate copies of patient wristbands so they could check the barcodes at the nursing station rather than in patient rooms. This shortcut significantly raised the potential for medication errors. Understanding what causes shortcuts is at the heart of knowing how to modify attitudes and behaviors. This is just as important as creating a more efficient process. Otherwise, people will lapse into the old way of doing things, and the new process will have no chance of becoming a habit.

Why don't people adopt desired process changes? Five main factors that affect performance are listed in exhibit 9.8.

EXHIBIT 9.8
Performance
Factors and
Possible
Interventions

Performance Factor	Possible Interventions
Expectations Do people know what they are supposed to do?	• Provide clear performance standards and job descriptions. • Create channels to communicate job responsibilities.
Feedback Do people know how well they are doing?	• Offer timely information about people's performance. • Use mistakes as learning opportunities.
Physical environment Does the work environment help or hinder performance?	• Make sure people are able to see, hear, touch, and feel what is necessary to do the job. • Correct problems causing environment, supply, or equipment complaints.
Motivation Do people have a reason to perform as they are asked to perform? Does anyone notice?	• Frequently provide reinforcement to people while they are learning new tasks. • Apply consequences (positive or negative) to change behaviors toward the desired direction.
Required skills and knowledge Do people know how to do the task?	• Ensure people have the skills needed to perform the work. • Provide access to learning opportunities.

Interventions to achieve compliance with process changes vary according to the performance issue, but the cause of failures must be understood before action is taken to correct them.

DON'T OVERLOOK EDUCATION

Knowledge, diligence, effort, focus, resources, and effective leadership are all essential to the achievement of performance improvement goals. Leaders would be unwise to announce improvement priorities and then expect the improvements to automatically materialize. This approach does not work. Just as cheerleading does not improve a football team's chances of winning, announcements from leadership alone do not create reliable quality. Project teams need encouragement from leaders, but everyone involved in process improvement also must be able to use basic quality tools and techniques such as those covered in this text.

CONCLUSION

Only recently has more attention been given to securing reliable healthcare quality through the application of human factors principles and reliability science. Rather than tinker with work systems and hope for the best, some healthcare organizations are applying improvement strategies that have been used successfully for years in other industries. High-reliability industries, such as aviation, air traffic control, and nuclear power, have long recognized that relying on human perfection to prevent accidents is a fallacy. These industries conduct training, enforce rules, and expect their high standards to be met, but they do not rely on people being perfect to prevent accidents. They look to their systems, as should healthcare organizations (Ghaferi et al. 2016).

Human factors and reliability design concepts should be required for all healthcare improvement projects. To reach higher levels of reliable performance, systems and processes must be designed to be more resistant to failure. Situations or factors likely to give rise to human error must be identified and process changes made to reduce the occurrence of failure or to minimize the impact of any errors on health outcomes. Efforts to catch human errors before they occur or to block them from causing harm are ultimately more fruitful than those seeking to somehow create flawless people.

The application of human factors principles and reliability science is long overdue in healthcare. As noted by Deming (1986), one of the founders of the contemporary quality movement, "It is not enough to do your best; you must know what to do, and then do your best."

For Discussion

1. What does reliability mean to you? In your experience, what healthcare process have you found to be reliable? What process have you found to be unreliable? Explain what is different about the reliable process versus the unreliable process.

2. Consider the failed improvement project in this chapter's case study when answering the following questions:

   a. What process changes could be implemented to achieve 80 to 90 percent reliability in preventing and managing heel ulcerations?

   b. What process changes could be implemented to reach 95 percent reliability in preventing and managing heel ulcerations?

   c. If process changes are made to achieve 80 to 90 percent reliability, how would you measure the effectiveness of these changes?

   d. If process changes are made to achieve 95 percent reliability, how would you measure the effectiveness of these changes?

Websites

- Agency for Healthcare Research and Quality (AHRQ) Innovations Exchange
www.innovations.ahrq.gov

- AHRQ, *Becoming a High Reliability Organization: Operational Advice for Hospital Leaders* (April 2008)
https://archive.ahrq.gov/professionals/quality-patient-safety/quality-resources/tools/hroadvice/hroadvice.pdf

- AHRQ Comprehensive Unit-Based Safety Programs (CUSP)
www.ahrq.gov/cusptoolkit/

- AHRQ Patient Safety Network: High Reliability
https://psnet.ahrq.gov/primers/primer/31/high-reliability

- American Hospital Association, Hospitals in Pursuit of Excellence
www.hpoe.org

- Clinical Human Factors Group
http://chfg.org

- The Dartmouth Institute Microsystem Academy
www.clinicalmicrosystem.org

- Grout, J. R. 2007. *Mistake-Proofing the Design of Health Care Processes.* AHRQ Publication No. 07-0020. Rockville, MD: Agency for Healthcare Research and Quality. https://archive.ahrq.gov/professionals/quality-patient-safety/patient-safety-resources/resources/mistakeproof/

- Healthcare Communities
  www.healthcarecommunities.org

- High Reliability Organizing
  http://high-reliability.org

- Home Health Quality Improvement
  www.homehealthquality.org

- Institute for Healthcare Improvement (IHI), "How to Improve" resources
  www.ihi.org/knowledge

- IHI, *Improving the Reliability of Health Care.* 2004.
  www.ihi.org/education/IHIOpenSchool/Courses/Documents/CourseraDocuments/08_ReliabilityWhitePaper2004revJune06.pdf

- Massachusetts Coalition for the Prevention of Medical Errors
  www.macoalition.org/

- Medical Group Management Association. *High Reliability Organization in the Healthcare Industry: A Model for Excellence, Innovation, and Sustainability.* Focus paper.
  www.mgma.com/practice-resources/articles/fellow-papers/2016/high-reliability-organization-in-the-healthcare-industry-a-model-for-excellence-innovation-and-sus

- Project Re-engineered Discharge, hospital discharge research from Boston University Medical Center
  www.bu.edu/fammed/projectred/index.html

- Society of Hospital Medicine's BOOSTing Care Transitions
  www.hospitalmedicine.org/ResourceRoomRedesign/RR_CareTransitions/CT_Home.cfm

REFERENCES

Agency for Healthcare Research and Quality (AHRQ). 2016. *2015 National Healthcare Quality and Disparities Report and 5th Anniversary Update on the National Quality Strategy.* Rockville, MD: Agency for Healthcare Research and Quality.

Amalberti, R., Y. Auroy, D. Berwick, and P. Barach. 2005. "Five System Barriers to Achieving Ultrasafe Health Care." *Annals of Internal Medicine* 142 (9): 756–64.

Bagian, J. P., B. J. King, P. D. Mills, and S. D. McKnight. 2011. "Improving RCA Performance: The Cornerstone Award and Power of Positive Reinforcement." *BMJ Quality & Safety* 20 (11): 974–82.

Baker, N., V. Crowe, and A. Lewis. 2009. "Making Patient-Centered Care Reliable." *Journal of Ambulatory Care Management* 32 (1): 6–13.

Bernstein, M., J. K. Hou, A. V. Weizman, J. Mosko, N. Bollegala, M. Brahmania, L. Liu, A. H. Steinhart, S. S. Silver, G. C. Nguyen, and C. M. Bell. 2016. "Quality Improvement Primer Series: How to Sustain a Quality Improvement Effort." *Clinical Gastroenterology and Hepatology* 14 (10): 1371–75.

Bodenheimer, T. 2008. "Coordinating Care—A Perilous Journey Through the Health Care System." *New England Journal of Medicine* 358 (10): 1064–71.

Bohmer, R. M. 2010. "Fixing Health Care on the Front Lines." *Harvard Business Review* 88 (4): 62–69.

Clinical Human Factors Group. 2016. "What Is Human Factors?" Accessed November 24, 2017. http://chfg.org/about-us/what-is-human-factors/.

Deming, W. E. 1986. *Out of the Crisis*. Cambridge, MA: MIT Press.

DeRosier, J. M., L. Taylor, and J. P. Bagian. 2007. "Root Cause Analysis of Wandering Adverse Events in the Veterans Health Administration." In *Evidence-Based Protocols for Managing Wandering Behaviors*, edited by A. Nelson and D. L. Algase, 161–80. New York: Springer.

Dlugacz, D., and P. L. Spath. 2011. "High Reliability and Patient Safety." In *Error Reduction in Health Care*, 2nd ed., edited by P. Spath, 35–56. San Francisco: Jossey-Bass.

Erasmus, V., T. J. Daha, H. Brug, J. H. Richardus, M. D. Behrendt, M. C. Vos, and E. F. van Beeck. 2010. "Systematic Review of Studies on Compliance with Hand Hygiene Guidelines in Hospital Care." *Infection Control and Hospital Epidemiology* 31 (3): 283–94.

Ghaferi, A. A., C. G. Myers, K. M. Sutcliffe, and P. Pronovost. 2016. "The Next Wave of Hospital Innovation to Make Patients Safer." *Harvard Business Review*. Published August 8. https://hbr.org/2016/08/the-next-wave-of-hospital-innovation-to-make-patients-safer.

Health and Safety Executive. 2014. "ALARP at a Glance." Accessed November 24, 2017. www.hse.gov.uk/risk/theory/alarpglance.htm.

Hopkinson, S. G., and B. M. Jennings. 2013. "Interruptions During Nurses' Work: A State-of-the-Science Review." *Research in Nursing & Health* 36 (1): 38–53.

Kochar, M. S., and B. A. Connelly. 2013. "Sleep Deprivation in Healthcare Professionals: The Effect on Patient Safety." In *Patient Safety Handbook*, 2nd ed., edited by B. J. Youngberg, 299–311. Burlington, MA: Jones & Bartlett Learning.

Koppel, R., T. Wetterneck, J. L. Telles, and B. Karsh. 2008. "Workarounds to Barcode Medication Administration Systems: Their Occurrences, Causes, and Threats to Patient Safety." *Journal of the American Medical Informatics Association* 15 (4): 408–23.

Luria, J. W., S. E. Muething, P. J. Schoettker, and U. R. Kotagal. 2006. "Reliability Science and Patient Safety." *Pediatric Clinics of North America* 53 (6): 1121–33.

McInnis, D. 2006. "What System?" *Dartmouth Medicine* 30 (4): 28–35.

Minnesota Department of Health. 2015. *Minnesota Adverse Health Events Measurement Guide*. Prepared by Stratis Health, Bloomington, MN. Revised December 2. www.stratishealth.org/documents/MN_AE_Health_Events_Measurement_Guide.pdf.

Nolan, T., R. Resar, C. Haraden, and F. A. Griffin. 2004. *Improving the Reliability of Health Care*. Institute for Healthcare Improvement Innovation Series white paper. Accessed November 24, 2017. www.ihi.org/education/IHIOpenSchool/Courses/Documents/CourseraDocuments/08_ReliabilityWhitePaper2004revJune06.pdf.

Patel, V. L., and T. G. Buchman. 2016. "Cognitive Overload in the ICU." WebM&M Spotlight Case. Published July/August. https://psnet.ahrq.gov/webmm/case/380/cognitive-overload-in-the-icu.

Peerally, M. F., S. Carr, J. Waring, and M. Dixon-Woods. 2016. "The Problem with Root Cause Analysis." *BMJ Quality & Safety* 26 (5): 417–22.

Resar, R. 2006. "Making Noncatastrophic Health Care Processes Reliable: Learning to Walk Before Running in Creating High-Reliability Organizations." *Health Services Research* 41 (4): 1677–89.

Sinai Hospital of Baltimore. 2017. "How We Prevent Elopements (Absconding) on Mount Pleasant One." Poster presentation at Patient Safety Conference sponsored by the Maryland Patient Safety Center, Baltimore, MD, March 17.

Spath, P. L. 2015. "High-Reliability Organizations." In *Handbook of Healthcare Management*, edited by M. D. Fottler, D. Malvey, and D. J. Slovensky, 38–65. Northampton, MA: Edward Elgar Publishing.

Stoelting, R. 2017. "About Anesthesia Patient Safety Foundation (APSF): Pioneering Safety." Accessed November 24. www.apsf.org/about_safety.php.

Ternov, S. 2011. "The Human Side of Medical Mistakes." In *Error Reduction in Health Care*, 2nd ed., edited by P. Spath, 21–33. San Francisco: Jossey-Bass.

US Department of Veterans Affairs, National Center for Patient Safety. 2016. "Root Cause Analysis." Accessed November 24, 2017. www.patientsafety.va.gov/professionals/onthejob/rca.asp.

Vincent, C., and R. Amalberti. 2016. *Safer Healthcare: Strategies for the Real World*. New York: Springer Open.

Wickens, C., J. Hollands, R. Parasuraman, and S. Banbury. 2012. *Engineering Psychology and Human Performance*, 4th ed. New York: Pearson.

Williams, L., and J. P. Bagian. 2014. "Humans and EI&K Seeking: Factors Influencing Reliability." In *Patient Safety: Perspectives on Evidence, Information and Knowledge Transfer*, edited by L. Zipperer, 224–36. Surrey, UK: Gower.

Zidel, T. G. 2012. *Lean Done Right: Achieve and Maintain Reform in Your Healthcare Organization*. Chicago: Health Administration Press.

CHAPTER 10

MANAGING THE USE OF HEALTHCARE RESOURCES

After reading this chapter, you will be able to

➤ describe the purpose of utilization management;

➤ discuss utilization management measurement, assessment, and improvement activities;

➤ recognize the role of physicians and nonphysicians in managing the use of healthcare resources;

➤ describe how clinical practice guidelines are used for utilization management purposes; and

➤ identify sources of comparative healthcare utilization data.

➤ Accountable care organizations (ACOs)

➤ Case managers

➤ Clinical paths

➤ Concurrent review

➤ Discharge planning

➤ Episode-based bundled payments

➤ Medically necessary

➤ Pay-for-performance systems

➤ Physician advisor

➤ Preadmission certification

➤ Prospective review

➤ Protocols

➤ Retrospective review

➤ Utilization

➤ Utilization management (UM)

➤ Utilization review

➤ Value-based reimbursement

Utilization management (UM)
Planning, organizing, directing, and, controlling healthcare products in a cost-effective manner while maintaining quality of patient care and contributing to the organization's goals.

Medically necessary
Appropriate and consistent with diagnosis and, according to accepted standards of practice in the medical community, imperative to treatment to prevent the patient's condition or the quality of the patient's care from being adversely affected.

Quality management is a broad term that encompasses many healthcare performance measurement, assessment, and improvement activities. Patient safety, the topic covered in chapter 8, is one component of quality management. This chapter introduces another component: utilization management. The activities involved in utilization management are somewhat different from those involved in patient safety and other performance improvement initiatives, as explained in this chapter.

UTILIZATION MANAGEMENT

In the early 1980s, the American Hospital Association defined **utilization management (UM)** as planning, organizing, directing, and controlling healthcare products in a cost-effective manner while maintaining quality of patient care and contributing to the organization's goals (Spath 2013). This definition is still relevant today. Providers use UM to eliminate underuse and overuse of **medically necessary** healthcare services. The UM activities of payers have a slightly different focus, as illustrated by the UM definition of the National Committee for Quality Assurance (NCQA): "Evaluating and determining coverage for and appropriateness of medical and behavioral health care services, as well as providing needed assistance to providers and patients, in cooperation with other parties, to ensure appropriate use of resources" (IOM 2011, 27).

Fundamentally, the purpose of UM is to ensure that patients receive necessary medical services at the lowest cost. In any business transaction, buyers do not want to pay for something they do not need, and they do not want to pay for top-shelf products when a less expensive product will work just as well. For instance, when your car needs an oil change, you don't want to buy extra parts or high-performance oil blends you do not need. You pay the entire bill in this transaction, so you decide what is necessary. You may consider the mechanic's recommendations, but you also know that the mechanic's desire for profit could motivate him to suggest unnecessary products or services.

In healthcare, the buyer–seller relationship is different. First, an insurance company often pays the majority of the bill, whereas the patient pays nothing or only a portion of expenses. Health insurers are the primary buyers of healthcare services, and like all buyers, insurers do not want to pay for unnecessary care. Healthcare customers—patients—rely almost solely on physicians and other providers to decide which services are necessary. Profit considerations could influence healthcare recommendations, as in other industries; however, the average patient cannot distinguish between necessary and unnecessary services, putting her at a disadvantage. Likewise, the average patient cannot recognize underuse of services—situations in which beneficial services are not provided. Fortunately, those in the best position to judge medical necessity—practitioners and healthcare organizations—actively evaluate services to prevent overuse and underuse.

> **? DID YOU KNOW?**
>
> The United States spends more on healthcare than on food or housing. In 2015, average per person spending on healthcare in the United States (including health insurance costs paid both by a third party and out-of-pocket) was $9,990 per person and accounted for 17.7 percent of the economy (CMS 2017c). By 2025, the Centers for Medicare & Medicaid Services projects health spending will be nearly one-fifth (19.9 percent) of the gross national product (CMS 2017d).

The importance of appropriate use of healthcare services was reiterated in the 2001 Institute of Medicine (IOM) report *Crossing the Quality Chasm: A New Health System for the 21st Century*. Effective healthcare—services developed on the basis of scientific knowledge and offered to all who may benefit but not to those not likely to benefit—is one of the six dimensions of quality described in the report.

DEFINING APPROPRIATE SERVICES

Many healthcare decisions are easily made. For instance, a patient with a broken arm needs bone realignment and a cast. Some medical decisions are not so obvious, however. To practice UM, purchasers and providers must have a way to judge the appropriateness of services.

Until relatively recently, only physicians decided whether services would benefit their patients. But in the early 1970s, researchers studying how physicians cared for patients with the same medical condition found a pattern. One of these researchers, John Wennberg, MD, a Dartmouth Medical School expert in geographic variation in healthcare delivery, uncovered substantial evidence of overuse—unneeded healthcare. In one analysis, for example, despite a lack of discernible improvements in health in the higher-spending locations, he found that 70 percent of children who grew up in Stowe, Vermont (higher spending), had tonsillectomies by age 15, compared with 10 percent of children from the neighboring town of Waterbury (lower spending) (Wennberg and Gittelsohn 1973). Similarly, approximately 50 percent of men in Portland, Maine, had prostate surgery by age 85, compared with about 10 percent of men in Bangor (Wennberg, Gittelsohn, and Shapiro 1975). These studies tended not to label **utilization** as appropriate or inappropriate, but the variability of the results suggested that many services were unnecessary. These findings caused purchasers to strengthen UM efforts.

Utilization
Use of medical services and supplies, commonly examined in terms of patterns or rates of use of a single service or type of service, such as hospital care, physician visits, and prescription drugs.

The concept of clinical practice guidelines is introduced in chapter 3 as the basis for creating evidence-based performance measures and as a means of standardizing clinical decision-making. Researchers found that in areas of treatment that enjoy strong professional consensus on the appropriate use of particular services (e.g., surgery for cancer of the bowel, hospitalization for hip fracture), utilization varies relatively little, whereas in areas with low consensus (e.g., the need for hysterectomy and prostatectomy), utilization varies more (Caper 1984). Health insurers encouraged the development of clinical practice guidelines and standardization of care for UM purposes, specifically to reduce the provision of unnecessary services.

To jump-start the guideline development effort, in 1990 the Agency for Healthcare Research and Quality (AHRQ)—then known as the Agency for Health Care Policy and Research—published a methodology for developing guidelines and began sponsoring clinical practice guideline development task groups (Field and Lohr 1990). Within a few years, medical, nursing, and allied health professional groups had developed their own practice guidelines, and the federally sponsored task groups were phased out. As of this writing, more than 1,700 clinical practice guidelines are catalogued on the AHRQ-sponsored National Guideline Clearinghouse (2017) website, www.guideline.gov/browse/. These guidelines help purchasers, healthcare organizations, practitioners, and consumers identify medically necessary services. For instance, in 2017 the American College of Physicians published a guideline addressing noninvasive treatments for acute, subacute, and chronic low back pain in adults. Authors of this guideline discourage clinicians from using spinal manipulation for patients with chronic low back pain as it has little effect on reducing pain (Qaseem et al. 2017).

Although hundreds of clinical practice guidelines are in place, for many conditions evidence is insufficient to use as a basis for judging treatment appropriateness. In these situations, physicians have considerable latitude in making treatment decisions. For this reason, variation in the services provided to patients with similar conditions is still evident (Wennberg, McPherson, and Goodman 2016). In theory, healthcare purchasers, including the Centers for Medicare & Medicaid Services (CMS), pay only for items and services that are reasonably necessary for the diagnosis and treatment of an illness or injury. In situations where no practice guidelines exist, decisions are made on the basis of the best available evidence and professional consensus (CMS 2015). CMS's legal authority to make coverage decisions stems from section 1862 of the Social Security Act, which states: "No payment may be made . . . for any expenses incurred for items or services . . . which are not reasonable and necessary for the diagnosis or treatment of illness or injury or to improve the function of a malformed body member" (US Social Security Administration 2017).

CMS and other purchasers of healthcare follow a rigorous process to determine whether services are appropriate and should be reimbursed (McCauley 2015). For example, Highmark Blue Cross Blue Shield (BCBS), one of the largest BCBS plans in the country, follows a thorough set of procedures for gathering information, assessing new technologies, and making coverage decisions. Highmark bases its coverage decisions on a definition of medical necessity of services that providers agree to in the payer–provider contract (Hill, Hanson, and O'Connell 2000). The service must

◆   be appropriate for symptoms, diagnosis, and treatment of a condition, illness, or injury;

◆   be provided for diagnosis, direct care, or treatment;

◆   be provided in accordance with standards of good medical practice;

◆   not be delivered primarily for the convenience of the member or member's provider; and

◆   constitute the most appropriate supply or level of treatment that can be safely provided to the member.

Purchasers and healthcare organizations also use clinical practice guidelines to identify underuse. For instance, evidence gathered by the American Association of Clinical Endocrinologists and the American College of Endocrinology for managing patients with diabetes points to the importance of annual dilated eye exams; foot exams by a healthcare professional; flu shots; and hemoglobin A1c (HbA1c) testing, which monitors blood sugar levels (Handelsman et al. 2015). According to the US Diabetes Surveillance System (2017), in 2015 the percentage of adult diabetic patients who received these preventive services ranged from a low of 61.9 percent for eye exams to a high of 71.6 percent for foot exams. As this example illustrates, underuse presents opportunities to improve the quality of medical care.

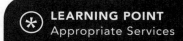

LEARNING POINT
Appropriate Services

The purpose of UM is to ensure that patients receive only medically necessary services at the lowest possible cost. Clinical practice guidelines, research evidence, and professional consensus are considered when identifying overuse and underuse of healthcare services.

Providers and purchasers encourage consumers to become familiar with clinical practice guideline recommendations and to consider them when making health-related decisions. Informed consumers can participate as partners in their own healthcare and help reduce overuse and underuse of services.

UTILIZATION MANAGEMENT FUNCTIONS

Utilization review
Process for monitoring and evaluating the use, delivery, and cost-effectiveness of healthcare services.

UM involves the three basic quality management activities: measurement, assessment, and improvement. **Utilization review** is the term typically used to describe the measurement and assessment tasks, whereas UM is a broad term that encompasses all three activities.

All healthcare organizations are engaged in or affected by one or more of these UM activities. Since the enactment of the Medicare and Medicaid programs in the mid-1960s, hospitals are required to have in place an internal process for evaluating the necessity of services and reducing unnecessary services. Requirements for this process are determined by the Medicare Hospital Conditions of Participation, which apply to most organizations that provide federally funded patient care. For Medicare and Medicaid patients, hospitals are currently required to assess the medical necessity of admission to the institution; the duration of stay; and the professional services furnished, including drugs and biologicals (CMS 2011).

For instance, long-term care facilities are required to evaluate each resident's drug regimen to ensure that only necessary medications are administered. The regulations define an unnecessary drug as any drug used (CMS 2017b)

◆ in excessive doses (including duplicate drug therapy),

◆ for excessive duration,

◆ without adequate monitoring,

◆ without adequate indications for its use,

◆ in the presence of adverse consequences that indicate the dose should be reduced or discontinued, or

◆ in any combination of the above-listed uses.

The Joint Commission accreditation standards do not specifically state that healthcare organizations must engage in UM activities, although they refer to certain UM functions. For instance, the hospital leadership standards encourage the use of clinical practice guidelines to improve quality and utilization (Joint Commission 2017c). Home health agencies accredited by The Joint Commission (2017b) are required to review physician orders and prescriptions for appropriateness and accuracy before providing care, treatment, or services.

Ambulatory surgery centers accredited by The Joint Commission (2017a) are required to collect and analyze data on the appropriateness of care. Health plans accredited by NCQA (2017) are required to conduct "fair and timely utilization evaluations using objective, evidence-based criteria," and the process should be done by "qualified health professionals."

Whether or not an organization is required to conduct internal UM, all providers are affected by the UM activities of health insurers. For instance, physicians may need to obtain prior payment approval from a patient's insurance company for expensive services or experimental treatments. Critical concept 10.1 lists examples of questions physicians must answer when requesting Medicare reimbursement for the cost of a semi-electric hospital bed for a patient who is living at home with a debilitating condition (CGS Administrators 2017).

Some insurers require hospitals to keep them informed of the condition of hospitalized health plan participants. Health plans want to ensure that patients are discharged as soon as they no longer need hospital services. All health insurers measure the cost and

---

① CRITICAL CONCEPT 10.1 Questions Determining Medicare Reimbursement for Use of a Semi-electric Hospital Bed

- Does the patient have a medical condition that requires positioning of the body in ways not feasible with an ordinary bed? (Elevation of the head/upper body less than 30 degrees does not usually require the use of a hospital bed.)

OR

- Does the patient require positioning of the body in ways not feasible with an ordinary bed in order to alleviate pain?

OR

- Does the patient require the head of the bed to be elevated more than 30 degrees most of the time due to congestive heart failure, chronic pulmonary disease, or problems with aspiration?

OR

- Does the patient require traction equipment, which can only be attached to a hospital bed?

Source: Adapted from CGS Administrators (2017).

Value-based reimbursement
Payment that requires healthcare providers to meet certain quality objectives and document compliance with best practices.

Pay-for-performance systems
Performance-based payment arrangements that control costs directly or indirectly by motivating providers to improve quality and reduce inappropriate utilization.

Accountable care organization (ACO)
A group of providers responsible for the quality and cost of care delivered to enrolled patients.

Episode-based bundled payments
A fixed, lump-sum payment for a patient's episode of care for a single illness or course of treatment, shared among all caregivers during and after hospitalization.

quality of care, and some use these data to select and contract only with cost-efficient, high-quality providers. Some large employers and health insurers employ a **value-based reimbursement** strategy. To get more value for their healthcare dollars, these purchasers require that healthcare providers meet certain quality objectives, including documenting how they are meeting best practices and achieving quality outcomes (NCQA 2007).

Similar to value-based reimbursement, Medicare uses **pay-for-performance systems**, which provide financial rewards to providers who achieve certain cost and quality performance expectations (Henkel and Maryland 2015). Medicare and some Medicaid programs are using alternative payment models such as **accountable care organizations (ACOs)** to reduce costs. In a shared-savings ACO model, a group of providers is held responsible for the quality and cost of care delivered to patients enrolled in the ACO. The providers share in any cost savings that may result from improved quality and reduction of unnecessary services.

Another alternative payment method that Medicare uses to reduce unnecessary costs is **episode-based bundled payments**. Hospitals, physicians, and post-hospital care providers are commonly paid separately for services occurring during and after a patient's hospital admission. With episode-based bundled payments, "a fixed, lump sum payment is shared among all caregivers, who also share savings when actual expenditures fall below the bundled payment amount" (Meara and Birkmeyer 2015, 815). For example, when a patient is admitted to the hospital for a total hip replacement, Medicare pays one bundled payment that is shared among the hospital, physicians, and any post-hospital care providers such as physical therapists. "Research has shown that bundled payments can align incentives for providers—hospitals, post-acute care providers, physicians, and other practitioners—allowing them to work closely together across all specialties and settings" (CMS 2017a).

Medicare value-based payment models such as ACOs and bundled payments are likely to expand. A recent study found that use of these models in 2015 at nearly 3,000 hospitals resulted in a net savings of $32 million (Castellucci 2017). More information about the current status of Medicare's alternative payment models can be found on the informational websites provided at the end of this chapter.

MEASUREMENT AND ASSESSMENT

The measurement and assessment component of UM—utilization review—examines the appropriateness of healthcare services. The purpose of these activities is to

◆ ensure services are medically necessary and appropriate, and

◆ promote delivery of services in the most cost-effective setting.

Utilization trends can be reviewed before a patient receives services through **prospective review**, during the delivery of services through **concurrent review**, or after the patient receives services through **retrospective review**.

PROSPECTIVE REVIEW

The purpose of prospective review is to judge the appropriateness of a service before it is rendered to prevent unnecessary use. For instance, an insurance company may refuse to authorize payment for a mammogram for a 37-year-old woman. According to current guideline recommendations, this study would not be considered medically necessary (US Preventive Services Taskforce 2016). The insurance company would likely request additional information about the woman's condition before agreeing to pay for the study. Hospitals and other providers often conduct prospective or **preadmission certification** reviews to determine whether a patient's condition warrants a service or admission to a facility.

CONCURRENT REVIEW

Nurses or other specially trained professionals perform concurrent reviews to assess what is happening in the moment. Such reviews ensure services are appropriate for the patient and are being provided in the least costly setting. In a hospital, a patient's condition and need for hospitalization are assessed at admission and throughout the hospital stay. When the patient no longer requires hospital services, discharge is arranged by the physician. Although nonphysicians are often involved in evaluating the medical necessity of hospital services, the patient's physician makes the final treatment decisions.

Exhibit 10.1 is a summary of a patient's hospital stay for an abdominal hysterectomy (removal of the uterus). Her hospital admission is considered medically necessary because this procedure could not be performed in an outpatient setting. The patient continues to stay in the hospital for several days after the surgery because, up to and including day 3, the patient receives services—intravenous (IV) fluids and pain medications—that she could not receive at home. Her postoperative condition also needs to be frequently evaluated because she may experience complications.

Say the patient has undergone a successful, routine hysterectomy. Her hospital stay up to and including day 3 is considered medically necessary. On day 4, the patient is able to eat, and her condition is improving. As expected, she is weak, but she is able to walk a short distance on her own. Her gastrointestintal function is recovering normally. At this point, the patient probably can be discharged safely.

On the morning of day 4, the nurse reviewer contacts the patient's physician to determine why the patient has not been scheduled for discharge on that day. The physician knows the patient's daughter will not be home to care for her until Saturday morning. He

Prospective review
A method of determining medical necessity and appropriateness of services before the services are rendered.

Concurrent review
An assessment of patient care services that is completed while those services are being delivered to ensure appropriate treatment and level of care.

Retrospective review
A method of determining medical necessity and appropriateness of services that have already been rendered.

Preadmission certification
Review of the need for medical care or services (e.g., inpatient admission, nursing home admission) that is completed before the care or services are provided.

Exhibit 10.1
Summary of
a Patient's
Hospitalization

Day 1 Monday	The patient is admitted for an abdominal hysterectomy. The surgery is performed the morning of admission. The patient is given IV fluids and pain medications postoperatively. The oral heart medications she was taking before surgery are restarted. Her temperature is 99.9 degrees in the late evening.
Day 2 Tuesday	The patient is receiving IV medication for pain control. She is started on a liquid diet at lunch but is also still on IV fluids. She is able to sit at the edge of the bed and can ambulate to the bathroom with assistance. Her temperature has returned to normal.
Day 3 Wednesday	In the morning, the patient's IV fluids are discontinued and she is switched to oral Vicodin for pain control. She is eating and tolerating a light soft diet. She is still weak and unable to walk more than six feet without tiring. She is passing flatus (gas) but has not had a bowel movement. Her temperature is normal.
Day 4 Thursday	The patient is eating and tolerating a light soft diet. Her bowel tones indicate activity and she is passing flatus, but she still has had no bowel movement. Her temperature is normal. She is able to walk by herself to the nursing station and back to her room.
Day 5 Friday	In the morning, the patient eats a regular meal and tolerates it well. She has a bowel movement after lunch. She is receiving her heart medications, and her pain is adequately controlled with Tylenol. She is able to walk without assistance, and her temperature is normal. Her physician writes an order for her to be discharged on Saturday.
Day 6 Saturday	The patient is medically stable, and she is discharged in the morning to her daughter's home.

does not want the patient to leave the hospital until then. While this justification is understandable, her stay beyond day 4 is not considered medically necessary. The patient can leave the hospital and be cared for at home by another family member or a home health aide. In this situation, the hospital may not be reimbursed by the patient's insurance company for days 5 and 6 of her stay.

Sending this patient home from the hospital before Saturday morning may seem mean-spirited, but considering that overuse of expensive medical services is one of the factors driving up healthcare expenditures, timely discharge is crucial. If everyone, including the patient and provider, does not do his or her part to reduce overuse, healthcare expenditures will continue to rise faster than inflation and consume an even larger part of the nation's resources.

The Medicare Conditions of Participation require hospitals and other healthcare facilities to review the medical necessity of patient admissions and continued stays (CMS 2011). Facilities also may be contractually obligated to conduct these reviews for other health insurers. When the patient is no longer receiving medically necessary services or when necessary services are being provided in a more costly setting, a nurse reviewer encourages the patient's physician to discontinue services or to provide them in a less expensive environment. For instance, patients with a condition that requires long-term IV medications do not necessarily require hospitalization. These services can be provided at a lesser cost in a long-term care facility or by a home health agency.

If the patient's physician does not agree with the reviewer's judgment, a **physician advisor** may become involved in the concurrent review process. Physician advisors are practicing physicians who care for patients in the same organization as the primary physician. They are appointed for utilization review purposes and charged with fostering cost-effective practice among other physicians. Concurrent review by a physician advisor creates an opportunity for peer-to-peer discussion about the best use of resources for a patient. If the nurse reviewer had asked a physician advisor on day 4 to become involved in the case described in exhibit 10.1, the patient might have been discharged sooner.

Concurrent reviews are conducted in all provider settings, but the process varies according to the setting. For instance, for Medicare to pay for home care services, patients must either need services that only a licensed nurse (either a registered nurse or a licensed practical nurse) can perform safely and correctly or need physical or speech-language therapy. Patients also must be homebound, meaning they are normally unable to leave home unassisted; when they leave home assisted, it must be to obtain medical care or for short, infrequent nonmedical reasons, such as to attend religious services (CMS 2014). Home health nurse reviewers periodically evaluate the medical needs and homebound status of patients receiving services to ensure they are following Medicare reimbursement guidelines.

Physician advisor
A practicing physician who supports utilization review activities by evaluating the appropriateness of admissions and continued stays, judging the efficiency of services in terms of level of care and place of service, and seeking appropriate care alternatives.

RETROSPECTIVE REVIEW

Retrospective review occurs after patients receive services. In a retrospective review, performance is measured to identify opportunities to reduce overuse and underuse of services. A portion of the review consists of system-level measures. For example, exhibit 10.2 is a line graph showing the average length of stay for Medicare patients at one hospital over a period of three years. The graph shows that for each year, the hospital's average length of stay is longer than the national average. This system-level measure suggests the hospital needs to examine its management of Medicare patients more closely.

The cost of care, another system-level measure, is also evaluated to determine whether it is within a reasonable range. Exhibit 10.3 is a line graph showing the cost of care over a period of three years for Medicare patients hospitalized for the treatment of pneumonia. The graph shows that the hospital's average cost of hospitalization was slightly higher than

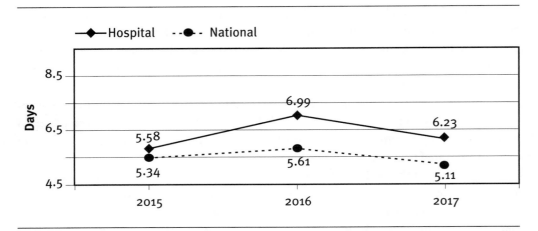

EXHIBIT 10.2
Line Graph
Showing Average
Length-of-Stay
Data for Medicare
Patients

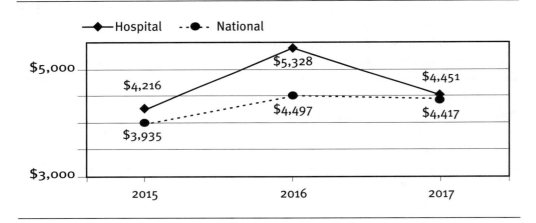

EXHIBIT 10.3
Line Graph
Showing Average
Cost-of-Care
Data for Medicare
Patients with
Pneumonia

the national average in 2015 and even higher in 2016. In early 2017, the hospital created an improvement team of physicians, nurses, pharmacists, and respiratory therapists to identify where costs could be reduced. By making some patient management changes, such as transferring patients to a regular nursing unit earlier in their hospitalization, the hospital was able to bring the overall cost of care closer to the national average in 2017.

Higher-than-expected costs are not always caused by overuse of services or inefficiencies. For example, one hospital discovered that its costs for treating Medicare patients with renal (kidney) failure were higher than other hospitals' costs. An improvement team of physicians, nurses, and other clinicians examined the treatment, looking for unnecessary services and inefficiencies. Instead, they found a quality concern. Their patients with renal failure had a higher complication rate than similar patients at other hospitals. In the complication index illustrated in exhibit 10.4, the national norm, or average complication rate, is expressed as the number 1. This hospital's complication rates for each year were above the norm, which explained the hospital's higher costs; more resources were needed to treat the complications. To reduce costs, the team needed to find and correct the cause of the high complication rate.

Comparison of patient cost and outcome data among facilities has become easier over the past few years because the amount of information available in the public domain continues to increase. The website of the AHRQ-sponsored Healthcare Cost and Utilization Project, www.hcup-us.ahrq.gov, contains the largest collection of healthcare utilization data in the United States and covers inpatient stays, emergency department

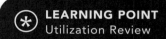

LEARNING POINT
Utilization Review

The purpose of utilization review is to ensure that services are medically necessary and appropriate and to promote delivery of patient care in the most cost-effective setting. Utilization is reviewed prospectively, concurrently, and retrospectively.

visits, and ambulatory care. Its nationwide and state-specific databases can be used to identify, track, and analyze trends in healthcare utilization, access, charges, quality, and outcomes (AHRQ 2017). The free HCUPnet online query system (https://hcupnet.ahrq.gov) provides immediate access to health statistics that are useful for performance comparison purposes.

CMS contracts with the TMF Health Quality Institute (2017b) to create provider-specific Medicare data statistics for discharges and services vulnerable to improper payments (e.g., potential overpayments or underpayments). These reports, known as PEPPER (Program for Evaluating Payment Patterns Electronic Report), can help a facility determine where it may be at risk for improper payments by comparing its billing statistics with national and state results for target areas identified by CMS. For example, one-day stays are a target area for hospitals because historically these stays have had high rates of unnecessary admissions,

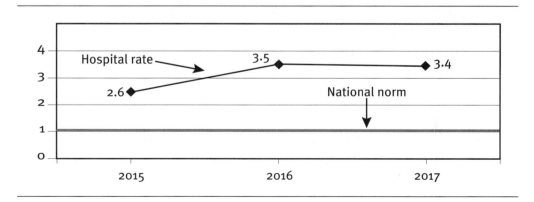

EXHIBIT 10.4
Line Graph Showing Complication Index for Patients with Renal Failure

Exhibit 10.5

Graph Showing a
Hospital's PEPPER
Report of One-Day
Stays for Patients
with Medical
Diagnoses

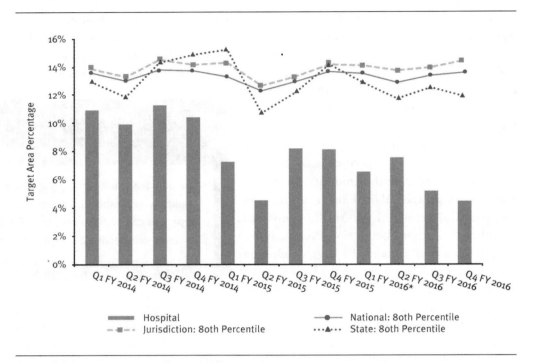

Note: Jurisdiction refers to the Recovery Audit Contractor (RAC) Program geographic area designated by CMS. There are five RAC jurisdictions in the United States.

* In fiscal year 2016, the coding system changed from ICD-9 to ICD-10.

with the stay being billed as inpatient when it should have been billed as an outpatient observation stay (TMF Health Quality Institute 2017a).

The PEPPER report of a hospital's one-day stays for patients with medical diagnoses is illustrated in exhibit 10.5. For 12 quarters, the hospital's percentage of one-day stays falls well below the 80th percentile rate at the national, jurisdictional, and state levels. This result indicates the hospital is most likely billing properly for one-day stays. If the hospital's rate is higher than the comparison rates, an internal investigation should be done to determine the cause of this variation.

UTILIZATION IMPROVEMENT

Providers use information gathered during concurrent and retrospective reviews to identify improvement opportunities. The purpose of the improvement initiative described in the previous section was to reduce the cost of care for patients with pneumonia, but not all utilization improvement activities are focused on cost reduction. For instance, one hospital found that inpatient rooms were not fully utilized. After patients were discharged, the empty rooms were not made available to new patients for up to three hours. Patients were being held in the emergency department until they could be accommodated, which is not a good use of hospital resources.

To address the problem, the hospital's utilization review committee chartered a rapid cycle improvement project. During the investigation, the improvement team discovered that the housekeeping department was not adequately staffed in the late afternoons, when most inpatients are discharged. Consequently, the number of untidy patient rooms was highest when the fewest housekeepers were on duty. A housekeeping discharge work team was created and scheduled to work from 10 a.m. to 8 p.m. The team's sole function was to clean the rooms of discharged patients. After implementing this change, the average time needed to clean a patient room decreased from 75 minutes to 45 minutes and emergency patients no longer had to wait as long for an inpatient bed to become available.

> **⊛ LEARNING POINT**
> **Utilization Improvement**
>
> Improving utilization of healthcare resources involves the same principles as any quality improvement initiative. Opportunities for improvement are identified and actions are taken to achieve utilization goals.

The improvement phase of UM is closely integrated with other quality management activities. Often, improving quality also reduces costs. For instance, the goal of a Lean improvement project is to eliminate waste from a process. Reduced waste means reduced costs. In the example above, moving patients quickly from the emergency department to inpatient beds not only improves utilization of hospital beds but also helps patients receive the inpatient services they need more quickly.

Utilization improvement also involves reducing underuse of needed services. Patients should be receiving care considered appropriate for their diagnosis, type of illness, or condition. To further this goal, job aids can be created for caregivers. Job aids are performance support tools used in all types of industries to provide information that helps people do their jobs. In healthcare, job aids can be designed to promote the use of evidence-based patient care practices. Job aids designed for this purpose usually take three forms: reminders, **clinical paths**, and standards of care.

Reminders are usually short forms or stickers attached to patient records to remind the healthcare provider to perform a certain task. Reminders are useful if underuse is the result of provider forgetfulness or focus on other tasks. For instance, stickers can be placed on the clinic records of patients with diabetes to remind physicians to perform annual eye and foot examinations and to order HbA1c tests. Pop-up alert reminders are often incorporated into electronic health records.

Clinical paths are descriptions of best practices for managing patients (Spath 2013). Also known as *critical paths* or *care paths*, these tools remind caregivers of interventions and

Clinical paths
Descriptions of key patient care interventions for a condition, including diagnostic tests, medications, and consultations, which, if completed as described, are expected to produce desired outcomes.

EXHIBIT 10.6

Inpatient
Appendectomy
Clinical Path
for Children
(nonruptured
appendix)

	Phase I Emergency Department to Immediately Prior to Surgery	Phase II Post-anesthesia Recovery Unit to Discharge
Consultations	• Anesthesia • Surgical	
Tests	• Complete blood count • Metabolic panel • Urinalysis, including pregnancy test per protocol • Abdominal ultrasound as indicated	
Treatments		• Give oxygen per nasal cannula to maintain oxygen saturation ≥92% • Pulse oximetry if receiving oxygen • Wean to room air as tolerated • Incentive spirometry every 1 hour x 24 hours, while awake, and then every 6 hours while awake • Remove surgical dressing 24 hours after surgery
Medications	• Cefoxitin 40 mg/kg/dose every 6 hours (maximum = 2 mg per dose) For pain: • Morphine sulfate 0.05 mg/kg IV every 2 hours as needed for moderate to severe pain • Morphine sulfate 0.1 mg/kg IV every 2 hours as needed for severe pain if pain is unrelieved by lower dose • Acetaminophen 15 mg/kg (maximum = 650 mg/dose) rectally or orally every 4 hours as needed for mild pain or temperature of >101.5°F (oral)	• Cefoxitin 40 mg/kg/dose every 6 hours (maximum = 2 mg per dose); discontinue after 4 doses • Arrangements made for home IV antibiotic therapy if IV antibiotic therapy not completed in hospital For mild pain: • Ketorolac 0.5 mg/kg (maximum = 30 mg per dose) IV times 1 (loading dose) then Ketorolac 0.25 mg/kg (maximum = 30 mg per dose) IV every 6 hours times 7 doses • If patient tolerates oral intake, discontinue Ketorolac and give ibuprofen 10 mg/kg (maximum = 600 mg per dose) orally every 6 hours for the remaining 7 doses, then every 6 hours as needed for pain; or • Acetaminophen 15 mg/kg (maximum = 650 mg/dose) rectally or orally every 4 hours as needed for pain or temperature of >101.5°F (oral) For moderate to severe pain: • Morphine sulfate 0.05 mg/kg IV every 2 hours as needed for moderate to severe pain • Morphine sulfate 0.1 mg/kg IV every 2 hours as need for severe pain if pain is unrelieved by lower dose; or • Acetaminophen with hydrocodone (500 mg/5 mg) ___ tabs orally every 4 hours as needed if tolerating oral fluids (maximum = 8 tabs in 24 hours) • Metoclopraminde 0.15 mg/kg (maximum = 10 mg/dose) IV every 6 hours as needed for nausea or vomiting
Activity	• Assist with care • Activity as tolerated	• Out of bed to chair in a.m. • Advance ambulation as tolerated • May resume bathing/showering 48 hours post-op
Nutrition/IV therapy	• Nothing by mouth • Lactated Ringer's 20 ml/kg IV over 30 minutes, then Dextrose 5 Lactated Ringer's (D5LR) at twice maintenance rate for weight _____ ml per hour	• Clear liquids if bowel sounds present, no abdominal distention, no nausea/emesis; no carbonated beverages • Advance to regular diet as tolerated • D5LR at 1½ maintenance rate for weight _____ ml per hour • IV bag/tubing change every 96 hours • Discontinue IV when oral intake adequate
Assessments	• Routine vital signs and pain assessment • Record intake and output each shift	• If patient develops a temperature of >100°F (oral), notify physician • If no urine output in 8 hours, without bladder distention, give IV bolus of Lactate Ringer's 20 mg/kg x1; if patient does not void within 4 hours, notify physician • Check incision • IV site inspection with dressing changes per protocol
Activity	• Assist with care • Activity as tolerated	• Out of bed to chair in a.m. • Advance ambulation as tolerated • May resume bathing/showering 48 hours post-op • Cough and deep breathe with vital signs
Teaching	• Explain diagnostic tests to patient/family • Begin teaching plan for appendectomy and general surgical care as indicated	• Continue teaching plan • Explain discharge instructions

Source: Spath (2013). Used with permission.

milestones expected to occur during an episode of care. Exhibit 10.6 shows a clinical path for pediatric patients admitted to the hospital for surgical removal of a nonruptured inflamed appendix. The episode of care is divided into two phases. Phase I begins at admission to the emergency department and ends at the time of surgery. Phase II begins at admission to the post-anesthesia recovery room after surgery and ends with the child's discharge from the hospital. The recommended actions for physicians, nurses, and other caregivers are sorted into the nine intervention categories listed in the first column.

    Standards of care are job aids that provide step-by-step instructions on how to perform tasks. These instructions are usually found in checklists, treatment **protocols**, and physician order sets. Critical concept 10.2 is a list of treatment recommendations for dentists prescribing antibiotics for patients. Caregivers are more likely to order services that are medically necessary when they are provided a preprinted list of recommendations.

Protocols
Formal outlines of care; treatment plans.

⚠ CRITICAL CONCEPT 10.2
Checklist for Antibiotic Prescribing in Dentistry

❏ Ensure evidence-based antibiotic references are readily available during patient visits.

❏ Avoid prescribing based on non-evidence-based historical practices, patient demand, convenience, or pressure from colleagues.

❏ Make and document the diagnosis, treatment steps, and rationale for antibiotic use (if prescribed) in the patient chart.

❏ Prescribe only when clinical signs and symptoms of a bacterial infection suggest systemic immune response, such as fever or malaise along with local oral swelling.

❏ Revise empiric antibiotic regimens on the basis of patient progress and, if needed, culture results.

❏ Use the most targeted (narrow-spectrum) antibiotic for the shortest duration possible (2–3 days after the clinical signs and symptoms subside) for otherwise healthy patients.

❏ Discuss antibiotic use and prescribing protocols with referring specialists.

Source: Adapted from Centers for Disease Control and Prevention (2017).

Job aids that encourage more cost-efficient care are often incorporated into the health information technology that is being used by an increasing number of healthcare providers. For instance, computer-generated reminders of appropriateness are part of some electronic medication prescription systems (Dlugacz 2011). Clinical decision aids for the treatment of hip and knee osteoarthritis incorporated into electronic health records at a large health system in Washington State resulted in 26 percent fewer hip replacement surgeries, 38 percent fewer knee replacements, and 21 percent lower costs over six months (Arterburn et al. 2012).

DISCHARGE PLANNING

Discharge planning
Evaluation of patients' medical and psychosocial needs for the purpose of determining the type of care they will need after discharge from a healthcare facility.

Most aspects of UM are invisible to healthcare consumers. Only occasionally are patients affected by prospective and concurrent review activities. The most visible aspect of UM is discharge planning. **Discharge planning** is a process by which patient needs are met as they transfer from one environment to another. The process may involve the patient, family, friends, caregivers, and agencies. For example, after leaving the hospital, patients may need in-home nurse visits or outpatient physical therapy. Discharge planning activities ensure that a patient's medical needs are anticipated and arranged before he leaves the hospital.

The care provided to patients as they transition from one environment to another can be fragmented and haphazardly coordinated. Two areas that are particularly problematic are communication between caregivers in different settings and patient education about medications and other therapies (Joint Commission 2012). Inadequate discharge planning can adversely affect the quality and cost of patient care. For this reason, accreditation groups and health insurers, including Medicare, have required for many years that healthcare organizations provide discharge planning services for patients. Often, organizations employ **case managers** (primarily nurses and social workers) to oversee discharge planning activities for patients. In some facilities, case managers perform utilization review tasks along with discharge planning duties. In other facilities, case managers work closely with utilization review staff but do not undertake specific utilization review responsibilities. The tasks involved in discharge planning are summarized in exhibit 10.7.

Case managers
Experienced healthcare professionals (e.g., doctors, nurses, social workers) who work with patients, providers, and insurers to coordinate medically necessary and appropriate healthcare services.

Discharge planning is a systematic approach to ensuring effective utilization of patient care resources and a smooth transition from one environment to the next. It includes the organization of care activities suited to the patient's needs. These features support the goal of patient-centered care—one of the healthcare quality characteristics identified as important by IOM (2001). The evaluation stage of discharge planning is the feedback loop through which effectiveness of the discharge process can be measured.

Activity	Tasks
Conduct initial patient assessment	• Gather history (social and medical) • Evaluate medical condition and treatment needs • Assess support systems (e.g., home environment, community resources, family needs)
Plan for continuing care	• Identify short- and long-term patient care needs • Prioritize needs according to input of patient and family • Consider available human, financial, and material resources • Update plan according to patient's condition
Implement plan	• Arrange for services and support that patient requires after discharge • Provide patient and family information about postdischarge treatment plan, services, and support
Evaluate results	• Follow up with patient or family after discharge to assess whether plan was successful and ensure that no problems arose after discharge that have not been addressed

EXHIBIT 10.7
Discharge Planning
Activities and
Related Tasks

CASE STUDY

The following case study illustrates discharge planning for a patient who will require posthospital medical services.

Mr. Jones, who is 78 years old, is scheduled for left total knee replacement surgery by his orthopedic surgeon. Because his hospitalization will be short, planning for his discharge begins before admission. The hospital preadmission nurse meets with Mr. Jones and his wife to educate them about the upcoming procedure and also gather information about Mr. Jones's medical condition, social situation, and potential posthospital needs. The hospital case manager then uses this information to answer the following questions to assess Mr. Jones's needs:

◆ Can Mr. Jones return to his preadmission situation?

◆ Will his ability to care for himself change after discharge?

◆ Will he need home care services?

◆ Will he need to go to a nursing care center or another facility at discharge?

◆   Which posthospital services will he need?

◆   Does he have behavioral health or social needs?

Before Mr. Jones arrives at the hospital, the case manager already has a good idea of his discharge needs. The information gathered through this initial assessment will be used to create a plan for his discharge, which is discussed with Mr. Jones and his wife in a phone call the day before his admission. The case manager anticipates that Mr. Jones will need physical therapy after leaving the hospital, which can be arranged through home health services. However, he may need to spend a few days in a nursing facility before going home. His wife is apprehensive about her husband going to a nursing facility, as she thinks people go there to die. The case manager reassures Mrs. Jones that patients who have had a knee replacement commonly stay at a nursing facility for only a short time to undergo physical therapy. Mrs. Jones would prefer that her husband return home after his surgery but understands that his physician knows what is best for him. The case manager meets with Mrs. Jones on the day of her husband's surgery and promises to keep her informed of any changes to the discharge plan they had previously discussed.

While Mr. Jones recovers from his surgery, the case manager discusses his posthospital needs with his surgeon, nurses, and other caregivers. The case manager needs to stay informed of Mr. Jones's status so that arrangements can be made for services he will require after discharge. Two days after his knee replacement, the surgeon tells the case manager that Mr. Jones can be discharged the next day. Mr. Jones's medical condition is stable, and his wife will be at home to care for him, so they decide against sending him to a nursing home. Physical therapy can be provided by a home health agency. The case manager discusses the discharge plans with Mr. Jones and his wife. Mrs. Jones expresses concern about being able to assist her husband with bathing and other routine activities. The case manager suggests that a home care aide help for a few days per week, in addition to the physical therapist's regular home visits.

By the end of Mr. Jones's two days in the hospital, all components of his discharge plan are in place. The case manager has arranged for physical therapy to start the day after he goes home. The case manager also provides the home health agency with information about Mr. Jones's medical condition, including his current medications and his tolerance of physical therapy treatments in the hospital.

Before leaving the hospital, Mr. Jones and his wife receive the following information from his nurse:

◆   A list of medications Mr. Jones will be taking (the dosage, times, and frequency) at home and the potential side effects of these medications

◆   The date of Mr. Jones's follow-up appointment with the surgeon

◆   Home care instructions, such as activity level, diet, restrictions on bathing, and wound care

◆ Signs of infection or worsening condition to watch for, such as pain, fever, bleeding, difficulty breathing, or vomiting

◆ An explanation of the physical therapy and home aide services that have been arranged

◆ The name of a person to contact in case of an emergency or if questions arise

While Mr. Jones was in the hospital, his surgeon was in charge of his care, so his primary care physician needs to know what occurred during the hospitalization. Within 48 hours of Mr. Jones's discharge, the hospital's health information management department provides his doctor with copies of pertinent hospital records. These records include

◆ a summary of the hospital stay, including tests and surgeries performed and results;

◆ a list of medications Mr. Jones will be taking, including the dosage and frequency;

◆ his discharge instructions; and

◆ the plan for home health services.

Three days after Mr. Jones's discharge, the hospital case manager telephones him to inquire about his progress and to answer any questions. The case manager discovers that physical therapy treatments began on the scheduled day and that the home care aide has visited once to help him with bathing and other self-care activities. Mr.

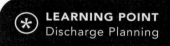

LEARNING POINT
Discharge Planning

Discharge planning streamlines patient care by coordinating healthcare services as patients move from one environment to another. Continuity of care is particularly important for patients who have ongoing medical needs.

Jones has no questions about his medications and reports that he has a follow-up appointment with his surgeon in one week. Mrs. Jones is satisfied with her husband's progress but would like the case manager to arrange with the Meals on Wheels program to deliver food for them to lessen her burden. The case manager takes care of this request later in the day.

UTILIZATION MANAGEMENT STRUCTURE

Healthcare organizations use several individuals and groups to accomplish UM goals. The Medicare Conditions of Participation require hospital boards to convene a utilization review committee to carry out utilization-related functions (CMS 2011). At least two committee members must be doctors of medicine or doctors of osteopathy. Physician advisors are usually members of this committee, as are nonphysician representatives from UM, case management, nursing, and fiscal services. All provider organizations that care for Medicare patients—hospitals, long-term care facilities, home health agencies, rehabilitation facilities, and so on—are required to conduct UM activities, but only some are required to designate a UM committee.

The Medicare Conditions of Participation also require hospitals to develop and follow a written UM plan, which details the UM functions that are carried out for each review (CMS 2011). Critical concept 10.3 describes the UM plan for a small hospital. The concurrent and retrospective review requirements in this plan reflect the requirements of the Medicare Hospital Conditions of Participation. At this small hospital, UM functions are delegated to individuals and committees that also have quality management responsibilities. More detail on the quality management structure in healthcare organizations is presented in chapter 12.

⓵ **CRITICAL CONCEPT 10.3**
Hospital Utilization Management Plan

OBJECTIVE

The purpose of the UM plan is to describe the hospital's process for ensuring that patient care is provided in the most efficient and cost-effective manner possible. To achieve this goal, professional services are reviewed to determine the medical necessity of (1) admissions and the appropriateness of the setting, (2) extended stays, and (3) services (e.g., medications, treatments, tests).

STRUCTURE AND SCOPE

1. The medical staff quality improvement committee oversees all UM functions. This committee is composed of six active physician members representing medical, surgical, and emergency services. Also represented on the committee are hospital administration, case management, quality management, and health information management. The committee meets monthly.

    1.1   No committee member shall have a direct financial interest in the hospital.

    1.2   No committee member may conduct a review of a case in which he or she was professionally involved in the care of the patient.

    1.3   At least two physician members will serve as physician advisors to assist with concurrent review activities and other UM support functions requiring physician input.

(continued)

> ! **CRITICAL CONCEPT 10.3**
> Hospital Utilization Management Plan *(continued)*

    1.4   Hospital staff to be delegated responsibilities for UM activities include case managers, social workers, and clinical documentation specialists.

2. The UM program includes review of patients with Medicare and Medicaid insurance as well as patients with any other health insurance for which the hospital is required to conduct UM. Reviews include an evaluation of the medical necessity of the admissions, duration of stays, adequacy of clinical documentation, and professional services furnished.

REVIEW AND SUPPORT ACTIVITIES

1. Preadmission review: Preadmission reviews shall be performed before admission to determine the appropriateness of the proposed admission.

    1.1   The case manager or preadmission reviewer will obtain information on the patient's admission diagnosis, vital signs, symptoms, and treatment plan to determine the medical necessity of admission and appropriateness of setting.

    1.2   Recommendations for alternative settings or other treatment options will be provided to the patient's physician when the patient does not meet medical necessity guidelines for inpatient admission.

2. Admission review: Admission reviews shall be completed within one working day of admission to determine the appropriateness of admission.

    2.1   The case manager will review the patient's medical record for documentation of diagnoses and procedures, vital signs, symptoms, orders, and plan of care to determine if medical necessity guidelines are met for inpatient admission.

    2.2   If the admission is medically necessary, the case is approved for admission and the next review date is assigned.

    2.3   If the admission is not medically necessary, the patient's physician is contacted for additional information.

        2.3.0.1   If the reason for inpatient admission is not apparent after contacting the patient's physician, the case is referred to a physician advisor for review.

(continued)

> ⓘ **CRITICAL CONCEPT 10.3**
> Hospital Utilization Management Plan *(continued)*

3. Continued stay review: The continued stay review is performed on a regular basis according to the assigned review date.

   3.1   The case manager reviews the patient's record for documentation supporting the need for continued hospital stay.

   3.2   If continued hospitalization is medically necessary, the case is approved and the next review date is assigned.

   3.3   If hospitalization does not appear to be medically necessary, the patient's physician is contacted.

      3.3.0.1   If the reason for continued hospitalization is not apparent after contacting the patient's physician, the case is referred to a physician advisor for review.

4. Physician advisor review: Physician advisors will review cases on referral from a case manager, social worker, or clinical documentation specialist. Reasons for referral include, but are not limited to, the following:

   4.1   Documentation in the patient's medical record does not support the need for admission or continued hospital stay.

   4.2   The treatment plan is not consistent with the patient's diagnosis.

   4.3   The patient's diagnosis is not adequately reflected in the record documentation.

   4.4   The services, treatments, tests, or medications ordered for the patient do not coincide with the patient's documented diagnosis or condition.

   4.5   Delay occurs in provision of services by the patient's physician.

   4.6   The hospital has received notice from the patient's health plan that the admission or continued stay may not be medically necessary.

5. Discharge planning: Discharge planning is a collaborative process among caregivers to ensure appropriate outcomes and continuity of care.

   5.1   The initial discharge planning assessment is documented by the patient's nurse within 12 hours of admission. The physician, the patient, the person acting on the patient's behalf, or any member of the healthcare team may identify discharge needs and make referrals to a case manager for more intense discharge planning.

(continued)

> ⚠ **CRITICAL CONCEPT 10.3**
> Hospital Utilization Management Plan *(continued)*
>
> 5.2   The formal discharge plan shall be developed and documented by a case manager or a social worker. The plan shall be developed in a timely manner to minimize delays in discharge. The plan shall be reassessed if other factors affect the continuing care needs and appropriateness of the discharge plan. The patient and/or caregiver shall participate in the discharge planning process, and final plans shall be communicated to the patient or caregiver.
>
> 5.3   The discharge plan will be implemented before the patient's actual discharge. Referrals shall be made as appropriate (e.g., home care, infusion, hospice, skilled nursing, rehabilitation, long-term acute, therapy). If the patient is referred to another facility, agency, or outpatient service, pertinent medical information is provided to allow for follow-up care.

HEALTH PLANS

All health plans accredited by NCQA (2016) and by URAC (2017)—the Utilization Review Accreditation Commission—must have a written UM plan, and many state regulations governing health plans have similar requirements. A health insurer's UM plan describes the policies and procedures used by UM staff to identify instances of overuse and underuse of healthcare services and the process for approving and denying payment for services. To meet NCQA and URAC accreditation standards, only clinical professionals who have appropriate clinical expertise in the treatment of a health plan member's condition or disease can deny or reduce payment for a service.

A health plan's UM committee is chaired by the plan's medical director. This committee is typically responsible for

◆   monitoring providers' requests to render healthcare services to its members;

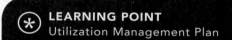

> ✱ **LEARNING POINT**
> Utilization Management Plan
>
> A UM plan defines the structure and function of an organization's UM activities. This document usually describes
>
> - the purpose and scope of UM activities;
> - the plan's structure and accountability;
> - procedures for evaluating medical necessity, access, appropriateness, and efficiency of services;
> - mechanisms for detecting underuse and overuse;
> - clinical practice guidelines and protocols used in decision-making; and
> - outcome and process measures for evaluating the effectiveness of UM activities.

◆ monitoring the medical appropriateness and necessity of healthcare services provided to its members;

◆ reviewing the effectiveness of the utilization review process and revising the process as needed; and

◆ writing UM policies and procedures that conform to industry standards, including methods, timelines, and individuals responsible for completing each task.

CONCLUSION

Provider utilization management requirements have been in place since the inception of Medicare in the 1960s. Although the function has changed, the goal remains the same: to provide appropriate patient care in the least costly setting.

UM is a component of an organization's quality management efforts. All healthcare organizations are involved in or affected by UM activities. UM applies the basic principles of performance measurement, assessment, and improvement to minimize costs and use healthcare resources effectively.

FOR DISCUSSION

1. Use the most current information in the Healthcare Cost and Utilization Project (https://hcupnet.ahrq.gov) database to answer the following questions:

   a. What are the nationwide average length of hospital stay and average hospital cost for patients with the following diagnoses? You will choose these diagnoses using ICD-9 or ICD-10 diagnosis codes. There are resources on the site to help you identify the correct code.

   • Abdominal pain

   • Acute myocardial infarction

   • Chronic obstructive pulmonary disease and bronchiectasis

   • Diabetes mellitus with complications

   b. What are the nationwide average length of hospital stay and average hospital cost for patients who undergo the following procedures? Again, choose these procedures using ICD-9 or ICD-10 procedure codes, referring to the resources on the site to help you identify the correct code.

- Cesarean section
- Hip replacement, total
- Hysterectomy, abdominal
- Percutaneous coronary angioplasty

c. If data are available for your state, what are your state's average length of hospital stay and average cost for patients with the diagnoses in question 1a and for patients who underwent the procedures in question 1b?

2. A hospital's UM committee discovers that the rate of cesarean section births at the hospital is higher than the rate at other hospitals in the region, where more women have vaginal deliveries. The UM committee wants to evaluate the medical necessity of cesarean section births at the hospital using clinical practice guidelines on this topic. Go to the website of the National Guideline Clearinghouse (www.guidelines.gov) to find the most current recommendations that address the indications for a cesarean section birth, and write a summary of the indications for the committee to consider.

3. What UM practices does your health insurance company follow to control costs and ensure the provision of medically necessary services? This information may be available in your insurance benefits booklet or on your health plan's website. If you do not have health insurance, go to the website of any major health insurance company and list the practices this company follows to control costs and to ensure the provision of medically necessary services.

WEBSITES

- American College of Physician Advisors
  www.acpadvisors.org
- *American Journal of Managed Care* Managed Markets Network
  www.ajmc.com
- Case Management Society of America
  www.cmsa.org
- Choosing Wisely
  http://choosingwisely.org
- Healthcare Cost and Utilization Project
  https://hcupnet.ahrq.gov

- Medicare Bundled Payments for Care Improvement Initiative
  https://innovation.cms.gov/initiatives/bundled-payments

- Medicare Conditions for Coverage & Conditions of Participations
  www.cms.gov/Regulations-and-Guidance/Legislation/CFCsAndCoPs/index.html

- Midwest Business Group on Health
  www.mbgh.org

- National Committee for Quality Assurance (NCQA)
  www.ncqa.org

- National Guideline Clearinghouse
  www.guidelines.gov

- Pacific Business Group on Health
  www.pbgh.org

- PEPPER Resources
  https://pepperresources.org

- URAC
  www.urac.org

References

Agency for Healthcare Research and Quality (AHRQ). 2017. "Healthcare Cost and Utilization Project (HCUP)." Accessed November 26. www.hcup-us.ahrq.gov.

Arterburn, D., R. Wellman, E. Westbrook, C. Rutter, T. Ross, D. McCulloch, M. Handley, and C. Jung. 2012. "Introducing Decision Aids at Group Health Was Linked to Sharply Lower Hip and Knee Surgery Rates and Costs." *Health Affairs* 31 (9): 2094–140.

Caper, P. 1984. "Variations in Medical Practice: Implications for Health Policy." *Health Affairs* 3 (2): 110–19.

Castellucci, M. 2017. "CMS Seeks Ideas on Creating Voluntary Pay Models, Cutting Regs." *Modern Healthcare* 47 (39): 10.

Centers for Disease Control and Prevention. 2017. "Checklist for Antibiotic Prescribing in Dentistry." Accessed November 25. www.cdc.gov/antibiotic-use/community/downloads/dental-fact-sheet-FINAL.pdf.

Centers for Medicare & Medicaid Services (CMS). 2017a. "Bundled Payments for Care Improvement (BPCI) Initiative: General Information." Updated November 20. https://innovation.cms.gov/initiatives/bundled-payments/.

————. 2017b. "Electronic Code of Federal Regulations, Title 42: Public Health, Part 483—Requirements for States and Long Term Care Facilities, Subpart B—Requirements for Long-Term Care Facilities, Section 483.45: Pharmacy Services." Updated September 12. www.ecfr.gov/cgi-bin/text-idx?c=ecfr&rgn=div5&view=text&node=42:5.0.1.1.2&idno=42.

————. 2017c. "National Health Expenditure Data: Historical." Accessed December 7. www.cms.gov/Research-Statistics-Data-and-Systems/Statistics-Trends-and-Reports/NationalHealthExpendData/NationalHealthAccountsHistorical.html.

————. 2017d. "National Health Expenditure Projections 2016–2025." Accessed December 7. www.cms.gov/Research-Statistics-Data-and-Systems/Statistics-Trends-and-Reports/NationalHealthExpendData/Downloads/proj2016.pdf.

————. 2015. "Medicare Coverage Determination Process." Updated April 8. www.cms.hhs.gov/DeterminationProcess.

————. 2014. *Medicare Basics: A Guide for Families and Friends of People with Medicare.* Revised November. www.medicare.gov/Pubs/pdf/11034.pdf.

————. 2011. "Electronic Code of Federal Regulations, Title 42: Public Health, Chapter IV, Part 482—Conditions of Participation for Hospitals, Section 482.30: Utilization Review." Accessed November 26, 2017. www.ecfr.gov/cgi-bin/text-idx?SID=f0255afacfa7296ac33e3447b701229c&mc=true&node=se42.5.482_130&rgn=div8.

CGS Administrators. 2017. *Hospital Beds & Accessories: Medical Review Documentation Checklist.* Accessed November 26. www.cgsmedicare.com/jc/mr/pdf/mr_checklist_hospital_beds.pdf.

Dlugacz, Y. D. 2011. "Medication Safety Improvement." In *Error Reduction in Health Care: A Systems Approach to Improving Patient Safety,* edited by P. Spath, 335–65. San Francisco: Jossey-Bass.

Field, M., and K. Lohr. 1990. *Clinical Practice Guidelines: Directions for a New Program.* Washington, DC: National Academies Press.

Handelsman, Y., Z. T. Bloomgarden, G. Grunberger, G. Umpierrez, R. S. Zimmerman, T. S. Bailey, L. Blonde, G. A. Bray, A. J. Cohen, S. Dagogo-Jack, J. A. Davidson, D. Einhorn, O. P. Ganda, A. J. Garber, W. T. Garvey, R. R. Henry, I. B. Hirsch, E. S. Horton, D. L. Hurley, P. S. Jellinger, L. Jovanovič, H. E. Lebovitz, D. LeRoith, P. Levy, J. B. McGill, J. I. Mechanick, J. H. Mestman, E. S. Moghissi, E. A. Orzeck, R. Pessah-Pollack, P. D. Rosenblit, A. I. Vinik, K. Wyne, and F. Zangeneh. 2015. "American Association of Clinical Endocrinologists and American College of Endocrinology—Clinical Practice Guidelines for Developing a Diabetes Mellitus Comprehensive Care Plan—2015." *Endocrine Practice*. Accessed November 26, 2017. www.aace.com/files/dm-guidelines-ccp.pdf.

Henkel, R., and P. Maryland. 2015. "The Risks and Rewards of Value-Based Reimbursement." *Frontiers of Health Services Management* 32 (2): 3–16.

Hill, H., A. Hanson, and B. O'Connell. 2000. "Using Evidence: Coverage Decisions." Agency for Healthcare Research and Quality workshop for state and local healthcare policymakers, Omaha, NE, May 8–10. Accessed November 26, 2017. https://archive.ahrq.gov/news/ulp/evidence/ulpevdnc5.htm.

Institute of Medicine (IOM). 2011. *Essential Health Benefits: Balancing Coverage and Cost*. Washington, DC: National Academies Press.

———. 2001. *Crossing the Quality Chasm: A New Health System for the 21st Century*. Washington, DC: National Academies Press.

Joint Commission. 2017a. *2017 Comprehensive Accreditation Manual for Ambulatory Health Care*. Oakbrook Terrace, IL: The Joint Commission.

———. 2017b. *2017 Comprehensive Accreditation Manual for Home Care*. Oakbrook Terrace, IL: The Joint Commission.

———. 2017c. *2017 Comprehensive Accreditation Manual for Hospitals*. Oakbrook Terrace, IL: The Joint Commission.

———. 2012. *Hot Topics in Health Care—Transitions of Care: The Need for a More Effective Approach to Continuing Patient Care*. Accessed November 26, 2017. www.jointcommission.org/hot_topics_toc/.

McCauley, J. L. 2015. "Guidelines and Value-Based Decision Making: An Evolving Role for Payers." *North Carolina Medical Journal* 76 (4): 243–46.

Meara, E., and J. D. Birkmeyer. 2015. "Medicare's Bundled Payments for Care Improvement (BPCI) Initiative: Expanding Enrollment Suggests Potential for Large Impact." *American Journal of Managed Care* 21 (11): 814–20.

National Committee for Quality Assurance (NCQA). 2017. "2018 Utilization Management Accreditation." Accessed November 26. www.ncqa.org/programs/accreditation /2018-utilization-management-um.

———. 2016. "States Using NCQA Commercial Managed Care Accreditation and Certification Programs." Published December. www.ncqa.org/Portals/0/Public%20Policy/ States%20Using%20NCQA%20Commercial%20managed%20care%20accreditation%20 and%20certification%20programs.pdf?ver=2016-12-06-103043-407.

———. 2007. *The Essential Guide to Health Care Quality*. Accessed November 26, 2017. www.ncqa.org/Portals/0/Publications/Resource%20Library/NCQA_Primer_web.pdf.

National Guideline Clearinghouse. 2017. "Browse by Organization." Accessed November 26. www.guideline.gov/browse/.

Qaseem, A., T. J. Wilt, R. M. McLean, and M. A. Forciea. 2017. "Clinical Guidelines Committee of the American College of Physicians. Noninvasive Treatments for Acute, Subacute, and Chronic Low Back Pain: A Clinical Practice Guideline from the American College of Physicians." *Annals of Internal Medicine* 166 (7): 514–30.

Spath, P. L. 2013. *Fundamentals of Health Care Quality Management*, 4th ed. Forest Grove, OR: Brown-Spath & Associates.

TMF Health Quality Institute. 2017a. *PEPPER: Short-Term Acute Care Program for Evaluating Payment Patterns Electronic Report: User's Guide*, 22nd ed. Accessed November 26. https://pepperresources.org/Portals/0/Documents/PEPPER/ST/STPEPPERUsers Guide_Edition22.pdf.

———. 2017b. "Welcome to PEPPER Resources." Accessed November 26. https://pepper resources.org.

URAC. 2017. "Health Plan Accreditation at a Glance." Accessed November 26. www.urac. org/wp-content/uploads/STDGlance_HealthPlan3.pdf.

US Diabetes Surveillance System, Centers for Disease Control and Prevention. 2017. "Diabetes Home: Data and Statistics." Accessed November 26. www.cdc.gov/diabetes/data/ index.html.

US Preventive Services Taskforce. 2016. "Breast Cancer: Screening." Released January. www.uspreventiveservicestaskforce.org/Page/Document/UpdateSummaryFinal/breast-cancer-screening1.

US Social Security Administration. 2017. "Compilation of the Social Security Laws." Accessed November 26. www.ssa.gov/OP_Home/ssact/title18/1862.htm.

Wennberg, J. E., and A. Gittelsohn. 1973. "Small Area Variations in Health Care Delivery." *Science* 182 (117): 1102–8.

Wennberg, J. E., A. Gittelsohn, and N. Shapiro. 1975. "Health Care Delivery in Maine I: Patterns of Use in Common Surgical Procedures." *Journal of the Maine Medical Association* 66 (9): 123–39, 149.

Wennberg, J. E., K. McPherson, and D. Goodman. 2016. "Small Area Analysis and the Challenge of Practice Variation." In *Health Services Research Series: Medical Practice Variations*, edited by A. Johnson and T. Stukel, 1–24. New York: Springer.

CHAPTER 11

MANAGING QUALITY IN POPULATION HEALTH CARE

After reading this chapter, you will be able to

➤ define population health care;

➤ recognize how reimbursement strategies influence provider involvement in population health care; and

➤ explain how quality measurement, assessment, and improvement activities are used to manage population health.

➤ Medical home model of care

➤ Population health

➤ Population health care

➤ Population health management

Chapter 1 of this book introduced the Institute of Medicine's definition of healthcare quality as "the degree to which health services for individuals and populations increase the likelihood of desired health outcomes and are consistent with current professional knowledge" (IOM 2001, 4). This wording recognizes the importance of the population component—the topic covered in this chapter. Kindig and Stoddart (2003, 381) define **population health** as "the health outcomes of a group of individuals, including the distribution of such outcomes within the group." The population can be any distinct group of individuals, such as patients recently hospitalized, kindergarten-age children, clinic patients seen for management of certain medical conditions (e.g., diabetes, asthma), or people enrolled in a particular health plan or residing in a specified geographic location.

Provision of services to improve population health has commonly been associated with the work of public health agencies. Today, financial incentives and demands for quality care are causing a growing number of healthcare provider organizations to also become involved in **population health care**, sometimes referred to as **population health management**. Population health care encompasses the use of information to surveil a group to identify health risks, prioritize interventions, and measure results. Individuals with known or predicted risk are targeted for interventions. The administrative and outcome aspects of this work are emphasized in Caron's definition of population health management: "The application of management strategies to improve the delivery of healthcare for populations, with an emphasis on achieving the highest quality at the lowest cost" (Caron 2017, 288).

Organizations traditionally involved in population health care include insurers, integrated health systems, and government providers such as the Veterans Health Administration and Indian Health Services. The transition toward value-based reimbursement for all providers has expanded interest in population health management.

Achieving the goal of population health care requires a multifaceted approach to address social factors. The social determinants of an individual's health and well-being fall into five key domains: (1) economic stability, (2) education, (3) health and healthcare, (4) neighborhood and built environment, and (5) social and community context (US Department of Health and Human Services 2017). Research has shown that access to and the quality of health services themselves only affect about 20 percent of an individual's health and well-being (Magnan et al. 2012). Thus, healthcare organizations involved in population health care must do more than improve the delivery of health services to manage the health of a population.

The National Association for Healthcare Quality (NAHQ) has identified essential competencies for quality professionals in the areas of population health and care transitions. According to NAHQ (2015), professionals in the fields of healthcare quality and care transitions should be able to perform various functions in the following dimensions:

Population health
"The health outcomes of a group of individuals, including the distribution of such outcomes within the group" (Kindig and Stoddart 2003, 381).

Population health care
Use of information to surveil a population to identify health risks, prioritize interventions, and measure results.

Population health management
"The application of management strategies to improve the delivery of healthcare for populations, with an emphasis on achieving the highest quality at the lowest cost" (Caron 2017, 288).

◆   Building the infrastructure for collaboration

◆   Innovatively planning and organizing for public and community health

◆   Identifying, describing, and trending cohorts

◆   Improving care processes and transitions

This chapter focuses on the quality management aspects of population health care. First, a brief overview of provider involvement and common population health care strategies will provide a foundation for this topic.

PROVIDER INVOLVEMENT IN POPULATION HEALTH CARE

Historically, providers enjoyed unlimited fee-for-service (FFS) reimbursement. But in the early 1970s, the rising costs of healthcare services prompted Medicare and other payers to experiment with various payment changes and utilization management tactics—yet these failed to achieve significant cost savings (see chapter 10). Payment mechanisms that reward providers for doing more do not incentivize the adoption of population health care strategies. When the health and well-being of individuals in a population are improved, use of health services declines—which translates into less revenue for providers getting FFS reimbursement. Likewise, until recently many consumers were not financially motivated to curtail their use of health services because insurers covered most of the costs.

The Health Maintenance Organization (HMO) Act of 1973 was a significant first step toward changing the FFS reimbursement model. An HMO provides "a comprehensive range of medical or health care services . . . to their subscribers in return for a fixed monthly or annual payment periodically determined and paid in advance" (SSA 1974, 35). The HMO fixed payment mechanism rewards providers for adopting population health care strategies to reduce use of

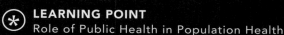

LEARNING POINT
Role of Public Health in Population Health

Public health agencies at the federal, state, and local levels are involved in the following population health initiatives:

• Collecting and analyzing population health status and health services utilization data

• Creating policies and recommendations to maintain and protect population health and respond to community values

• Sharing analyses of population health data and health service improvement recommendations with the public and with policy makers

• Engaging with stakeholders to develop consensus on needed actions

• Ensuring that necessary population health and personal health services are provided to all

Source: Adapted from American Public Health Association (1995).

services. Kaiser Permanente, an HMO founded in 1945, has built a reputation on population health care by stressing early detection and disease management to improve the health and well-being of its members.

In the early 1990s, the American Hospital Association (AHA) proposed a restructured healthcare delivery system—community care networks—that was intended to improve access, encourage economic discipline, and improve quality. The AHA hoped adoption of their recommendations would increase public ownership of and accountability for the local community's health status (Granatir 1995). Several community care networks were formed throughout the United States, but FFS reimbursement continued to discourage providers from adopting significant population health care initiatives.

An incentive intended to encourage provider engagement in population health management strategies is found in the federal tax regulations. To maintain their tax-exempt status, nonprofit hospitals are required to provide community benefit in response to identified community health and wellness needs. The Robert Wood Johnson Foundation (2012) reports that "nationwide, about 2,900 hospitals (60 percent of hospitals) are nonprofit, and the financial benefit to these hospitals from being tax-exempt is estimated to be worth $12.6 billion annually." During fiscal year 2009, nonprofit hospitals spent an average of 7.5 percent of their operating expenses on community benefit (James 2016). Most of the community benefit expenditures covered the costs of charity care and revenue losses associated with low reimbursement by government programs. Only 15 percent of community benefit expenditures were for programs or activities that affect population health, such as education and the support of health-related community groups (James 2016). Health policy experts have called for more accountability among tax-exempt hospitals to improve regional population health (Corrigan, Fisher, and Heiser 2015).

Different aspects of the 2010 Affordable Care Act (ACA) expanded incentives for provider involvement in population health care (Kaiser Family Foundation 2013). In addition to strengthening the community benefit requirements for tax-exempt hospitals, the ACA accelerated the development and testing of several alternative payment models to replace traditional FFS reimbursement. This included expanding bundled payment options for some medical conditions and procedures, creating the **medical home model of care**, and making special payments to physicians for care coordination (Fried and Sherer 2016). The Medicare Access and CHIP Reauthorization Act of 2015, better known as MACRA, created the Merit-Based Incentive Payment System and Advanced Payment Models, which link physician reimbursement with quality and resource use measures and clinical practice improvement activities such as care coordination and population health care (Wynne 2016). An increasing number of commercial insurers and other government health insurance programs are adopting similar alternative payment mechanisms that link reimbursement to cost containment and quality improvements.

Medical home model of care
A healthcare delivery model in which patient treatment is coordinated through the primary care physician and facilitated by partnerships with other providers and health information exchanges to ensure patients get indicated care when and where they need it.

The reimbursement landscape is changing with new payment models that motivate providers to become involved in population health care initiatives. For example, at Community Hospital of the Monterey Peninsula (CHOMP) almost 75 percent of payments come from public or government sources, which required a shift in philosophy several years ago to population health care. The first step for CHOMP was to reach out to other providers, community groups, staff, patients, employers, health plans, and other interested parties to build and implement population health care capabilities (Ananth 2016). One of the initiatives involved intensive population health care training for case managers and care managers in the various clinical settings.

PROVIDER STRATEGIES FOR POPULATION HEALTH CARE

The Health Research & Educational Trust (HRET) of the American Hospital Association maintains that population health depends on effective initiatives that "(1) increase the prevalence of evidence-based preventive health services and preventive health behaviors, (2) improve care quality and patient safety, and (3) advance care coordination across the health care continuum" (HRET 2012, 4).

Exhibit 11.1 illustrates a framework for providers seeking to implement population health care. This framework is similar to the continuous improvement models described in chapter 5. First, a provider defines its population health challenges and selects one or more target populations. Next, it conducts an assessment of internal and external strengths related to managing health in the target populations. It sets measurable goals for each target population before developing and implementing action strategies for achieving those goals. Progress toward achieving the goals is measured, and successful initiatives are continued while unsuccessful initiatives are revised or ended. Finally, the continuous improvement cycle resumes with the provider reassessing its population health challenges and selecting the same or other target populations.

Addressing the social determinants of health is a priority for organizations involved in population health care. Providers may facilitate housing, transportation, and educational offerings to meet population health care goals. For example, in 2016 five hospitals in Portland, Oregon, along with CareOregon, a nonprofit health plan, pledged a combined $21.5 million toward the construction of nearly 400 housing units for the homeless and low-income population (Flaccus 2016). Studies have shown that stress related to food insecurity and unstable housing adversely affects an individual's health outcomes (AHIP 2017). Easing some of this stress by increasing housing access is expected to improve population health and ultimately drive down emergency department visits and other reactive care at Portland hospitals and clinics.

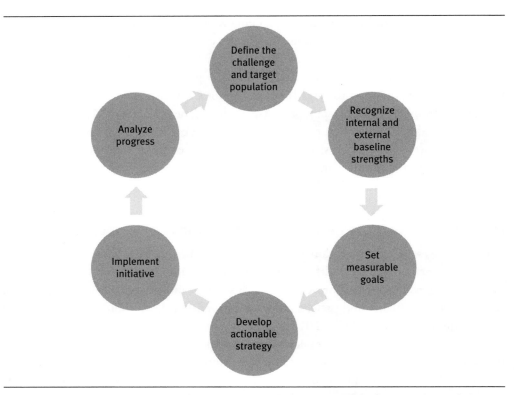

CASE STUDY

The following case study uses the framework steps illustrated in exhibit 11.1 to describe how a hospital-based primary care clinic in a rural area implemented a population health care initiative.

Step 1: Define the challenge and target population

The managed care health plan that insures the majority of the clinic's patients notified clinic leadership that only 58 percent of the children and adolescents seen in the clinic are receiving recommended immunizations. The challenge for the clinic is ensuring the target population—children and adolescents—gets these recommended vaccines.

Step 2: Recognize internal and external baseline strengths

◆   Most children and adolescents are seen at least once a year in the clinic.

◆   The clinic information system has a patient portal where a parent or guardian
    can access immunization status information for family members.

◆   The hospital hosts annual vaccine education classes for the public.

◆   The county public health department offers free immunizations for children
    and adolescents at the mobile clinic and at the health department office.

Step 3: Set measurable goals

The managed care health plan reports that 71 percent of children and adolescents receive
recommended immunizations statewide, and that the national rate is a bit higher at 77
percent. The primary care clinic providers determine they want to achieve an 80 percent
immunization rate within one year.

Step 4: Develop an actionable strategy

◆   Identify preventable immunization barriers by reviewing clinic procedures and
    talking with parents/guardians.

◆   Determine whether inadequate documentation practices are affecting the
    clinic's reported immunization rate.

◆   Partner with the county public health department to discover whether there is
    sufficient public awareness of recommended immunizations for children and
    adolescents.

Step 5: Implement the initiative

◆   Change clinic procedures to improve the integration of immunization records
    from the health department and other providers into patient electronic health
    records (EHRs) at the clinic.

◆   Change the immunization page on the clinic's patient portal to enable
    parents/guardians to add immunization records from other providers that will
    then be confirmed by clinic staff and added to the patient's EHR.

◆   Add patient-specific immunization reminders to the EHR so physicians and
    staff are alerted when a patient is due for a vaccine.

◆   Give immunizations at any visit when due, not just during annual health
    maintenance visits.

◆   Change clinic policies to allow immunization of children and adolescents who only have a "cold."

◆   Have clinic nurses partner with public health nurses to visit local schools at least every six months to discuss the importance of immunizations and distribute educational coloring books to children.

◆   Put immunization awareness posters and educational coloring books in the clinic's pediatric patient waiting room.

◆   Include in the hospital's new mother class a session on recommended immunizations and the services offered by the county public health department.

Step 6: Analyze progress

◆   Monitor compliance with clinic policy/procedure changes and share results with clinic staff.

◆   Gather and analyze feedback from public health nurses regarding the success of school educational visits and the use of free immunization services.

◆   Measure the percentage of children and adolescents with documentation in their clinic electronic records that they received the recommended immunizations.

By the end of 12 months, the managed care health plan reported that 81.5 percent of the children and adolescents seen in the clinic had received recommended immunizations.

QUALITY MANAGEMENT IN POPULATION HEALTH CARE

According to Derose and Petitti (2003, 363), the purpose of population health care is to "maximize the health and well-being of persons in a defined population." The quality management cycle of measurement, assessment, and improvement helps support this purpose.

John Muir Health, an integrated health system in Walnut Creek, California, has been involved in population health care initiatives for several years (Ananth 2016). System leaders gather and analyze measurement data to understand the population it serves and this group's barriers to care. This information is used to identify the improvements needed to enhance the quality of care and the health of the population and to reduce costs. Measurement data are further analyzed to determine whether initiatives aimed at achieving these goals have been successful.

Information technology (IT) and data analytics capabilities are vital to the success of quality management in population health care. Organizations must have access to current information about target populations to identify and understand the needs of high-risk individuals and evaluate the effect of interventions.

MEASUREMENT

To answer the question "How are we doing?" as it relates to population health care requires measurements more encompassing than those used to evaluate performance within a department or facility. For instance, the average time a patient waits before being seen by a physician is a measure of access in a primary care clinic. A measure of access from a population health perspective is the average wait time for anyone within the population of interest to get an appointment with a primary care provider. For the population health care measure, the entire population, not just those receiving care, is being evaluated.

> **(?) DID YOU KNOW?**
>
> The earliest forms of medical records were narratives written by ancient Greeks to document observations about symptoms and outcomes and to teach others using case studies. Some of these records were advice to patients about diet and recipes while others were testimonials of successful or remarkable cures, autopsies, or lessons for surgeons.

As described in chapter 3, quality can be measured based on structure, process, outcome, and patient experience. The same types of measures are useful for population health care purposes. Structural measures evaluate aspects of the resources in the population. These can be healthcare resources such as access to 24-hour urgent care services or social determinants such as availability of adequate housing and transportation. Process measures evaluate the clinical interventions for certain populations, such as provision of recommended immunizations for children and adolescents. Outcome measures evaluate results such as percentage of hospitalized patients (a population) readmitted within 30 days or incidence of opioid addiction in high-risk populations. Patient experience measures evaluate factors such as whether patients feel they have a say in decisions about their care and whether questions are answered in a way patients understand.

The Healthcare Effectiveness Data and Information Set (HEDIS) measurement project was established by the National Committee for Quality Assurance in 1991. This project, described in chapter 3, was originally developed to compare population health care performance among HMOs. The HEDIS measures are now used by many different public and private health plans to evaluate care provided to its members and also by health systems involved in population health care initiatives. Exhibit 11.2 lists examples of HEDIS measures used to evaluate access/availability of care in a defined population.

Population health care measurements are focused on prevention, long-term health improvement, cost avoidance, and the ability of individuals to lead an active lifestyle.

- Percent of population reporting language interpretation services are available when needed for healthcare encounters.
- Percent of population between 2 and 20 years of age with an annual dentist visit.
- Percent of children and young adults (12 months to 19 years of age) with at least one visit with a primary care physician in the past year.
- Percent of patients hospitalized for mental illness who had a follow-up appointment within 7 days of hospital discharge.
- Percent of children who had 6 or more well-child visits with a primary care physician within the first 15 months of life.
- Percent of population reporting it is easy to get care after regular clinic hours.

Source: Adapted from CMS (2016).

HRET (2014) recommends that providers involved in population health use several process and outcome measurements to evaluate whether patient and community health are improving. Examples of HRET's suggested measurements are listed by category in exhibit 11.3.

Obtaining data for many population health care measures requires a comprehensive electronic information system that is fully integrated and capable of capturing various data types (clinical, financial, demographic, patient experience, etc.) from a variety of settings (providers, pharmacies, community groups, public health databases, etc.). Sophisticated data analytics capabilities help organizations identify populations that would benefit from healthcare management initiatives. Real-time access to measurement data allows for prompt interventions if needed. For example, data linkages with area pharmacies let providers know if patients are not picking up their prescribed medications.

Creating the information system needed to fully support the purpose of population health care is technically challenging as well as fraught with privacy concerns and other legal hurdles. When data sharing among all stakeholders becomes less problematic, measurement capabilities will more fully support the goals of population health care.

Assessment

The assessment phase of quality management involves analysis of measurement data to determine whether an acceptable level of quality has been achieved. This involves comparing current performance to previous levels or to a quality goal. Performance measurement data display formats described in chapter 4 also are used to display population health care measurement results.

A challenge in assessing measurement results for population health care initiatives is obtaining comparative data for the target population. For instance, consider an integrated health system that decides to target its population health care initiatives on patients with

Category	Measurement
Summary measures	• Health-adjusted life expectancy at birth (years) • Years of healthy life • Disability-adjusted life years
Inequality measures	• Geographic variation in age-adjusted mortality rate (AAMR) among counties in a state (standard deviation of county AAMR/state AAMR) • Mortality rate stratified by sex, ethnicity, income, education level, social class or wealth • Life expectancy stratified by sex, ethnicity, income, education level, social class or wealth
Health status	• Percentage of adults who self-report fair or poor health • Percentage of children reported by their parents to be in fair or poor health • Percentage of children aged 3–11 years exposed to secondhand smoke
Psychological state	• Percentage of adults with serious psychological distress (score ≥ 13 on the K6 scale) • Percentage of adults who report joint pain during the past 30 days (adults self-report) • Percentage of adults who are satisfied with their lives
Ability to function	• Percentage of adults who report a disability (for example, limitation of vision or hearing, cognitive impairment, lack of mobility) • Mean number of days in the past 30 days with limited activity due to poor mental or physical health (adults self-report)
Access to health care	• Percent of population that is insured • Percentage of the population that has a designated primary care physician
Clinical preventive services	• Percentage of adults who receive a cancer screening based on the most recent guidelines • Percentage of adults with hypertension whose blood pressure is under control • Percentage of children aged 19–35 months who receive the recommended vaccines
Cost of care	• Percentage of unnecessary emergency department (ED) visits • Percentage decrease in ED costs • Percentage decrease in cost of care per patient, per year

EXHIBIT 11.3
Sample Population Health Measurements

Source: Reprinted with permission from Health Research & Educational Trust, *The Second Curve of Population Health*. Copyright © 2014.

congestive heart failure (CHF). This population was selected when data showed a significant variation in management of these patients by health system physicians. The physicians agree to follow the current CHF clinical practice guidelines recommended by the American College of Cardiologists. Uniform patient management flowsheets are integrated into the systemwide EHR to remind physicians and nurses of appropriate treatment and follow-up practices for patients with CHF. A CHF community support group facilitated by a cardiac nurse practitioner is formed by one of the system hospitals. The hospital contracts with a vendor to provide remote daily weight telemonitoring services for high-risk patients. Patients reporting clinically significant weight variations are referred to a cardiac nurse practitioner for follow-up.

Six months after implementation of these various initiatives, the health system assesses its performance and finds the readmission rate for the CHF population has decreased by more than 20 percent. After one year, there is improved prescription of recommended CHF medications and closer monitoring of high-risk patients. This results in continued decreases in hospital admissions and readmissions.

While the health system is able to evaluate its own experiences, comparing its performance with other health systems is difficult due to differences in information systems and data definitions. In chapter 4, exhibit 4.20 shows a list of online sources of performance

EXHIBIT 11.4
Sources of Data on Population Counts and Characteristics

- City Health Dashboard
  www.cityhealthdashboard.com
- County Health Rankings
  www.countyhealthrankings.org
- 500 Cities: Local Data for Better Health
  www.cdc.gov/500cities
- HealthData.gov
  www.healthdata.gov
- Human Mortality Database
  www.mortality.org
- National Center for Health Statistics
  www.cdc.gov/nchs/index.htm
- State Health Access Data Assistance Center (SHADAC) Data Center
  http://statehealthcompare.shadac.org
- US Census Bureau
  www.census.gov

comparison data. Some of these data sources may contain information useful for evaluating population health care results. Exhibit 11.4 contains sources of data on population counts and characteristics that could also be useful for comparative purposes and for selecting at-risk target populations. For example, a recent analysis of statistics from three of these data sources found that "the counties with the highest mortality rates from asthma are located along the southern half of the Mississippi River and in Georgia and South Carolina" (Dwyer-Lindgren et al. 2017, 1139). Health organizations in these geographic areas have an opportunity to reduce these mortality rates by initiating population health care for asthma target populations in their local community.

IMPROVEMENT

Population health care improvement activities follow the same steps as any improvement project: Define the improvement goal, analyze current practices, design and implement improvements, and measure success. See chapter 5 for descriptions of various models used to improve performance. To achieve population health care improvement goals, initiatives require a team approach, with representatives from all stakeholder groups. Chapter 7 covers the topic of improvement project teams.

Successful population health care improvements rely on the collection and effective use of data to identify at-risk target populations and select the best strategies for achieving goals. A substantial financial investment by organizations is required to create and support information systems that can be used to better manage the care of large populations (Connelly and Sykes 2016).

CASE STUDY

The following case study demonstrates how a population health care initiative was enacted in an accountable care organization (ACO) using the Plan-Do-Study-Act improvement model.

A Medicaid ACO composed of 13 private and public affiliates annually studies diabetes care for its enrollees. The most recent study shows that during the previous year only 31 percent of enrollees with diabetes had at least one glycemic test (hemoglobin A1c), and only 16 percent had retinal examinations. Because these annual exams are recommended by national guidelines, the ACO decides to target enrollees with diabetes for population health care initiatives.

PLAN: The first step is to determine the prevalence of diabetes among the ACO's 32,100 enrollees. By analyzing ambulatory encounter, inpatient, emergency department, pharmacy, and laboratory data, the ACO finds that 16 percent of its enrollees have diabetes—exceeding the national prevalence rate of 9.4 percent.

A multidisciplinary improvement team is formed. It includes representatives from several stakeholder groups: affiliated clinics, health education sponsors, local retail pharmacies, quality and case management, data/informatics support, and public health. The team sets the project goal of meeting the American Diabetes Association's current clinical practice guidelines within one year. Based on these guideline recommendations, the team defines the following process and outcome measures of success:

◆ Annual hemoglobin A1c testing rate

◆ Percent of patients whose hemoglobin A1c test results are acceptable

◆ Annual rate of retinal examinations

◆ Patient perceived quality of life (as measured by a diabetes-specific survey)

◆ Patient and practitioner satisfaction

The team develops several interventions aimed at patients with diabetes to meet the goals, including the following:

◆ Create preventive care flowsheets for clinics that detail diabetes care and treatment requirements based on guideline recommendations.

◆ Incorporate patient-specific preventive care schedules into clinic electronic records with mailings or e-mail reminders to patients alerting them to services that are due.

◆ Refer patients to case management if more intensive interventions are needed.

◆ Strengthen the discussion of preventive care measures and the guidelines' diabetes management recommendations in provider-sponsored and public health diabetes education classes.

◆ Contract with a vendor to conduct quality-of-life and satisfaction surveys.

◆ Identify better ways to identify patients not filling prescriptions for diabetes medications. Retail pharmacies will create a team to discuss how to best accomplish this.

DO: All physicians caring for ACO enrollees with diabetes review and agree to follow the American Diabetes Association clinical practice guidelines. Once agreement is obtained, the IT changes are initiated. These include construction of an electronic preventive care flowsheet for clinic health records, creation of electronic preventive care reminders, and design of electronic alerts for case managers to notify them when a patient is overdue for preventive services or has uncontrolled hemoglobin A1c levels. These IT changes take five months to complete—longer than had been anticipated. Because of this delay, the goal of meeting guidelines is revised to 18 months from the start of the project from the original 12 months.

A brochure about preventive care and management is developed and disseminated to health educators for use in diabetes education classes. The brochure is also made available to local retail pharmacies. A request for proposal is sent to three survey vendors and one is chosen. Surveys are to be conducted annually in March. All population health care interventions are completed six months after the start of the project, except for better communication linkages with retail pharmacies. The pharmacy team continues to look into ways of sharing patient medication compliance with clinics.

STUDY: At 18 months, the ACO re-measures and analyzes data. The retinal examination rate of 32 percent represents significant improvement. The hemoglobin A1c testing rate also shows significant improvement: 69 percent of enrollees with diabetes had at least one hemoglobin A1c test during the measurement year. However, 43 percent of those tested had results greater than 7 percent, indicating poor glycemic control. Only 70 percent of these patients had been contacted by case managers to discuss diabetes management strategies.

ACT: The ACO provides information and feedback from these analyses to their private and public affiliates and recognizes the people who helped make the improvements possible. The previous interventions are continued. Education on the importance of glycemic control to delay the onset of diabetes-related complications is added for enrollees and practitioners. Improving communication between local retail pharmacies and the clinic is an ongoing issue that has yet to be resolved.

CONCLUSION

Population health care involves the use of information and targeted interventions to maximize the health and well-being of persons in a defined population.

Health maintenance organizations and providers such as the Veterans Health Administration have traditionally implemented population health care initiatives. Alternative payment models that replace FFS reimbursement have increased providers' incentives to be involved in population health care. While any organization that delivers health care services to a defined group of individuals can practice population health management, integrated health systems are more likely to be involved in these initiatives.

The steps of quality management—measurement, assessment, and improvement—can be applied to population health care initiatives. Data are used to measure structural aspects such as health-related community resources. Process measures enable providers to determine if best practices are being followed. Outcome measures report end results, such as the distribution of hemoglobin A1c test results in the diabetic population. The individual's perspective of quality is evaluated using patient experience measures.

Measurement data are periodically reviewed to determine if improvement goals are being met and where targeted population health care initiatives should be focused. Measurement data are instrumental in identifying high-risk groups that would benefit from population health management interventions. The development and implementation of these initiatives follow the same steps as commonly used improvement models.

FOR DISCUSSION

Go to the County Health Rankings website (www.countyhealthrankings.org) and explore the health outcomes and health factors data for the county where you reside.

1. Describe one or more population health care initiatives that could improve health outcomes or reduce factors that affect health outcomes in your county.

2. Create a population health care improvement project charter for an initiative in the county where you live. (Improvement project charters are discussed in chapter 7.) Provide as much information as possible in your charter.

WEBSITES

*   American Hospital Association, *Next Generation of Community Health* (2016)
    www.aha.org/content/17/committee-on-research-next-gen-community-health.pdf

*   America's Health Insurance Plans, Population Health Resources
    https://www.ahip.org/issues/population-health/

*   Canadian Institute of Population and Public Health
    www.cihr-irsc.gc.ca/e/13777.html

*   Centers for Disease Control and Prevention, *Implementation Guide for Public Health Practitioners: The Shands Jacksonville Patient-Centered Medical Home Diabetes and Hypertension Self-Management Education Model* (2015)
    www.cdc.gov/dhdsp/docs/shands-implementation-guide.pdf

*   Centers for Disease Control and Prevention, Social Determinants of Health: Know What Affects Health
    www.cdc.gov/socialdeterminants/index.htm

- Health Research & Educational Trust Community Health Resources
www.hpoe.org/communityhealth

- Healthy People 2020, Social Determinants of Health
www.healthypeople.gov/2020/topics-objectives/topic/social-determinants-of-health

- Improving Population Health
www.improvingpopulationhealth.org

- Institute for Population Health
http://ipophealth.org/

- Medicare Alternative Payment Models
http://innovation.cms.gov/initiatives/index.html#views=models

- Population Health Alliance
www.populationhealthalliance.org/

- Robert Wood Johnson Foundation, Better Data for Better Health
www.rwjf.org/en/library/collections/better-data-for-better-health.html

- Stroudwater, *Introduction to Population Health* (video)
www.stroudwater.com/?resources=introduction-to-population-health-part-1-of-8

- UC Davis Health, Institute for Population Health Improvement
www.ucdmc.ucdavis.edu/iphi/

- Wyoming Institute of Population Health
www.cheyenneregional.org/location/wyoming-institute-of-population-health/

REFERENCES

American Public Health Association. 1995. "The Role of Public Health in Ensuring Healthy Communities." Published January 1. www.apha.org/policies-and-advocacy/public-health-policy-statements/policy-database/2014/07/30/10/48/the-role-of-public-health-in-ensuring-healthy-communities.

America's Health Insurance Plans (AHIP). 2017. *Beyond the Boundaries of Health Care: Addressing Social Issues.* Published July. www.ahip.org/wp-content/uploads/2017/07/SocialDeterminants_IssueBrief_7.21.17.pdf.

Ananth, S. 2016. "Tackling Contradictions of Population Health, and Five Key Success Factors." *H&HN Daily.* Published September 1. www.hhnmag.com/articles/7536-achieving-success-in-pop-health-management.

Caron, R. M. 2017. *Population Health: Principles and Applications for Management*. Chicago: Health Administration Press.

Centers for Medicare & Medicaid Services (CMS). 2016. *2017 Quality Rating System Measure Technical Specifications*. Accessed December 8, 2017. www.cms.gov /Medicare/Quality-Initiatives-Patient-Assessment-Instruments/QualityInitiatives GenInfo/Downloads/2017_QRS-Measure_Technical_Specifications.pdf.

Connelly, M. D., and R. Sykes. 2016. "Big Data: Central to the Population Health Journey." *Frontiers of Health Services Management* 32 (4): 40–45.

Corrigan, J., E. Fisher, and S. Heiser. 2015. "Hospital Community Benefit Programs: Increasing Benefits to Communities." *Journal of the American Medical Association* 313 (12): 1211–12.

Derose, S. F., and D. B. Petitti. 2003. "Measuring Quality of Care and Performance from a Population Health Care Perspective." *Annual Review of Public Health* 24: 363–84.

Dwyer-Lindgren, L., A. Bertozzi-Villa, R. W. Stubbs, C. Morozoff, S. Shirude, M. Naghavi, A. H. Mokdad, and C. J. L. Murray. 2017. "Trends and Patterns of Differences in Chronic Respiratory Disease Mortality Among US Counties, 1980–2014." *Journal of the American Medical Association* 318 (12): 1136–49.

Flaccus, G. 2016. "6 Portland Health Providers Give $21.5M for Homeless Housing." *U.S. News & World Report*. Published September 23. www.usnews.com/news/news/ articles/2016-09-23/6-portland-health-providers-give-215m-for-homeless-housing.

Fried, B. M., and J. D. Sherer. 2016. "Value Based Reimbursement: The Rock Thrown into the Health Care Pond." *Health Affairs Blog*. Posted July 8. http://healthaffairs.org/ blog/2016/07/08/value-based-reimbursement-the-rock-thrown-into-the-health-care -pond/.

Granatir, T. 1995. "Quality and Community Accountability: A View of the American Hospital Association." In *The Epidemiology of Quality*, edited by V. A. Kazandjian, 253–68. Gaithersburg, MD: Aspen Publishers.

Health Research & Educational Trust (HRET). 2014. *The Second Curve of Population Health*. Published March. www.hpoe.org/Reports-HPOE/SecondCurvetoPopHealth2014.pdf.

———. 2012. *Managing Population Health: The Role of the Hospital.* Published April. www. hpoe.org/Reports-HPOE/managing_population_health.pdf.

Institute of Medicine (IOM). 2001. *Crossing the Quality Chasm: A New Health System for the 21st Century.* Washington, DC: National Academies Press.

James, J. 2016. "Health Policy Brief: Nonprofit Hospitals' Community Benefit Requirements." *Health Affairs.* Published February 25. http://healthaffairs.org/healthpolicy briefs/brief_pdfs/healthpolicybrief_153.pdf.

Kaiser Family Foundation. 2013. "Summary of the Affordable Care Act." Published April 25. www.kff.org/health-reform/fact-sheet/summary-of-the-affordable-care-act/.

Kindig, D., and G. Stoddart. 2003. "What Is Population Health?" *American Journal of Public Health* 93 (3): 380–83.

Magnan, S., E. Fisher, D. Kindig, G. Isham, D. Woods, M. Eustis, C. Backstrom, and S. Leitz. 2012. "Achieving Accountability for Health and Health Care." *Minnesota Medicine* 95 (11): 37–39.

National Association for Healthcare Quality (NAHQ). 2015. *Essential Competencies: Population Health and Care Transitions.* Chicago: National Association for Healthcare Quality.

Robert Wood Johnson Foundation. 2012. "What's New with Community Benefit?" *Health Policy Snapshot.* Published October. www.rwjf.org/content/dam/farm/reports/ issue_briefs/2012/rwjf402124.

US Department of Health and Human Services, Office of Disease Prevention and Health Promotion. 2017. "Social Determinants of Health." Accessed December 8. www.healthy people.gov/2020/topics-objectives/topic/social-determinants-of-health.

US Social Security Administration (SSA). 1974. "Notes and Brief Reports: Health Maintenance Organization Act of 1973." *Social Security Bulletin.* Published March. www.ssa. gov/policy/docs/ssb/v37n3/v37n3p35.pdf.

Wynne, B. 2016. "Moops? A Roadmap to MIPS." *Health Affairs Blog.* Posted February 26. http://healthaffairs.org/blog/2016/02/26/moops-a-roadmap-to-mips/.

CHAPTER 12

ORGANIZING FOR QUALITY

After reading this chapter, you will be able to

➤ identify groups responsible for quality in a healthcare organization,

➤ describe typical participants in healthcare quality management activities,

➤ explain the purpose and content of a quality management plan,

➤ recognize aspects of organizational culture that influence the effectiveness of quality management, and

➤ discuss strategies for overcoming environmental characteristics inhospitable to quality improvement.

High-performing healthcare organization
An organization that is committed to success and continuously produces outstanding results and high levels of customer satisfaction.

Governing body
The individuals, group, or agency with ultimate legal authority and responsibility for the overall operation of the organization; often called the *board of trustees*, *board of governors*, or *board of directors*.

Quality management system
A set of interrelated or interacting elements that organizations use to direct and control the implementation of quality policies and achieve quality objectives.

Quality does not happen by accident. Organizations must make an intentional effort to measure, assess, and improve performance. Not only must an organization's board of trustees and senior management be committed to quality, but they also must create a framework for accomplishing quality activities and an environment that supports continuous improvement. Active and personal board involvement in quality and patient safety oversight contributes to building a **high-performing healthcare organization** (Jiang et al. 2009).

An organization's **governing body**—the board of trustees—is ultimately responsible for the quality of healthcare services (Wagonhurst and Habte 2008). The board exercises this duty through oversight of quality management activities. If a healthcare provider does not have a board of trustees (e.g., in the case of a limited partnership physician clinic), the legal owners of the business assume this responsibility.

Although the day-to-day activities of measurement, assessment, and improvement are delegated to senior leaders, physicians, managers, and support staff, the board's oversight role can greatly influence quality. For example, board members set the approach to handling quality issues. In addition, the questions trustees raise can lead to new insights or inform the board and management of actions they need to take (Zastocki 2015).

To accomplish quality management functions, healthcare organizations create a **quality management system** or framework that defines and guides all measurement, assessment, and improvement activities. This infrastructure can be organized in many ways. Variables that affect the organization of the quality framework include

◆ the type of organization,

◆ the size of the organization,

◆ available resources,

◆   the number and type of externally imposed quality requirements, and

◆   internal quality improvement priorities.

Small independent healthcare providers, such as outpatient clinics and university student health centers, typically have informal quality management infrastructures; the clinic manager performs most, if not all, quality management activities and reports information directly to the clinic owner or medical director. Large health systems that include several hospitals as well as nonhospital providers have formal, well-defined quality frameworks.

Many healthcare organizations are required by accreditation standards or government (federal and state) regulations to have a plan that explains their method of fulfilling quality management activities. Some standards and regulations have explicit requirements regarding plan content and the structure of improvement activities. For instance, hospitals in Pennsylvania must have a patient safety committee that includes two residents of the community, who are served by—but are not agents, employees, or contractors of—the facility (Commonwealth of Pennsylvania 2002). Laboratories that voluntarily comply with the standards of the Clinical and Laboratory Standards Institute (2017) must have a quality manual that documents the quality management structure and activities. The Joint Commission (2016) accreditation standards do not require a written plan, but they do require that organizations take a systematic approach to performance improvement.

> **(?) DID YOU KNOW?**
>
> Avedis Donabedian, physician and professor of public health at the University of Michigan from 1966 to 1989, became internationally known for his research on healthcare improvement. Before his death on November 9, 2000, he identified "the determination to make it work" as the most important prerequisite to ensuring quality of care: "If we are truly committed to quality, almost any mechanism will work. If we are not, the most elegantly constructed of mechanisms will fail" (Eldar 2001, 92).

Although written plans may not be required, most accredited organizations have them in place to illustrate that they have organized their internal quality management activities. Good business sense dictates the importance of having a written, board-approved **quality management plan** that describes the organization's quality infrastructure and required quality management activities.

QUALITY MANAGEMENT SYSTEM

Healthcare organizations' quality management systems vary according to the entity's governance and management structure. In general, the following six groups typically fulfill quality management roles:

1.   The board, which oversees and supports measurement, assessment, and improvement activities

Quality management plan
A formal document that describes the organization's quality management system in terms of organizational structure, responsibilities of management and staff, lines of authority, and required interfaces for those planning, implementing, and assessing quality activities.

2. Administration, which is responsible for the organization and management of measurement, assessment, and improvement activities

3. The coordinating committee (or individual), which directs measurement, assessment, and improvement activities

4. The medical staff, which develops and participates in measurement, assessment, and improvement activities related to the performance of physicians and other medical professionals who practice independently

5. Departments, which develop and participate in measurement, assessment, and improvement activities related to nonphysician performance

6. Quality support services, which assist all groups in the organization with measurement, assessment, and improvement activities

THE BOARD

The governing body or board—usually called the *board of trustees*, *board of governors*, or *board of directors*—is a group of people who have ultimate legal authority and responsibility for the operation of the healthcare organization, including its quality management activities. The board of trustees' involvement in quality management activities includes, but is not limited to, the following responsibilities:

◆ Defining the organization's commitment to continuous improvement of patient care and services in the organization's mission statement

◆ Prioritizing the organization's quality goals (with administration and the medical staff)

◆ Incorporating the results of assessment and improvement activities into strategic planning

◆ Learning approaches to and methods of continuous improvement

◆ Providing financial support for measurement, assessment, and improvement activities

◆ Promoting healthcare quality improvement

◆ Evaluating the organization's progress toward its quality goals

◆ Reviewing the effectiveness of the quality management program

ADMINISTRATION

The responsibility for implementing quality management activities throughout the organization lies with administration—the chief executive officer, the chief operating officer, the vice presidents, and other senior leaders. In contrast to the board's high-level role, administration ensures that day-to-day quality management operations are meeting the organization's needs.

Administration's involvement in quality management activities includes, but is not limited to, the following responsibilities:

◆ Defining the organization's quality management infrastructure

◆ Assigning quality management responsibilities and holding people accountable for fulfilling them

◆ Allocating the resources necessary to support quality management activities

◆ Encouraging those who use or provide the organization's services to participate in quality management activities

◆ Promoting physician and employee education about the concepts and techniques of quality management

◆ Using performance data for strategic planning purposes and to design and evaluate new services or programs

◆ Identifying opportunities for performance improvement and helping to achieve these improvements (with the medical staff)

◆ Keeping the board informed of quality and patient safety issues

THE COORDINATING COMMITTEE

The quality coordinating committee, often called the *quality council, performance improvement committee,* or *quality and patient safety committee,* guides all measurement, assessment, and improvement activities. In small organizations, an individual, rather than a committee, may fill this role. The coordinating committee's involvement in quality management activities includes, but is not limited to, the following responsibilities:

◆ Meeting periodically to direct the activities of the organization's quality management program

◆ Setting expectations; developing plans; ensuring implementation of processes to measure; and assessing and improving the quality of the organization's governance, management, clinical, and support processes

◆ Analyzing summary reports of system- and activity-level measures of performance and performance improvement activities, and providing reports of these analyses to the board of trustees

◆ Setting improvement priorities and chartering interdepartmental, multidisciplinary improvement teams

◆ Directing resources necessary for measurement, assessment, and improvement activities

◆ Establishing quality goals for the organization, with board approval

◆ Coordinating and communicating all quality management activities throughout the organization

◆ At least annually, overseeing evaluation of the quality management program's effectiveness in meeting the organization's quality goals, and revising strategy where necessary

◆ Communicating quality management activities to the board of trustees

◆ Ensuring that the quality management infrastructure and activities meet accreditation and regulatory requirements

Typically, the quality coordinating committee is made up of physicians, nurses, other clinicians, and administrative representatives, but its composition depends in part on the size of the healthcare organization. Most important, the people who oversee and are accountable for quality in the organization should be included. Exhibit 12.1 lists examples

EXHIBIT 12.1
Composition
of Quality
Coordinating
Committee in Two
Organizations

Teaching Hospital	Neighborhood Health Clinic
• Chief operating officer • Vice president of medical affairs • Vice president of nursing • Vice president of clinical support services • Medical staff president • Director of quality and patient safety	• Medical director • Senior staff nurse • Clinic manager • Director of health information management

of committee members for two types of organizations—a major teaching hospital and a neighborhood health clinic.

THE MEDICAL STAFF

The Medicare Conditions of Participation (CoPs) for Hospitals, along with The Joint Commission accreditation standards, require that hospitals have an **organized medical staff**. A hospital's medical staff is composed of physicians, dentists, and other professional medical personnel who provide care to the hospital's patients independently. The theory behind the quality role of the organized medical staff is that lay members of the board are neither trained nor competent to judge the performance of physicians and other medical professionals. Therefore, they delegate to the medical staff the responsibility of evaluating the quality of patient care provided by physicians and other medical professionals and advising the board of the results. The board retains legal authority to make final decisions.

The Medicare CoPs and Joint Commission standards require that medical personnel have bylaws and rules or regulations that establish mechanisms by which they accomplish their tasks. The medical staff infrastructure for accomplishing its quality management responsibilities is found in these documents. The Joint Commission (2016) standards require, at a minimum, the formation of a medical staff executive committee to represent physicians in the organization's governance, leadership, and performance improvement functions. Additional medical staff committees or groups may be formed to fulfill other quality management functions. For instance, chapter 3 introduced the concept of clinical decision-making—the process by which physicians and other clinicians determine which patients need what and when. The medical staff is responsible for evaluating the appropriateness of physicians' clinical decisions.

Critical concept 12.1 is an excerpt from one hospital's medical staff regulations that describes the quality management duties of the pharmacy and therapeutics committee. One duty of this committee is to evaluate whether physicians are overusing, underusing, or misusing medications.

In organizations that lack an organized medical staff, the medical director or the governing board assumes physician-related quality management responsibilities. For instance, the Medicare CoPs for freestanding ambulatory surgery centers (ASCs) require the facility to have "a governing body that assumes full legal responsibility for determining, implementing, and monitoring policies governing the ASC's total operation. The governing body has oversight and accountability for the quality assessment and performance improvement program, ensures that facility policies and programs are administered so as to provide quality health care in a safe environment, and develops and maintains a disaster preparedness plan" (CMS 2016).

> **Organized medical staff**
> A formal organization of physicians, dentists, and other professional medical personnel with the delegated responsibility and authority to maintain proper standards of medical care and plan for continued betterment of that care.

> **(!) CRITICAL CONCEPT 12.1** Quality Management Responsibilities of a
> Hospital's Pharmacy and Therapeutics Committee
>
> Medical staff involvement in quality management activities includes, but is not limited to,
> the following responsibilities:
>
> • Providing leadership oversight for the physician-related aspects of quality
>   management
>
> • Measuring, assessing, and improving clinical aspects of patient care
>
> • Evaluating the clinical competence of physicians and other medical professionals
>   who care for patients independently in the organization
>
> • Identifying, within all departments in the organization, opportunities to improve
>   patient care, and helping to achieve these improvements
>
> • Reporting the results of quality management activities to the medical staff, oversight
>   committees, and the board

DEPARTMENTS

All departments and services in a healthcare organization participate in quality management activities. Managers of these departments and services are responsible for overseeing performance in their respective areas. Manager involvement in quality management activities includes, but is not limited to, the following responsibilities:

◆ Providing leadership oversight for departmental quality management activities

◆ Measuring, assessing, and improving clinical and operational performance

◆ Ensuring the competence of people working in the department

◆ Identifying opportunities to improve performance in the department and throughout the organization, and helping to achieve these improvements

◆ Reporting the results of departmental quality management activities to departmental staff, oversight committees, and the board

QUALITY SUPPORT SERVICES

Many individuals in a healthcare organization assist with quality management activities. Their job titles and areas of expertise vary considerably among organizations. In smaller organizations, the responsibilities may be combined. In some cases, only one or two employees may support all of the organization's quality management activities. A discussion of common quality-related positions follows. Several of these offer certification examinations. The websites for their certifying agencies are found at the end of this chapter.

Quality director. The quality director is the administrative head of quality management functions and may be a member of the organization's senior administrative team. The quality director serves as an internal consultant and assists the organization with measurement, assessment, and improvement activities. The director often manages a department of data analysts and other staff who support quality management functions.

Patient safety coordinator. In response to the increased emphasis on patient safety improvement (covered in chapter 8), some healthcare organizations have appointed a patient safety coordinator or patient safety officer. Oversight of patient safety improvement activities may include evaluating patient incident data, facilitating root cause analyses and other patient safety improvement projects, and coordinating the flow of patient safety information throughout the organization.

Physician quality advisor. Some organizations appoint a physician as a full- or part-time advisor to the quality management program. Organizations that have a medical director may assign quality advisor duties to that position. The physician quality advisor provides input to the senior administrative team and to the medical staff on issues related to physician performance measurement and improvement activities. The quality advisor works closely with the quality director and the president of the medical staff to ensure appropriate medical staff participation in quality management activities. The physician quality advisor may also provide guidance for utilization management (UM) activities.

Case manager/utilization reviewer. Case managers and utilization reviewers are responsible for facility-wide UM activities (covered in chapter 10). These individuals conduct prospective, concurrent, and retrospective reviews to determine appropriateness of medical care and to gather information on resource use. In addition, they assist with discharge planning to coordinate patient services between caregivers and provider sites.

Patient advocate. The patient advocate is the primary customer service contact for patients and staff members for the resolution of customer service problems related to a patient's healthcare experience. The patient advocate, sometimes called the *patient representative* or *ombudsman*, participates at all levels of the quality management program.

Risk manager. The risk manager coordinates the organization's **risk management** activities. The goal of risk management is to protect the organization from financial losses that may result from exposure to risk. This goal is achieved through initiatives aimed at

Risk management
The act or practice of dealing with risk, which includes planning for risk, assessing (identifying and analyzing) risk areas, developing risk-handling options, monitoring risks to determine how they have changed, and documenting the overall risk management program.

preventing harm to patients, visitors, and staff. In addition to other duties, the risk manager may be responsible for maintaining the organization's patient incident report system and may serve as the organization's patient safety officer.

Infection control coordinator. The infection control coordinator, usually a nurse, provides surveillance, education, and consulting services for physicians and staff in matters related to preventing patient infections. The infection control coordinator gathers data for infection-related performance measures and is also responsible for facilitating the implementation of government regulations and accreditation standards relevant to infection control.

Medical staff services coordinator. This medical staff services professional is primarily responsible for supporting the administrative and medical–legal components of the medical staff organization, including peer review and credentialing of physicians and allied health practitioners.

Compliance officer. In recent years, some healthcare organizations have added a compliance officer to the quality team. This person interprets accreditation standards and government regulations pertaining to quality management and helps physicians and staff adhere to all standards and regulations.

Data analyst. Data analysts are responsible for gathering and reporting performance measurement information. These individuals may have a clinical background (e.g., nursing, therapy) or a nonclinical background (e.g., health information management). Some data analysts may report to the quality director, and some may be employed in other departments, such as nursing or surgical services. Several data analysts are needed to support quality management activities in large healthcare organizations. Reporting and analysis of measurement results will continue to require the services of data analysts even when electronic data sources make data collection less burdensome.

A growing number of the data elements necessary for measurement purposes can be captured electronically; however, these measures require staff resources as well to ensure the data "accurately reflect the clinical picture" (Panzer et al. 2013, 1974). As the data for some quality measures are not routinely documented in the patient's electronic health record (EHR), staff may need to collect some of the data (Panzer et al. 2013). Hybrid methods of data collection, involving EHR-derived data and medical record reviews, are still needed. For instance, a 2014 national survey of 394 randomly selected physician practices found that physicians and support staff spent 15.1 hours per week tracking quality metrics for Medicare and other payers and regulators (Casalino et al. 2016).

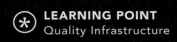

LEARNING POINT
Quality Infrastructure

Every healthcare organization has a quality infrastructure designed to fulfill the goals of quality management. As the complexity of the organization increases, so does the need for a formal, well-defined quality infrastructure. Six groups typically involved in an organization's quality management activities are the board of trustees, administration, the coordinating committee, the medical staff, all departments, and quality support services.

Providers are not the only group adding support staff to meet quality management expectations. More than 90 percent of health plans produce and submit performance data to the National Committee for Quality Assurance (NCQA 2017). These health plans invest significant resources in data collection and have hired additional staff to review patient records. State and national groups that receive data from providers and health plans have added support staff to analyze and report aggregate results for the growing number of quality measures. Nearly all state health agencies have increased staffing to conduct performance management activities aimed at improving the quality and outcomes of public health services.

QUALITY MANAGEMENT PLAN

The document describing the organization's structure and process for measuring, assessing, and improving performance may be called a *quality management plan*, a *performance improvement plan*, a *quality and patient safety plan*, or one of a number of other descriptive titles. For simplicity, the term *quality management plan* will be used throughout this chapter. The purpose of the plan is to serve as a blueprint for quality and patient safety in the organization. At a minimum, the plan includes the following elements:

- ◆ A quality statement

- ◆ A description of the quality management infrastructure

- ◆ Details of performance measurement, assessment, and improvement activities

- ◆ An evaluation of the effectiveness of quality management activities

QUALITY STATEMENT

The quality statement describes the goal to which all quality management activities are directed. The statement reflects the organization's ideals—what it wants for patients and the community. An organization's quality statement often incorporates its mission, vision, and values. For example, this is the quality statement of St. Hope Foundation (2017), a patient-centered medical home in Texas:

> Our goal is to serve you with high quality, culturally compassionate and accessible health care so that you get the care you need in a way that works best for you.

The board and administration jointly develop the quality statement. In facilities with an organized medical staff, physicians are also involved in its creation.

QUALITY MANAGEMENT INFRASTRUCTURE

The plan describes each quality management stakeholder and its responsibilities. Some plans describe infrastructure and stakeholder activities in great detail and are several pages long. Plans do not need to describe every element, however. Quality management responsibilities are often specified in employee job descriptions, and duplicating these statements in the quality plan is redundant. In general, the quality management plan should be sufficiently detailed to convey the organization's approach to quality management. At a minimum, the description of the infrastructure should include the following:

◆ Major stakeholders (individuals and groups) and expectations for their participation in quality management functions

◆ Committee structure (e.g., committees involved, committee chairs and members, meeting frequency, methods of communicating quality management activities throughout the organization)

Drawing an organizational structure diagram may help depict the relationships and flow of information among individuals, groups, and committees. Exhibit 12.2 illustrates the flow of performance information in a hospital.

PERFORMANCE MEASUREMENT, ASSESSMENT, AND IMPROVEMENT ACTIVITIES

Variables to be measured and the execution of assessment and improvement activities are detailed in the quality management plan. The improvement model also may be documented, as well as the groups that charter and participate in improvement projects. In some

EXHIBIT 12.2

Flow of Performance Information in a Hospital

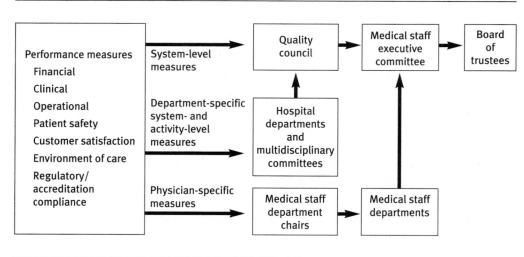

> **⚠ CRITICAL CONCEPT 12.2** 2016–17 Quality Goals and Objectives for Nevada Medicaid and Nevada Check Up Members
>
> **Goal 2:** Increase use of evidence-based practices for members with chronic conditions.
>
> **Objective 2.1:** Increase rate of HbA1c testing for members with diabetes.
>
> **Objective 2.2:** Decrease rate of HbA1c poor control (⋯⟩9.0%) for members with diabetes.
>
> **Objective 2.3:** Increase rate of HbA1c good control (⟨⋯8.0%) for members with diabetes.
>
> **Objective 2.4:** Increase rate of eye exams performed for members with diabetes.
>
> **Objective 2.5:** Increase medical attention for nephropathy for members with diabetes.
>
> **Objective 2.6:** Increase blood pressure control (⟨⋯140/90 mm Hg) for members with diabetes.
>
> **Objective 2.7a:** Increase medication management for people with asthma—medication compliance 50 percent.
>
> **Objective 2.7b:** Increase medication management for people with asthma—medication compliance 75 percent.
>
> *Source*: Reprinted from Nevada Department of Health and Human Services, *Quality Assessment and Performance Improvement Strategy (Quality Strategy): 2016–2017*, pages 1–12. Copyright © 2016.

organizations, the quality plan does not change often—each year it is reviewed and updated slightly to reflect infrastructure changes and new regulatory or accreditation requirements, but the fundamentals remain the same.

Elements of the quality program that frequently change, such as quality improvement goals and objectives, measures of performance, and sources of performance data, are described in appendixes to the plan or in other organizational documents. Critical concept 12.2 lists an example of one of the six 2016–17 quality goals and related objectives established by the Nevada Department of Health and Human Services (2016) for Nevada Medicaid and Nevada Check Up members. New or updated goals and objectives are set for the following year and the document is revised to reflect those changes. The organization's performance measures and information sources are also frequently updated.

EVALUATION OF THE EFFECTIVENESS OF QUALITY MANAGEMENT ACTIVITIES

Periodically (usually annually), the coordinating committee evaluates overall quality management performance by (1) determining whether the quality infrastructure has improved organizational performance and (2) making changes as necessary. The coordinating committee also determines whether the organization has met the year's quality goals and uses its findings to plan the following year's quality improvement activities.

Critical concept 12.3 is a quality plan template that can be customized to suit the needs of a healthcare organization that lacks an organized medical staff structure, such as an outpatient clinic, a freestanding ASC, or a nursing home.

> **(!) CRITICAL CONCEPT 12.3** Quality Plan Template for Organizations That Do Not Have an Organized Medical Staff
>
> **Quality Statement**
>
> The purpose of quality management activities is to improve clinical and operational processes and outcomes through continuous measurement, assessment, and improvement activities. The quality program of *(insert organization name)* strives to ensure that all aspects of healthcare service, whether clinical or nonclinical, are designed for optimal performance and patient safety and delivered consistently across the organization.
>
> **Quality Infrastructure and Responsibilities**
>
> The governing body of *(insert organization name)* has overall responsibility for the quality program and delegates operational responsibilities through the management structure.
>
> The objectives of the quality program are to
>
> - establish a system for ongoing monitoring of performance to identify problems or opportunities to improve patient care, operational performance, and customer satisfaction;
>
> - resolve identified problems and improve performance using quality improvement principles and techniques;
>
> - ensure that performance improvement actions are taken and the effectiveness of the actions is evaluated;
>
> - refer unresolved performance deficiencies to the medical director (or management structure, as appropriate) for resolution; and
>
> - maintain a consistent and systematic approach to quality improvement that involves planning activities, enacting plans, monitoring performance, and acting on improvements and deficiencies.
>
> *(continued)*

> (!) **CRITICAL CONCEPT 12.3** Quality Plan Template for Organizations
> That Do Not Have an Organized Medical Staff *(continued)*
>
> A quality management committee, consisting of *(insert the number and type of positions reflective of the organizational structure)*, is responsible for coordinating and integrating all measurement, assessment, and improvement efforts. The committee reports its findings to the medical director and management for review or implementation and problem resolution at that level, or for referral to the governing body, if indicated.
>
> Other organizational representatives involved directly and indirectly in quality management activities include managers, members of the clinical and nonclinical staffs, and administrative support staff. Appropriate staff members are involved in activities within the sphere of their responsibilities and expertise.
>
> The quality management committee is responsible for identifying measures of performance for important aspects of patient and operational services. Organizational representatives are responsible for ongoing monitoring and evaluation of performance and resolution of problems affecting their areas of responsibility. These activities are reported at least quarterly to the quality management committee for analysis, further study, or implementation (as necessary).
>
> Recommendations and actions of the quality management committee are documented and forwarded to the governing body.
>
> The quality management committee periodically reviews organization-wide quality management activities to ensure the goals of the quality program are being met and performance is continuously improving. At least annually, the quality plan is reviewed and revised as necessary.

A HOSPITABLE ENVIRONMENT

To improve quality, an organization must have the will to improve, the capacity to translate that will into positive change, the infrastructure necessary to support improvement, and an environment hospitable to quality. The last factor—environment—relates to the organization's culture. *Culture* is a system of shared actions, values, and beliefs that guides the behavior of an organization's members. The corporate culture of a business setting is one example of such a system. Edgar H. Schein (1986), a clinical psychologist turned organizational theorist, identified three levels of **organizational culture**:

Organizational culture
Prevalent patterns of shared beliefs and values that provide behavioral guidelines or establish norms for conducting business.

  Level 1: Observable culture—the way things are done in the organization

Level 2: Shared values—awareness of organizational values and recognition of their importance

Level 3: Common assumptions—realities that members take for granted and share as a result of their joint experiences

The organizational culture at all three levels is pivotal to successful continuous improvement. Culture influences the manner in which quality management is implemented and executed. Cultural tone—whether trust or fear, collaboration or isolation, interdependency or autonomy—affects the way senior leaders, managers, physicians, and employees interact in the quality management process. Quality leaders have long recognized the importance of culture as a driver of **performance excellence**. The term *performance excellence* was introduced by Peters and Waterman in 1982 to refer to an overall way of working that balances stakeholder concerns and increases the probability of long-term organizational success.

Several of the 14 quality principles espoused by W. Edwards Deming (1986) more than 25 years ago (see chapter 2) address the cultural aspects of quality improvement:

◆ Help people do a better job

◆ Drive out fear

◆ Break down barriers

◆ Restore pride of workmanship

◆ Make quality everyone's job

Performance excellence
Term introduced by Tom Peters and Robert Waterman in their book *In Search of Excellence* (1982) to refer to an overall way of working that balances stakeholder concerns and increases the probability of long-term organizational success.

⊛ LEARNING POINT
Planning for Quality

Every healthcare organization has a quality management infrastructure. An effective infrastructure begins at the board level and cascades vertically and horizontally to levels throughout the organization. The size, function, and number of components that support quality management activities vary according to the size of the organization and the types of healthcare services it provides. A healthcare organization's quality management infrastructure is often documented in a quality management plan.

In a culture committed to quality, senior leaders and managers lead by example and encourage an environment of open, candid dialogue and continuous improvement. The people who do the work are actively involved; management seeks their views and listens to what they have to say (Sherwood 2013). Everyone in the organization is clear on the expected level of performance and receives feedback on progress. Staff members are acknowledged and recognized for the contributions they make to further the organization's quality goals. People trust and have confidence in leadership's determination to continuously improve organizational performance.

The relationship between a supportive quality culture and an organization's ability to achieve aggressive improvement goals has been substantiated numerous times (Mannion, Davies, and Marshall 2005; Shortell et al. 2005; Nembhard et al. 2009; Mardon et al. 2010; Carney 2011; Sorra et al. 2012; Berry et al. 2016; Joint Commission 2017). In 2004, for instance, the Commonwealth Fund published the results of a study that identified supportive quality culture as a key factor contributing to the success of four high-performing US hospitals. The top-performing hospitals demonstrated a high degree of motivation and commitment to ensuring quality patient care. This commitment was reflected in and nurtured by the following elements (Meyer et al. 2004):

◆ Active leadership and personal involvement on the part of the senior team and the board of trustees

◆ An explicit quality-related mission and best-in-industry quality improvement targets

◆ Standing and ad hoc quality committees

◆ Regular reporting of performance measures with accountability for improved results

◆ Promotion of a safe environment for reporting errors

A study of home health agencies found the overarching characteristic of high-performing agencies is an engrained culture of commitment to the quality of patient care and continuous self-review and improvement (University of Colorado, Denver 2011).

In 2009, The Joint Commission revised its leadership standards to reflect the need for a culture that supports quality performance. Leaders in accredited organizations are expected to "create and maintain a culture of safety and quality throughout the organization" (Joint Commission 2017, 5). Compliance with these standards requires leaders to

◆ regularly evaluate the organization's culture of safety and quality,

◆ define and encourage acceptable work behaviors that support a culture of safety and quality, and

◆ identify and manage behaviors that undermine a culture of safety and quality.

There is no "correct" culture. A culture that works in one organization may not work in another. A culture's suitability depends on how well it supports the organization's quality management goals. Is the culture undermining quality improvement efforts? Some red flags that signal incompatibility are as follows:

◆ Tolerance of poor communication, corner-cutting, and poor performance

◆ Acceptance of improper procedures, complacency, and inefficiency

◆ Lack of trust

◆ Sacrifice of quality or patient safety to save money or time

◆ Comments heard such as, "Nobody ever listens to me" or "This is the way we do things around here"

Organizational culture is the root of many performance problems. If any of these red flags is evident, the organization's leaders must identify inhospitable attributes of the culture and modify the values, beliefs, and actions that affect the success of quality management activities. By nurturing the culture to an appropriate level, the organization will reap the rewards of quality management. Aspects of culture often found in high-performing organizations are summarized in critical concept 12.4.

(!) CRITICAL CONCEPT 12.4
Characteristics of a High-Performing Culture

- Senior leaders and managers communicate and support high-quality performance through words and actions.

- Open communication is practiced; people are free to voice opinions, share ideas, and make decisions.

- Conflict and disagreement are dealt with openly.

- People are dedicated to continuous improvement; higher quality goals are set once initial goals are met.

- People know what they are accountable for, take ownership of their responsibilities, and continuously strive to perform better.

- People support one another; the concept of teamwork is apparent throughout the organization.

- Individual and collective performance is monitored, reinforced, and corrected on an ongoing basis.

- Individual and team successes are acknowledged and celebrated.

- Individual competencies are systematically developed on an ongoing basis.

- Employees constantly learn from the best practices of top-performing organizations.

- Performance excellence is pursued for its own sake.

Cultural change can be difficult and time consuming to achieve because culture is rooted in the collective history of an organization and in the subconscious of its staff. In general, cultural change is instituted through the following steps:

◆ Uncover core values and beliefs, including both stated goals and goals embedded in employee behaviors. Two sources of healthcare organization culture surveys are listed in the website resources at the end of the chapter.

◆ Look for cultural characteristics that are undermining the organization's capacity to continuously improve. Conduct a series of focus groups with a representative sample of survey participants to identify areas needing change and practical interventions that will make a difference. Turn this information into a comprehensive cultural-change action plan.

◆ Establish new behavioral norms that demonstrate desired values.

◆ Repeat these steps over a long period. Emphasize to new hires the importance of the organization's culture. Reinforce desirable behavior.

Throughout most of his life, nineteenth-century French chemist Louis Pasteur insisted that germs—not the body—were the cause of disease. Not until the end of his life did he come to believe the opposite. After reaching this conclusion, he declined treatment for potentially curable pneumonia, reportedly saying, "It is the soil, not the seed" (Spath and Minogue 2008). In other words, a germ (the seed) causes disease when our bodies (the soil) provide a hospitable environment. This bacteriology lesson is relevant to the performance improvement efforts in healthcare organizations. The organization's culture (the soil) must provide

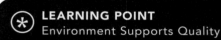

LEARNING POINT
Environment Supports Quality

An organization's environment—its culture—influences the success of quality management activities. Leaders must create a culture that supports their organization's goals and, when necessary, change that culture to encourage continuous improvement.

a hospitable environment for quality management activities (the seeds) to succeed.

CONCLUSION

Healthcare quality is not only dependent on the efforts of well-meaning frontline employees. The organization's leaders must systematically channel and manage the efforts to achieve optimal organizational performance. Healthcare organizations should have an appropriate quality management structure that operates at all levels and has the power to evaluate and improve all aspects of patient care and services.

Defining the quality management infrastructure and activities in a written document demonstrates the organization's formal commitment to quality. A written plan clearly communicates to employees the organization of quality management activities and the groups or individuals responsible for quality components.

Organizing for quality also involves creating a supportive organizational culture in which performance can flourish. Culture—the collective values, beliefs, expectations, and commitments that affect behavior at all levels—should further the quality goals of the organization. A culture built on trust and support will achieve high performance. Organizations will reap the most benefits from quality management when managers and employees value the process; encourage open, candid dialogue; support career growth; and pursue improved personal and organizational performance.

In the 2001 report *Crossing the Quality Chasm: A New Health System for the 21st Century*, the Institute of Medicine identified six dimensions of US healthcare that need improving. Not only did the report provide a basis for defining healthcare quality, but it also created a significant challenge for the healthcare industry. How can we make healthcare safer, more effective, patient centered, timely, efficient, and equitable? National policy changes and new regulations and standards have limited influence on what actually happens on the front lines of patient care. Addressing the challenge of improving healthcare quality requires that every organization continuously measure, assess, and improve performance.

For Discussion

1. Some healthcare organizations post their quality plan on the web. Search the Internet for quality plans from two different types of healthcare organizations (e.g., hospital, long-term care facility, ambulatory clinic, health plan). You may need to use search terms other than *quality management plan*, such as *performance improvement plan*, *patient safety plan*, or *quality plan*. Summarize the similarities and differences between the two plans.

2. Consider the cultural assumptions and beliefs underlying a perfectionist mentality: Perfection is always expected; mistakes are not allowed. This assumption can create an environment inhospitable to quality improvement. How would you change that perception?

3. Consider the organization you now work in, or if you are not currently employed, consider your last employer. What three words or phrases would you use to describe the company or department culture? Does the culture prompt or inhibit quality performance?

CERTIFICATION INFORMATION FOR QUALITY SUPPORT PROFESSIONALS

- Case manager certification
  https://ccmcertification.org
  www.acmaweb.org/acm

- Healthcare compliance officer certification
  www.aapc.com/certification/cpco.aspx
  www.compliancecertification.org/CHC/CertifiedinHealthcareCompliance.aspx

- Health Care Quality & Management Certification
  www.abqaurp.org/ABQMain/Certification

- Health data analyst certification
  www.ahima.org/certification/chda

- Healthcare quality certification
  http://nahq.org/certification/certified-professional-healthcare-quality

- Healthcare risk manager certification
  www.ashrm.org/education/cphrm.dhtml

- Medical staff services certification
  www.namss.org/Certification.aspx

- Patient advocate certification
  https://pacboard.org
  www.patientadvocatetraining.com/certificate-programs

- Patient safety certification
  www.npsf.org/?page=aboutcbpps

- Physician advisor certification
  www.abqaurp.org/ABQMain/Certification

WEBSITES

- Agency for Healthcare Research and Quality, Surveys on Patient Safety Culture
  www.ahrq.gov/professionals/quality-patient-safety/patientsafetyculture/index.html

- American College of Healthcare Executives and IHI/NPSF Lucian Leape Institute,
  Leading a Culture of Safety: A Blueprint for Success
  www.npsf.org/page/cultureofsafety

- American Hospital Association, Trustee Services
  http://trustees.aha.org/

- American Society for Healthcare Risk Management, *Different Roles, Same Goal: Risk and Quality Management Partnering for Patient Safety*
  www.ashrm.org/pubs/files/white_papers/Monograph.07RiskQuality.pdf

- Center for Healthcare Quality and Safety, University of Texas Health Science Center, Safety Attitude Questionnaires and Safety Climate Surveys
  https://med.uth.edu/chqs/surveys/safety-attitudes-and-safety-climate-questionnaire/

- Center for Rural Health, *The Board's Role in Quality*
  https://ruralhealth.und.edu/projects/flex/mbqip/pdf/boards_role.pdf

- ECRI Institute, "Patient Safety, Risk, and Quality"
  www.ecri.org/components/HRC/Pages/RiskQual4.aspx

- Health Resources and Services Administration, *Developing and Implementing a QI Plan*
  www.hrsa.gov/sites/default/files/quality/toolbox/508pdfs/developingqiplan.pdf

- Lucian Leape Institute, *Through the Eyes of the Workforce: Creating Joy, Meaning, and Safer Health Care*
  www.npsf.org/?page=throughtheeyes

- Office of Inspector General, compliance education materials for healthcare providers, practitioners, and suppliers
  https://oig.hhs.gov/compliance/101/index.asp

- Office of Inspector General, compliance resource materials
  https://oig.hhs.gov/compliance/compliance-guidance/compliance-resource-material.asp

- Washington State Hospital Association, *Patient Safety: Transforming Culture*
  www.wsha.org/wp-content/uploads/Transforming_Culture_Toolkit.pdf

REFERENCES

Berry, J. C., J. T. Davis, T. Bartman, C. C. Hafer, L. M. Lieb, N. Khan, and R. J. Brilli. 2016. "Improved Safety Culture and Teamwork Climate Are Associated with Decreases in Patient Harm and Hospital Mortality Across a Hospital System." *Journal of Patient Safety* (e-pub ahead of print), doi:10.1097/PTS.0000000000000251.

Carney, M. 2011. "Influence of Organizational Culture on Quality Healthcare Delivery." *International Journal of Health Care Quality Assurance* 24 (7): 523–39.

Casalino, L. P., D. Gans, R. Weber, M. Cea, A. Tuchovsky, T. Bishop, Y. Miranda, B. A. Frankel, K. B. Ziehler, M. M. Wong, and T. B. Evenson. 2016. "US Physician Practices Spend More Than $15.4 Billion Annually to Report Quality Measures." *Health Affairs* 35 (3): 401–6.

Centers for Medicare & Medicaid Services (CMS). 2016. *42 CFR, Ch. IV, §416.41: Condition for Coverage—Governing Body and Management.* Accessed December 9, 2017. www.ecfr.gov/cgi-bin/text-idx?SID=a0a569dfbb9be549ac73ca843c68c0a0&mc=true&node=pt42.3.416&rgn=div5.

Clinical and Laboratory Standards Institute. 2017. *Handbook for Developing a Laboratory Quality Manual.* Wayne, PA: Clinical and Laboratory Standards Institute.

Commonwealth of Pennsylvania. 2002. "Medical Care Availability and Reduction of Error (MCARE) Act of Mar. 20, 2002, P. L. 154, No. 13, Cl. 40, Chapter 3, Section 310." Published March 20. www.legis.state.pa.us/cfdocs/legis/li/uconsCheck.cfm?yr=2002&sessInd=0&act=13.

Deming, W. E. 1986. *Out of the Crisis.* Cambridge, MA: MIT Press.

Eldar, R. 2001. "In Memoriam Avedis Donabedian (1919–2000)." *Croatian Medical Journal* 42 (1): 92.

Institute of Medicine. 2001. *Crossing the Quality Chasm: A New Health System for the 21st Century.* Washington, DC: National Academies Press.

Jiang, H. J., C. Lockee, K. Bass, I. Fraser, and E. P. Norwood. 2009. "Board Oversight of Quality: Any Differences in Process of Care and Mortality?" *Journal of Healthcare Management* 54 (1): 15–30.

Joint Commission. 2017. *Sentinel Event Alert, Issue 57.* Published March 1. www.jointcommission.org/assets/1/18/SEA_57_Safety_Culture_Leadership_0317.pdf.

———. 2016. *2017 Comprehensive Accreditation Manual for Hospitals.* Oakbrook Terrace, IL: The Joint Commission.

Mannion, R., H. Davies, and M. Marshall. 2005. "Cultural Characteristics of 'High' and 'Low' Performing Hospitals." *Journal of Health Organization and Management* 19 (6): 431–39.

Mardon, R. E., K. Khanna, J. Sorra, N. Dyer, and T. Famolaro. 2010. "Exploring Relationships Between Hospital Patient Safety Culture and Adverse Events." *Journal of Patient Safety* 6 (4): 226–32.

Meyer, J. A., S. Silow-Carroll, T. Kutyla, L. S. Stepnick, and L. S. Rybowski. 2004. *Hospital Quality: Ingredients for Success—Overview and Lessons Learned*. New York: Commonwealth Fund.

National Committee for Quality Assurance (NCQA). 2017. "HEDIS® and Quality Compass®." Accessed December 9. www.ncqa.org/HEDISQualityMeasurement/WhatisHEDIS.aspx.

Nembhard, I. M., J. A. Alexander, T. J. Hoff, and R. Ramanujam. 2009. "Why Does the Quality of Health Care Continue to Lag? Insights from Management Research." *Academy of Management Perspectives* 23 (1): 24–42.

Nevada Department of Health and Human Services. 2016. *Quality Assessment and Performance Improvement Strategy (Quality Strategy): 2016–2017*. Accessed December 9, 2017. http://dhcfp.nv.gov/uploadedFiles/dhcfpnvgov/content/Members/BLU/NV2016-17_QAPIS_Report_F1.pdf.

Panzer, R. J., R. S. Gitomer, W. H. Greene, P. R. Webster, K. R. Landry, and C. A. Riccobono. 2013. "Increasing Demands for Quality Measurement." *Journal of the American Medical Association* 310 (18): 1971–80.

Peters, T. J., and R. H. Waterman. 1982. *In Search of Excellence: Lessons from America's Best-Run Companies*. New York: HarperCollins.

Schein, E. H. 1986. "What You Need to Know About Organizational Culture." *Training and Development Journal* 40 (1): 30–33.

Sherwood, R. 2013. "Employee Engagement Drives Health Care Quality and Financial Returns." *Harvard Business Review*. Published October 30. https://hbr.org/2013/10/employee-engagement-drives-health-care-quality-and-financial-returns.

Shortell, S. M., J. Schmittdiel, M. C. Wang, R. Li, R. R. Gillies, L. P. Casalino, T. Bodenheimer, and T. G. Rundall. 2005. "An Empirical Assessment of High-Performing Medical Groups: Results from a National Study." *Medical Care Research and Review* 62 (4): 407–34.

Sorra, J., K. Khanna, N. Dyer, R. Mardon, and T. Famolaro. 2012. "Exploring Relationships Between Patient Safety Culture and Patients' Assessments of Hospital Care." *Journal of Patient Safety* 8 (3): 131–39.

Spath, P. L., and W. Minogue. 2008. "The Soil, Not the Seed: The Real Problem with Root Cause Analysis." Patient Safety Network. Published July. https://psnet.ahrq.gov/perspectives/perspective/62/.

St. Hope Foundation. 2017. "Patient Centered Medical Home (PCMH)." Accessed December 9. http://offeringhope.org/patient-resource/.

University of Colorado, Denver, Division of Health Care Policy and Research. 2011. *Evaluation of the Home Health Pay for Performance Demonstration*. Accessed December 9, 2017. www.cms.gov/Research-Statistics-Data-and-Systems/Statistics-Trends-and-Reports/Reports/Downloads/HHP4P_Demo_eval_Final_Vol2.pdf.

Wagonhurst, C. L., and M. L. Habte. 2008. "Health Care Boards of Directors' Legal Responsibilities for Quality." *Compliance Today* 10 (12): 9, 11–13, 56.

Zastocki, D. K. 2015. "Board Governance: Transformational Approaches Under Healthcare Reform." *Frontiers of Health Services Management* 31 (4): 3–17.

GLOSSARY

Accident: An unplanned, unexpected event, usually with an adverse consequence.

Accountable care organization (ACO): A group of providers responsible for the quality and cost of care delivered to enrolled patients.

Accreditation: A self-assessment and external assessment process used by healthcare organizations to gauge their level of performance in relation to established standards and implement ways to continuously improve.

Accreditation standards: Levels of performance excellence that organizations must attain to become credentialed by a competent authority.

Activity-level measures: Data describing the performance of one process or activity.

Adverse event: An event that results in unintended harm to the patient and is related to the care or services provided to the patient, rather than to the patient's underlying medical conditions.

Affinity diagrams: Charts used by improvement teams to organize ideas and issues, gain a better understanding of a problem, and brainstorm potential solutions. (An example of an affinity diagram is shown in exhibit 6.2.)

Agency for Healthcare Research and Quality (AHRQ): The health services research arm of the US Department of Health and Human Services; the lead federal agency for research on healthcare quality, costs, outcomes, and patient safety.

Analytic tools: Qualitative (language) and quantitative (numeric) tools used during an improvement project; often called *quality improvement tools*.

Appropriate: Suitable for a particular person, place, or condition.

Assessment: Use of performance information to determine whether an acceptable level of quality has been achieved.

A3 report form: A summary of Lean or kaizen project results presented on a one-page standard letter-sized A3 sheet of paper. (An A3 report form template is shown in exhibit 6.19.)

Average: The numerical result obtained by dividing the sum of two or more quantities by the number of quantities; sometimes called an *arithmetic mean*.

Balanced scorecards (BSCs): Frameworks for displaying system-level performance measures; components of structured performance management systems that align an organization's vision and mission with operational objectives.

Baldrige National Quality Award: Recognition conferred annually by the Baldrige Performance Excellence Program to US organizations, including healthcare organizations, that demonstrate performance excellence.

Bar graphs: Graphs used to show the relative size of different categories of a variable, with each category or value of the variable represented by a bar; also called a *bar chart*. (Examples of bar graphs are found in exhibits 4.9 and 4.10.)

Benchmarking: Learning about the best practices in other companies for the purpose of using them in your own organization.

Brainstorming: An interactive decision-making technique designed to generate a large number of creative ideas.

Case managers: Experienced healthcare professionals (e.g., doctors, nurses, social workers) who work with patients, providers, and insurers to coordinate medically necessary and appropriate healthcare services.

Catastrophic processes: Processes with a high likelihood of patient death or severe injury immediately or within hours of a failure (e.g., identification of correct surgery site, administration of compatible blood for a transfusion).

Cause and effect diagrams: Graphic representations of the relationship between outcomes and the factors that influence them; sometimes called *Ishikawa* or *fishbone diagrams*. (Examples of cause and effect diagrams are shown in exhibits 6.3 and 6.4.)

Central tendency: A measure of the middle or expected center value of a dataset. The most common measures of central tendency are the arithmetic mean, the median, and the mode.

Charter: A written declaration of an improvement team's purpose. (An example of an improvement project charter is found in exhibit 7.2.)

Check sheet: A form on which data can be sorted into categories for easier analysis.

Clinical paths: Descriptions of key patient care interventions for a condition, including diagnostic tests, medications, and consultations, which, if completed as described, are expected to produce desired outcomes.

Clinical practice guidelines: "Statements that include recommendations intended to optimize patient care that are informed by a systematic review of evidence and an assessment of the benefits and harms of alternative care options" (Graham et al. 2011, 4; see chapter 3).

Common cause variation: Variation in performance that does not result from a specific cause but is inherent in the process being measured.

Concurrent review: An assessment of patient care services that is completed while those services are being delivered to ensure appropriate treatment and level of care.

Conditions of Participation: Federal regulations that determine an entity's eligibility for involvement in a particular activity.

Continuous improvement: Analyzing performance of various processes and improving them repeatedly to achieve quality objectives.

Control chart: A line graph that includes statistically calculated upper and lower control limits. (Examples of control charts are found in exhibits 4.22–4.25.)

Corrective action plan: A proposed solution to fix a problem or a process.

Cost-effectiveness: The minimal expenditure of dollars, time, and other elements necessary to achieve a desired healthcare result.

Criteria: Standards or principles by which something is judged or evaluated.

Critical failures: The most important process failures to prevent, according to criticality scoring results.

Criticality: Ranking of potential failures according to their combined influence of severity and frequency and probability of occurrence.

Customer service: A series of activities designed to attend to customers' needs.

Dashboard: A set of performance measures displayed in a concise manner that allows for easy interpretation.

Data: Numbers or facts that are interpreted for the purpose of drawing conclusions.

Data analytics: The science of examining raw data with the purpose of drawing conclusions about that information.

Data visualization: The communication of information clearly and effectively through graphical means.

Decision matrix: A chart used to identify, analyze, and rate the strength of relationships between sets of information; it is especially useful for looking at large numbers of decision factors and assessing each factor's relative importance. (Exhibit 6.5 is an example of a decision matrix.)

Defensive medicine: Diagnostic or therapeutic interventions conducted primarily as a safeguard against malpractice liability.

Denominator: The number written below the line in a common fraction, which functions as the divisor of the numerator.

Discharge planning: Evaluation of patients' medical and psychosocial needs for the purpose of determining the type of care they will need after discharge from a healthcare facility.

Electronic clinical quality measures (eCQMs): Data from EHR and/or health information technology systems to measure healthcare quality. These data are used by CMS in a variety of quality-reporting and incentive programs (CMS 2017a; see chapter 3).

Episode-based bundled payments: A fixed, lump-sum payment for a patient's episode of care for a single illness or course of treatment, shared among all caregivers during and after hospitalization.

Evidence-based measures: Data describing the extent to which current best evidence is used in making decisions about patient care.

Facilitator: An individual knowledgeable about group processes and team interaction as well as performance improvement principles and techniques.

FADE model: Performance improvement model developed by Organizational Dynamics Inc.

Failure: Compromised function or intended action.

Failure mode and effects analysis (FMEA): Systematic assessment of a process to identify the location, cause, and consequences of potential failure for the purpose of eliminating or reducing the chance of failure; also called *failure mode, effects, and criticality analysis*

(FMECA) and *healthcare failure mode and effects analysis* (HFMEA). (An example of a completed FMEA is shown in exhibit 8.7.)

Failure modes: Different ways a process step or task could fail to provide the anticipated result.

Faulty system design: Work system failures that set up individuals who work in that system to fail.

Five Whys: A form of analysis that delves into the causes of problems by successively asking *what* and *why* until all aspects of the situation, process, or service are reviewed and contributing factors are considered. (An example of a Five Whys analysis is shown in exhibit 6.6.)

Flowcharts: Graphic representations of a process. (Examples of flowcharts are shown in exhibits 6.8 through 6.11.)

Force field analysis: A technique for identifying and visualizing the relationships between significant forces that influence a problem or goal. (An example of a force field analysis is shown in exhibit 6.15.)

Gantt charts: Graphic representations of a planning matrix. (Exhibit 6.17 is an example of a Gantt chart.)

Governing body: The individuals, group, or agency with ultimate legal authority and responsibility for the overall operation of the organization; often called the *board of trustees*, *board of governors*, or *board of directors*.

Ground rules: Established guidelines for how an improvement team wants to operate; norms for behavior. (Examples of ground rules are found in critical concept 7.1.)

Harm: An outcome that negatively affects a patient's health or quality of life.

Hazard analysis: The process of collecting and evaluating information on hazards associated with a process.

Hazards: Events, actions, or things that can cause harm.

Healthcare Effectiveness Data and Information Set (HEDIS): Health plan performance measurement project sponsored by the National Committee for Quality Assurance.

Healthcare quality: "Degree to which health services for individuals and populations increase the likelihood of desired health outcomes and are consistent with current professional knowledge" (IOM 2001, 4; see chapter 1).

Health maintenance organization (HMO): Public or private organization providing comprehensive medical care to subscribers on the basis of a prepaid contract.

High-performing healthcare organization: An organization that is committed to success and continuously produces outstanding results and high levels of customer satisfaction.

High-reliability organizations (HROs): Entities or businesses with systems in place that are exceptionally consistent in accomplishing their goals and avoiding potentially catastrophic errors.

High-risk activities: Tasks or processes known to be error-prone or that have the potential for causing significant patient harm should an error occur.

High-value healthcare: Low-cost, high-quality healthcare.

Histograms: Bar graphs used to show the center, dispersion, and shape of the distribution of a collection of performance data. (An example of a histogram is found in exhibit 4.11.)

Horizontal axis: The x-axis on a graph.

Human factors: "The environmental, organizational and job factors, and individual characteristics which influence behavior at work" (Clinical Human Factors Group 2016; see chapter 9).

IHI Triple Aim framework: A framework developed by the Institute for Healthcare Improvement (IHI) that encourages implementation of strategies for simultaneously enhancing the experience and outcomes of the patient, improving the health of the population, and reducing per capita cost of care for the benefit of communities (IHI 2017; see chapter 1).

Improvement: Planning and making changes to current practices to achieve better performance.

Improvement plan: A plan to eliminate the cause of undesirable performance or to make good performance even better.

Improvement project: An initiative set up to achieve a performance improvement objective within a certain time frame.

Improvement team: A group of individuals organized to work together to accomplish a specific improvement objective.

Incident reports: Instruments (paper or electronic) used to document occurrences that could have led or did lead to undesirable results. (An example of an incident report is shown in exhibit 8.5.)

Incidents: Events or occurrences that could have led or did lead to undesirable results.

Independents: Improvement team members who have little or no knowledge of the process under consideration and have no vested interest in the outcome of the project.

Inputs: Products, services, or information flowing into a process.

Institute for Healthcare Improvement (IHI): An independent, nonprofit organization driving efforts to improve healthcare throughout the world.

Interrater reliability: The probability that a measurement is free from random error and yields consistent results regardless of the individuals gathering the data. (For example, a measure with high interrater reliability means that two or more people working independently will gather similar data.)

Interviews: Formal discussions between two parties in which information is exchanged.

Judgment: Formation of an opinion after consideration or deliberation.

Kaizen event: "A focused, short-term project aimed at improving a particular process" (McLaughlin and Olson 2017, 413; see chapter 5).

Leadership: An organization's senior leaders or decision makers.

Lean: A performance improvement approach aimed at eliminating waste; also called *Lean manufacturing* or *Lean thinking*.

Lean principles: The five Lean principles are (1) value—identify what is really important to the customer and focus on that, (2) value stream—ensure all activities are necessary and add value, (3) flow—strive for continuous processing through the value stream, (4) pull—drive production with demand, and (5) perfection—prevent defects and rework.

Lean Six Sigma: A process improvement model that combines the techniques of Lean and Six Sigma.

Line graph: A graph in which trends are highlighted by a line connecting data points.

Lower control limit: The lower boundary above which data plotted on a control chart can vary without the need for change or correction.

Measurement: Collection of information for the purpose of understanding current performance and seeing how performance changes or improves over time.

Measures: Instruments or tools used to gather information.

Medical errors: Preventable adverse events or near misses during the provision of healthcare services.

Medical home model of care: A healthcare delivery model in which patient treatment is coordinated through the primary care physician and facilitated by partnerships with other providers and health information exchanges to ensure patients get indicated care when and where they need it.

Medically necessary: Appropriate and consistent with diagnosis and, according to accepted standards of practice in the medical community, imperative to treatment to prevent the patient's condition or the quality of the patient's care from being adversely affected.

Medication error: Any preventable event that may cause or lead to inappropriate medication use or patient harm while the medication is in the control of the healthcare professional, patient, or consumer.

Metrics: Any type of measurement used to gauge a quantifiable component of performance.

Mistake proofing: Improving processes to prevent mistakes or to make mistakes obvious at a glance; also called error proofing.

Misuse: Incorrect diagnoses, medical errors, and other sources of avoidable complications.

Muda: The Japanese term for waste, a concept taken from Lean manufacturing. (Muda is anything that does not add value to the customer. Although some muda is inevitable, the goal of a Lean project is to reduce it as much as possible.)

Multivoting: A group decision-making technique used to reduce a long list of items to a manageable number by taking a series of structured votes.

National Academy of Medicine: A private, nonprofit organization created by the federal government to provide science-based advice on matters of medicine and health. Formerly called the Institute of Medicine (IOM).

National Quality Forum (NQF): A public–private partnership formed in 1999 to develop and implement a national strategy for improving healthcare quality.

National Quality Strategy: Document prepared by the Agency for Healthcare Research and Quality on behalf of the US Department of Health and Human Services that helps healthcare stakeholders across the country—patients; providers; employers; health insurance companies; academic researchers; and local, state, and federal governments—prioritize quality improvement efforts, share lessons, and measure collective success.

Near miss: Any process variation that does not affect the outcome or result of an adverse event but carries a significant chance of an adverse outcome if it were to recur; also known as a *close call*.

Nominal group technique: A structured form of multivoting used to identify and rank issues.

Noncatastrophic processes: Processes that do not generally lead to patient death or severe injury within hours of a failure (e.g., hand hygiene, administration of low-risk medications).

Normal distribution: A spread of information (such as performance data) in which the most frequently occurring value is in the middle of the range and other probabilities tail off symmetrically in both directions; sometimes called the *bell-shaped curve.*

Numerator: The number written above the line in a common fraction, which signifies the number to be divided by the denominator.

Opportunity for improvement: A problem or performance failure.

Organizational culture: Prevalent patterns of shared beliefs and values that provide behavioral guidelines or establish norms for conducting business.

Organized medical staff: A formal organization of physicians, dentists, and other professional medical personnel with the delegated responsibility and authority to maintain proper standards of medical care and plan for continued betterment of that care.

ORYX performance measurement: Performance measurement project sponsored by The Joint Commission.

Outcome measures: Used to judge the results of patient care and support functions.

Outputs: Products, services, or information flowing out of a process.

Overuse: Provision of healthcare services that do not benefit the patient, are not clearly indicated, or are provided in excessive amounts or in an unnecessary setting.

Pareto charts: Special types of bar graphs that display the most frequent problem as the first bar, the next most frequent as the next bar, and so on; also called *Pareto diagrams.* (An example of a Pareto chart is found in exhibit 4.12.)

Pareto Principle: Originally, the Pareto Principle referred to the observation that 80 percent of Italy's wealth belonged to only 20 percent of the population. The principle conveys the notion that the majority of results come from a minority of inputs (an 80/20 rule of thumb).

Patient experience measures: Patient-reported information used to judge "whether something that should happen in a health care setting (such as clear communication with a provider) actually happened or how often it happened" (AHRQ 2016; see chapter 3).

Patient safety: Actions undertaken by individuals and organizations to protect healthcare recipients from being harmed by the effects of healthcare services; also defined as freedom from accidental or preventable injuries produced by medical care.

Patient safety organizations (PSOs): Groups that have expertise in identifying risks and hazards in the delivery of patient care, determining the underlying causes, and implementing corrective and preventive strategies.

Pay-for-performance systems: Performance-based payment arrangements that control costs directly or indirectly by motivating providers to improve quality and reduce inappropriate utilization.

Performance: The way in which an individual, a group, or an organization carries out or accomplishes its important functions and processes.

Performance comparison: Examination of similarities or differences between one organization's performance and the performance of other organizations.

Performance excellence: Term introduced by Tom Peters and Robert Waterman in their book *In Search of Excellence* (1982) to refer to an overall way of working that balances stakeholder concerns and increases the probability of long-term organizational success.

Performance expectations: Minimum acceptable or desired level of quality.

Performance gap: The difference between actual and expected performance.

Performance improvement: A method for analyzing performance problems and enacting improvements to ensure good performance.

Performance improvement models: Systematic approaches for conducting improvement projects.

Performance measures: Quantitative tools used to evaluate an element of patient care; also called *quality measures*.

Performance targets: Desired performance.

Performance trends: Patterns of gradual change in performance; the average or general tendency of performance data to move in a certain direction over time.

Physician advisor: A practicing physician who supports utilization review activities by evaluating the appropriateness of admissions and continued stays, judging the efficiency of services in terms of level of care and place of service, and seeking appropriate care alternatives.

Pie charts: Graphs in which each unit of data is represented as a pie-shaped piece of a circle. (An example of a pie chart is found in exhibit 4.6.)

Plan-Do-Check-Act (PDCA) cycle: The Shewhart performance improvement model.

Plan-Do-Study-Act (PDSA) cycle: The Deming performance improvement model. (An example of a PDSA improvement project is found in exhibit 5.3.)

Planning matrix: A diagram that shows tasks needed to complete an activity, the persons or groups responsible for completing the tasks, and an activity schedule with deadlines for task completion.

Population health: "The health outcomes of a group of individuals, including the distribution of such outcomes within the group" (Kindig and Stoddart 2003, 381; see chapter 11).

Population health care: Use of information to surveil a population to identify health risks, prioritize interventions, and measure results.

Population health management: "The application of management strategies to improve the delivery of healthcare for populations, with an emphasis on achieving the highest quality at the lowest cost" (Caron 2017, 288; see chapter 11).

Preadmission certification: Review of the need for medical care or services (e.g., inpatient admission, nursing home admission) that is completed before the care or services are provided.

Proactive risk assessment: An improvement model that involves identifying and analyzing potential failures in healthcare processes or services for the purpose of reducing or eliminating risks that are a threat to patient safety.

Problem statement: A description of the performance problem that needs to be solved. Sometimes called the *aim statement*.

Process capability: A quantitative or qualitative description of what a process is capable of producing.

Process diagram: A visual representation of the flow of individual steps or activities in a process.

Process measures: Used to judge whether patient care and support functions are properly performed.

Process owners: Individuals ultimately responsible for a process, including its performance and outcomes.

Process variation: Fluctuation in process output.

Prospective review: A method of determining medical necessity and appropriateness of services before the services are rendered.

Protocols: Formal outlines of care; treatment plans.

Providers: Individuals and organizations licensed or trained to give healthcare.

Purchasers: Individuals and organizations that pay for healthcare services either directly or indirectly.

Qualitative tools: Analytic improvement tools used for generating ideas, setting priorities, maintaining direction, determining problem causes, and clarifying processes.

Quality: Perceived degree of excellence.

Quality assurance: Evaluation activities aimed at ensuring compliance with minimum quality standards. (*Quality assurance* and *quality control* may be used interchangeably to describe actions performed to ensure the quality of a product, service, or process.)

Quality Assurance and Performance Improvement (QAPI) program: This CMS requirement for nursing homes involves the coordinated application of two mutually reinforcing aspects of a quality management system: quality assurance (QA) and performance improvement (PI).

Quality circles: Small groups of employees organized to solve work-related problems.

Quality control: Operational techniques and activities used to fulfill quality requirements. (*Quality control* and *quality assurance* may be used interchangeably to describe actions performed to ensure the quality of a product, service, or process.)

Quality improvement organizations: Groups of health quality experts, clinicians, and consumers organized to improve the quality of care delivered to people with Medicare.

Quality indicators: Measures used to determine the organization's performance over time; also called *performance measures.*

Quality management: A way of doing business that continuously improves products and services to achieve better performance.

Quality management plan: A formal document that describes the organization's quality management system in terms of organizational structure, responsibilities of management and staff, lines of authority, and required interfaces for those planning, implementing, and assessing quality activities.

Quality management system: A set of interrelated or interacting elements that organizations use to direct and control the implementation of quality policies and achieve quality objectives.

Quality planning: Setting quality objectives and specifying operational processes and related resources needed to fulfill the objectives.

Quality storyboard: A tool that visually communicates the major elements of an improvement project. (A mock-up of a quality storyboard is shown in exhibit 6.18.)

Quantitative tools: Analytic improvement tools used for measuring performance, collecting and displaying data, and monitoring performance.

Questionnaires: Forms containing questions to which subjects respond. (Exhibit 6.13 is an example of a questionnaire.)

Radar charts: Graphs used to display the differences between actual and expected performance for several measures; also called *spider charts* or *spider diagrams* because of their shape.

Rapid cycle improvement (RCI): An improvement model that supports repeated incremental improvements in a practice to optimize performance.

Ratio: One value divided by another; the value of one quantity in terms of the other.

Reliability: The measurable capability of a process, procedure, or health service to perform its intended function in the required time under commonly occurring conditions.

Reliability science: A discipline that applies scientific know-how to a process, procedure, or health service activity so that it will perform its intended function for the required time under commonly occurring conditions.

Reliable: Yielding the same or compatible results in different situations.

Reportable events: Incidents, situations, or processes that contribute to—or have the potential to contribute to—a patient injury or that degrade the provider's ability to provide safe patient care.

Response rate: The number of respondents who complete a survey out of the number who received the survey, usually expressed as a percentage; can also apply to individual questions.

Response scales: Ranges of answers from which the survey respondent can choose.

Retrospective review: A method of determining medical necessity and appropriateness of services that have already been rendered.

Risk: The possibility of loss or injury.

Risk analysis: The process of defining, analyzing, and quantifying the hazards in a process, which typically results in a plan of action undertaken to prevent the most harmful risks or minimize their consequences.

Risk management: The act or practice of dealing with risk, which includes planning for risk, assessing (identifying and analyzing) risk areas, developing risk-handling options, monitoring risks to determine how they have changed, and documenting the overall risk management program.

Root cause analysis (RCA): A structured process for identifying the underlying factors that caused an adverse event.

Root causes: Primary and fundamental origins of undesirable performance.

Safeguards: Physical, human, or administrative controls incorporated into a process to identify and correct errors before a patient is harmed.

Safety: The quality or condition of being safe; freedom from danger, injury, or damage.

Sample: A representative portion of a larger group.

Scatter diagrams: Graphs used to show how two variables may be related. (Examples of scatter diagrams are found in exhibits 4.7 and 4.8.)

Sentinel event: An adverse event involving death or serious physical or psychological injury (or the risk thereof) that signals the need for immediate investigation and response.

Six Sigma: A disciplined methodology for process improvement that deploys a wide set of tools following rigorous data analysis to identify sources of variation in performance and ways of reducing the variation. (An example of a Six Sigma project is found in exhibit 5.7.)

Six Sigma quality: Rate of less than 3.4 defects per 1 million opportunities, which translates to a process that is 99.99966 percent defect free.

Special cause variation: Unexpected variation in performance that results from a non-random event.

Sponsor: An individual or a group that supports, guides, and mentors an improvement project team; serves as a link to the organization's leadership; removes barriers; and acquires the resources a team needs to achieve successful outcomes.

Stakeholder analysis: A tool used to identify groups and individuals who will be affected by a process change and whose participation and support are crucial to realizing successful outcomes.

Standard deviation: A measure of the dispersion of a collection of values.

Standards: Performance expectations established by individuals or groups.

Statistical process control (SPC): Application of statistical methods to identify and control performance.

Statistical thinking: A philosophy of learning and action based on the following fundamental principles: All work occurs in a system of interconnected processes, variation exists in all processes, and understanding and reducing variation are keys to success.

Structure measures: Used to judge the adequacy of the environment in which patient care is provided.

Surveys: Questionnaires or interviews used to obtain information from a group of individuals about a process, product, or service.

Survey sample: A subgroup of respondents derived from the target population.

System: A set of interdependent elements that interact to achieve a common aim.

Systematic: Conducted using step-by-step procedures.

System-level measures: Data describing the overall performance of several interdependent processes or activities.

Tampering: Doing something in reaction to a particular performance result without knowing whether it was caused by natural variation or some unusual occurrence.

Underuse: Failure to provide appropriate or necessary services, or provision of an inadequate quantity or lower level of service than that required.

Upper control limit: The upper boundary below which data plotted on a control chart can vary without the need for change or correction.

Utilization: Use of medical services and supplies, commonly examined in terms of patterns or rates of use of a single service or type of service, such as hospital care, physician visits, and prescription drugs.

Utilization management (UM): Planning, organizing, directing, and controlling healthcare products in a cost-effective manner while maintaining quality of patient care and contributing to the organization's goals.

Utilization review: Process for monitoring and evaluating the use, delivery, and cost-effectiveness of healthcare services.

Valid: Relevant, meaningful, and correct; appropriate to the task at hand.

Validity: The degree to which data or results of a study are correct or true.

Value: A relative measure that describes a product's or service's worth, usefulness, or importance.

Value-based reimbursement: Payment that requires healthcare providers to meet certain quality objectives and document compliance with best practices.

Vertical axis: The *y*-axis on a graph.

Vigilant: Carefully observant or attentive; on the lookout for possible problems.

Workflow diagram: An illustration of the movement of employees or information during a process. (An example of a workflow diagram is shown in exhibit 6.12.)

Work systems: Sets of interdependent elements, both human and nonhuman (e.g., equipment, technologies), that interact to achieve a common aim.

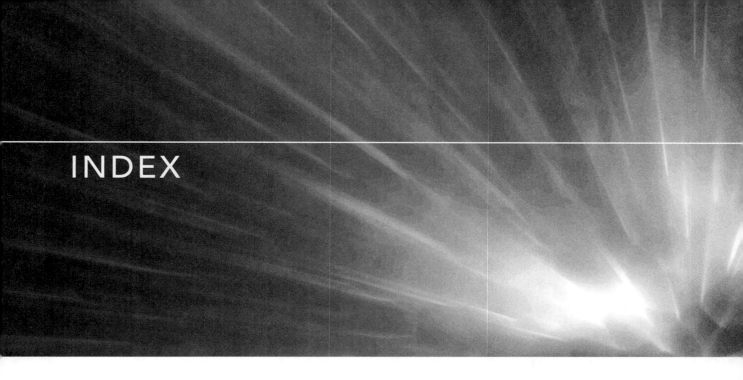

INDEX

Medicare (*continued*)
259, 269, 270, 307; Joint Commission accreditation standards and, 23; pay-for-performance systems, 256; provider quality requirements, 23; reimbursement for use of semi-electric hospital bed, 255; third-party payers' effects on, 5; utilization management requirements, 254

Medicare Access and CHIP Reauthorization Act (MACRA): Merit-Based Incentive Payment System and Advanced Payment Models, 284; Quality Payment Program, 51

Medicare patients: average hospital length of stay, 259, *260*; pneumonia and renal failure treatment in, 259–61, *260, 261*

Medication: hospital administration process, *199*; unnecessary use of, 254

Medication errors: definition of, 211

MedWatch: FDA Safety Information and Adverse Event Reporting Program website, 221

Meetings: of improvement project teams, 183–87; agendas, 187; ground rules for, 183, *184,* 185; leader's responsibilities, 185, 187; length of improvement project, 185; minutes, 185; organization and leadership, 185, 187; recorders and timekeepers of, 182; timeline of improvement project, *186*

Merit-Based Incentive Payment System and Advanced Payment Models, 284

Metrics: definition of, 37. *See also* Performance measures

MGMA. *See* Medical Group Management Association

Midwest Business Group on Health: website, 276

Minnesota Adverse Health Events Measurement Guide: website, 221

Minnesota Department of Health: Patient Safety website, 221

Minnesota Department of Public Health Quality Improvement Resources & Tools: website, 173

Mistake proofing (error proofing), *133,* 197–99; definition of, 197; examples of, 197–98

Mistake-Proofing the Design of Health Care Processes (Grout): AHRQ website, 245

Misuse of healthcare services: definition of, 15

Monitoring: of action plans, 238–39; of healthcare costs, 251; of performance, 15, 238–40; of process change, 242–43

Motorola, 134

Muda (waste): categories and examples of, *131*; definition of, 130

Multivoting, *145, 146–47, 148*

NAHQ. *See* National Association for Healthcare Quality

NASA Aviation Safety Reporting System, 203

National Academy of Medicine: definition of, 7; website, 11

National Alliance of Healthcare Purchaser Coalitions: website, 31

National Association for Healthcare Quality (NAHQ): on competencies for quality professionals, 282

National Association of County and City Health Officials: website, 31

National Cardiovascular Data Registry, 102

National Center for Health Statistics: website, 292

National Commission on Correctional Health Care: organizations and programs accredited by, *27*

National Committee for Quality Assurance (NCQA), 68, 255, 311; accreditation standards, 273; Healthcare Effectiveness Data and Information Set measurement project, 289; organizations and programs accredited by, *28*; as performance comparison data source, *104*; utilization management defined by, 250; website, 53, 74, 276

National Database of Nursing Quality Indicators (NDNQI), 102, 103

National Guideline Clearinghouse: website, 252, 275, 276

National Healthcare Quality Report, 2016 (Agency for Healthcare Research and Quality), 194

National Institute of Standards and Technology, 19

National League for Nursing Education, 22

National Network of Public Health Institutes: website, 138

National Physicians Alliance, 68

National Public Health Performance Standards: website, 31

National Quality Center: Quality Academy Useful Quality Improvement Tools tutorial, website, 174; Quality Academy: Using Teams to Improve Quality tutorial website, 191; Quality Improvement Resources website, 138

National Quality Forum (NQF): definition of, 66; website, 74

National Quality Measures Clearinghouse: Agency for Healthcare Research and Quality sponsorship of, 69; website, 74

National Quality Strategy, 48; adaptation of Institute for Healthcare Improvement Triple Aim framework, 9; aims of, 9; definition of, 8; priorities in advancement of aims of, 9; purpose of, 8–9; website, 11

NCQA. *See* National Committee for Quality Assurance

NDNQI. *See* National Database of Nursing Quality Indicators

Near miss (close call), 209

Negative correlation: in scatter diagrams, 87, *87,* 88, 89

Nevada Medicaid and Nevada Check Up members: quality goals and objectives for (2016–17), 313

Nightingale, Florence, 105

Nominal group technique, *145,* 147–48; definition of, 147; steps in, 147–48

Noncatastrophic processes, 228

Nonprofit hospitals: tax-exempt status of, 284

Normal distribution, 106

Norming stage: in improvement team dynamics, 188, *189*

NQF. *See* National Quality Forum

Numerators, 57, 59

Nurses: work problems encountered by, 196, 228

Observation: as performance data source, 62

Occupational Safety and Health Administration: radiation exposure regulations, 100; Regulations for Healthcare Facilities website, 32

Occurrence reports. *See* Incident reports

Office of Inspector General: compliance materials: website, 322

Ohno, Taiichi, 130

100 Hospital Patient Safety Benchmarks: website, 221

Opportunity for improvement, 120

Oregon Patient Safety Commission: website, 221

Organizational culture: definition of, 196, 315; incompatibility with quality management efforts, 317–18; levels, 315–16; performance problems and, 318

Organizational Dynamics Inc., 129

Organizational structure diagrams, 312, *312*

Organized medical staff, 307

ORYX performance measurement, 52

Outcome measures, 43, 44, *45,* 46–47, 289; of action plans, 240; for clinical decision making, 67; for Medicare-certified home health agencies, *50;* as performance reliability measure, 226; of process reliability, 226

Outliers, 40

Outputs: process, 179

Overuse of healthcare services, 5, 68; definition of, 14; healthcare expenditures associated with, 252

Pacific Business Group on Health: website, 276

Pareto, Vilfredo, 92

Pareto charts, 84, *92,* 92–93, 99, *145,* 151

Pareto Principle, 92

Pasteur, Louis, 319

Patient advocates, 309

Patient-centered care: definition of, 7; discharge planning in, 266

Patient centeredness: as healthcare quality attribute, *7,* 48; radiology services, *57*

Patient experience measures, 43, 44, *45,* 46, 47

Patient records: as performance data source, 62, *63*

Patient safety, 193–222; definition of, 194; as healthcare quality attribute, 7, *7,* 9, 48; improvement projects in, 205–17; measurement of, *200,* 200–201, 203–4; mistake proofing for, 197–99, *198;* patient's role in, 217–19; quality management and, 201; radiology services, *57;* websites, 220–22

Patient Safety and Quality Improvement Act (Patient Safety Act): passage of, 204

Patient safety committees, 305

Patient safety coordinators, 309

Patient safety organizations (PSOs): definition of, 204

Patient satisfaction: measurement and assessment, 38–39

Pay-for-performance systems, 256

ABOUT THE AUTHOR

Patrice L. Spath, MA, RHIT, is a health information management professional with a master's degree in management and broad experience in healthcare quality and safety improvement. She is president of Brown-Spath & Associates (www.brownspath.com), a healthcare publishing and training company based in Forest Grove, Oregon. During the past 35 years, Patrice has presented more than 400 educational programs on healthcare quality management topics and has completed numerous quality and patient safety program consultations for healthcare organizations.

Patrice has authored and edited many books and peer-reviewed articles for Health Administration Press, Health Forum/AHA Press, Jossey-Bass, AHC Media, Brown-Spath & Associates, and other groups. Her recent books include *Fundamentals of Health Care Quality Management*, 5th ed. (Brown-Spath & Associates, 2018); *Applying Quality Management in Healthcare: A Systems Approach*, 4th ed. (Health Administration Press, 2017); *Error Reduction in Health Care*, 2nd ed. (Jossey-Bass, 2011); and *Engaging Patients as Safety Partners* (AHA Press, 2008). Her 2005 book, *Leading Your Healthcare Organization to Excellence*, received the James A. Hamilton Book of the Year Award. This award is given annually to the author of a management or healthcare book judged outstanding by the American College of Healthcare Executives Book of the Year Committee.

Patrice is an adjunct assistant professor in the Department of Health Services Administration at the University of Alabama, Birmingham, where she currently teaches online graduate-level patient safety courses. She also has current and past quality management and patient safety teaching responsibilities in the health information technology program at Missouri Western State University in St. Joseph, in the graduate certificate program in health information management at Oregon Health & Science University in Portland, in the School of Healthcare Administration and Leadership at Pacific University in Forest Grove, Oregon, and in the Master of Science in Medical and Healthcare Simulation Program at Drexel University College of Medicine in Philadelphia.

Patrice currently serves as consulting editor for *Hospital Peer Review* and is an active member of the American Health Information Management Association, the National Association for Healthcare Quality, and the American Society for Healthcare Risk Management.